PRAISE FOR

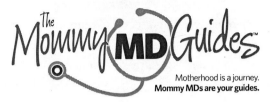

Motherhood is a journey.
Mommy MDs are your guides.

It is fascinating to find the real experiences of physician moms interposed with solid data about healthy pregnancy and delivery. *The Mommy MD Guide to Pregnancy and Birth* is an enjoyable and enlightening book that will "hold hands" with women through their pregnancies.

> —*Joanna M. Cain, MD, Chace/Joukowsky Professor and chair, assistant dean of women's health at the Warren Alpert Medical School of Brown University, and obstetrician and gynecologist-in-chief at Women & Infants Hospital, both in Providence, RI*

The Mommy MD Guide to Your Baby's First Year is fun, easy to read, and informative. I love that the advice from physicians is practical and based on experience, in addition to medical expertise.

Since it is a series of vignettes, it's easy to read and pick up in between other activities, which is ideal for busy people like me and new moms.

> —*Jennifer Arnold, MD, a neonatologist and the medical director of the Pediatric Simulation Center at Texas Children's Hospital and an assistant professor at Baylor College of Medicine, both in Houston, and the star of TLC's* The Little Couple

The Mommy MD Guide to the Toddler Years is a great testament to the fact that no two kids or parents are exactly alike. I am always looking for new ideas for entertaining, disciplining, teaching, and loving on my kids because what worked with my first child doesn't always work with the other five! I love that this book accepts, appreciates, and addresses the fact that there isn't just one answer to any question or concern parents have with their children. For me, the more suggestions I can get, the better!

—*Casey Jones, a mom of a 9-year-old daughter and 4-year-old quintuplets and costar of* Quints by Surprise, *in Austin, TX*

❧

I found a quiet corner in the living room and flipped open *The Mommy MD Guide to Pregnancy and Birth*, about a topic I last experienced 10 years ago. The more I read, the more I kept thinking to myself, "I wish this book had been *around* 10 years ago." I would have devoured every word if I'd read it 20 years ago, as I plodded through my very first experience with the baffling world of pregnancy. This book really is different from every other pregnancy book I've read.

The Mommy MD Guide to Pregnancy and Birth has advice from 60 doctors who are moms. Aside from the great medical advice, I was drawn to the anecdotal feeling of this book. As I read, I felt like I was sitting in the living room with these women as they shared their personal stories. I'm a person who loves to hear a good birth story, and I was really drawn to the personal nature of the advice. Instead of feeling like it was coming from a textbook, the advice feels like it's coming from a girlfriend who's just navigated the road herself. But it went beyond "just" a girlfriend's guide, because it was a girlfriend's guide times 60.

I highly recommend *The Mommy MD Guide to Pregnancy and Birth*. I have a feeling many dads wouldn't mind reading it either since it's not long chapters of information, but short snippets of advice, gathered in a very logical way.

I enjoyed the website that's hosted by the authors and look forward to the series this team is working on, covering the other stages of parenting, from newborn sleep issues to elementary school struggles. It's a great idea that was truly done right.

—*Judy Berna, a mom of four and writer for GeekMom.com*

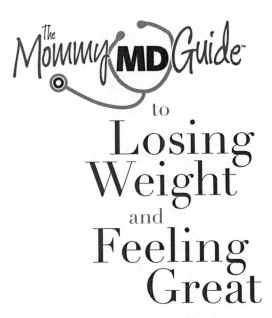

The Mommy MD Guide

to Losing Weight and Feeling Great

The Mommy MD Guide

to
Losing Weight
and
Feeling Great

More Than 700 Tips That 50 Doctors
Who Are Also Mothers
Use to Slim Down, Shape Up,
Fight Fatigue, Boost Mood,
Look Great, and Live Better

By Rallie McAllister, MD, MPH
and Jennifer Bright Reich

MOMOSA PUBLISHING

This book is intended as a reference volume only, not as a medical manual. The information given here is designed to help you make informed decisions about your health. It is not intended as a substitute for any treatment that might have been prescribed by your doctor. If you suspect that you have a medical problem, we urge you to seek competent medical help.

Internet addresses given in this book were accurate at the time it went to press.

© 2014 by Momosa Publishing LLC

Printed in the United States of America

Illustrations by Carrie Wendel

Book design by Leanne Coppola

Library of Congress Control Number 2013912373

ISBN 978–0–9844804–6–3

2 4 6 8 10 9 7 5 3 1 paperback

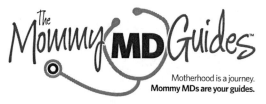

Motherhood is a journey.
Mommy MDs are your guides.

MommyMDGuides.com

To Monica, Every day is an adventure!
—RM

To Mike, Tyler, and Austin
—JBR

Contents

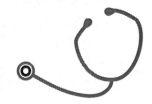

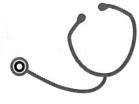

Acknowledgments

The books in the Mommy MD Guides series are proof positive that if we dream big, work hard, and believe in ourselves, we can accomplish anything we feel passionate about. If we're lucky enough to have the help and support of friends and family while we're at it, the process is a whole lot easier, and a lot more fun.

I feel incredibly blessed to have Jennifer as a friend, coauthor, and business partner. Although it's roughly 600 miles from my desk to hers, she's as close to me as a sister. Jennifer and I are both passionate about helping moms carry out one of the most important jobs in the world—raising healthy, happy children. We couldn't do this without the help of our awesome team at the Mommy MD Guides or the incredible physicians who generously shared the stories of their lives. I'm grateful to each of them.

I'm also grateful to my family—Robin, Oakley, Gatlin, Chad, Lindsey, Bella, and Cam—and very thankful for all the love and laughter we share.

—*Rallie McAllister, MD, MPH*

✿

First and foremost, thank you so very much to Rallie. You make every day at Momosa Publishing a great day, and your energy, optimism, ideas, and vision always amaze me. I will forever be grateful to you!

Thank you to the dozens of Mommy MD Guides who shared their stories and experiences with us for this book. The best part of my job is meeting and talking with smart, funny, fascinating, and kind people like you! Thank you for sharing your tips and wisdom with us.

Many thanks also to the Mommy MD Guides team. I'm so fortunate to work with such a talented group: editor Amy Kovalski, consultant Jennifer Goldsmith, writer Marie Suszynski, designer Leanne Coppola, researcher Jennifer Kushnier, layout designer Susan Eugster, illustrator Carrie Wendel, indexer Nanette Bendyna, and Magnum Offset Printing sales manager Alice Fan.

I am very grateful to Drew Frantzen, our logo designer, who has helped to establish the very tone and style of our brand.

Thank you to my mentors and friends who have shared their wisdom and advice: Susan Berg, Elly Phillips, Chris Krogermeier, Anne Egan, Joey Green, Tim Foster, Colleen Krcelich, Andrew K. Gonsalves, and Buddy Lesavoy.

Most of all, thank you to my family—Mike, Tyler, and Austin Reich and John R. Bright, Mary L. Bright, Robyn Swatsburg, and Judy Beck—for all of your support, encouragement, and love and for making my life so rich, rewarding—and fun.

—*Jennifer Bright Reich*

Introduction

Some things in life are universal. If you asked 100 women if they'd like to lose weight and feel great, it's a pretty good bet you'd get 100 yeses.

Wouldn't it be great to look and feel your best—every day? Wouldn't you love to slim down, shape up, boost your energy levels, improve your mood, and feel better? No matter what your size, *everyone* deserves to feel great—at your current weight, at your goal weight, and at every ounce in between.

To create this book, we spoke with 50 Mommy MD Guides—doctors who are also mothers. Some of these Mommy MD Guides have ongoing struggles with their weight, energy, esteem, and mood. Others have faced challenges only at particular points in their lives.

These smart, funny, fascinating women opened their hearts and lives to us. They shared their challenges with weight, energy, esteem, and mood. They also talked with us about celebrating meeting their goals, shopping for clothes, choosing makeup, optimizing their hairstyles, and recharging their batteries.

The more than 700 tips and stories in this book are presented in the Mommy MD Guides' own words, and each tip is clearly attributed to the doctor who *lived* it. Most of these stories contain kernels of advice. This is what doctors did to lose weight and feel great. Other stories in this book are just that—true stories. The implied advice is: I made it through this pesky problem, and you can too!

As a special bonus, we've included Take Five! The Mommy MD Guide's Program for Maximum Weight Loss Success! This program has been proven to work for women who needed to lose both small and large amounts of weight. It's simple, and it's effective.

Even though this book is filled with advice from a select group—all Mommy MD Guides—you'll find that they hold vastly differing opinions. We've presented many different viewpoints—but not with the intent to confuse or to offer conflicting advice. Instead, these diverse voices are presented so that you can choose what's best for you on your own weight loss journey.

As you read this book, keep in mind that every *body* is different. Women face different challenges with their weight, energy, esteem, and mood, and these things improve at different speeds for everyone. Not all progress is the same, and not all progress is linear. You might have some ups and downs. You might experience some plateaus—even some setbacks. Try to remember that your weight is not a measure of your self-worth. Smart, talented, and attractive people come in all shapes and sizes. Love yourself for who you are, not for what you look like.

As Lao-Tzu said, "The journey of a thousand leagues begins with a single step." We hope you celebrate your first step, the step when you meet your goals, and every step in between.

Welcome to the Mommy MD Guides! Best wishes for your health and happiness!

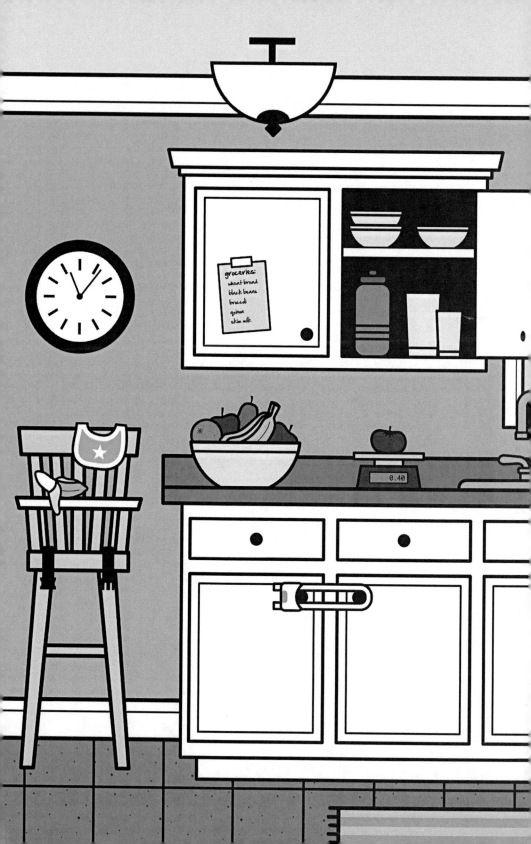

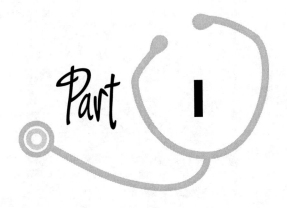

Part I

LOSING WEIGHT

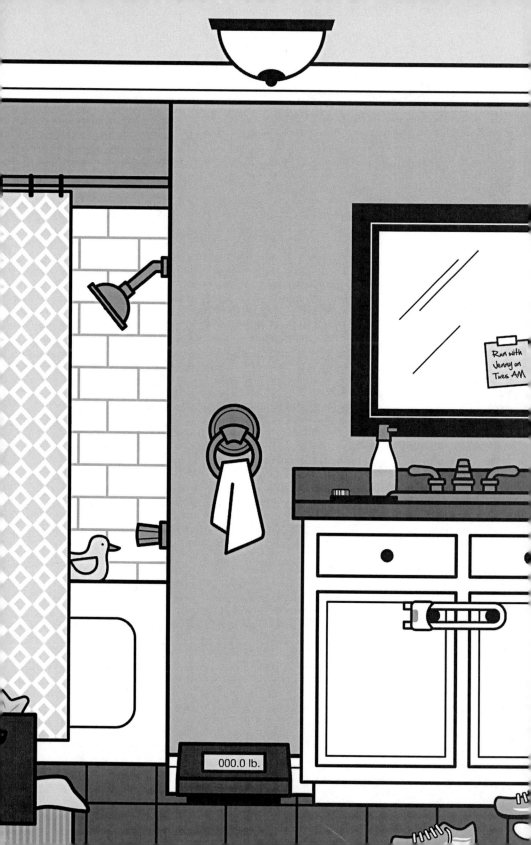

Run with
Jenny on
Tues AM

000.0 lb.

Chapter 1
Losing Weight

YOUR BODY

Like so many of us, you're probably thinking about losing weight. You have plenty of company! According to a Gallup poll from 2012, 54 percent of people surveyed said they would like to lose weight. (And we question the honesty of much of the other 46 percent. . .) Among them, 25 percent were seriously trying to lose weight. Of the women, 33 percent were working on dropping pounds, while 16 percent of the men were trying to get slimmer.

We certainly have good reason to want to lose weight. More than two-thirds of U.S. adults are overweight or obese. Obesity has reached epidemic proportions in the United States. The prevalence of obesity in children has increased markedly, with approximately 20 to 25 percent of children either overweight or obese. The problem of obesity has also been increasing rapidly throughout the world, and the incidence of obesity nearly doubled from 1991 to 1998. Worldwide, more than 1.5 billion people are overweight.

All of those extra pounds bring weighty complications and risks. Being overweight or obese can heighten your risk for type 2 diabetes, heart disease and stroke, sleep apnea, osteoarthritis, some types of cancer, complications with pregnancy, fatty liver disease, and gallbladder disease.

Losing just 5 to 10 percent of your weight can lower your blood pressure, reduce your LDL ("bad") cholesterol, improve your blood sugar, and lower your risk for heart disease. Experts say that 90 percent of all cases of diabetes, 80 percent of heart disease, and 60 percent of cancers are preventable with healthier lifestyles and normal body weights.

Losing weight and achieving a healthier body can bring so many other benefits not measured in a lab. You'll have more energy to play at the park with your family, more strength to hug and carry your children, and a better mood to enjoy every part—every day—of your life.

JUSTIFICATION FOR A CELEBRATION

As you begin your weight loss journey and start to take steps toward a healthier you—toward a healthier life—celebrate the small victories that bring you closer to your goal. Did you say yes to a healthy snack, lace up your running shoes, cook a nutritious new recipe, or pop in an exercise DVD? Celebrate your positive choices! Way to go!

> **The secret of getting ahead is getting started.**
> **The secret of getting started is breaking your complex overwhelming tasks into small manageable tasks, and then starting on the first one.**
> —*Mark Twain*

Setting Goals

A dream might be a wish that your heart makes, but a goal is a wish that your *brain* makes.

What is your weight loss goal? For most of us, that goal is a *number*. It might be a number you remember fondly—such as what you weighed in college, when you got married, or before you got pregnant. Or it might be a size, such as the size of your wedding gown or of your favorite pair of jeans.

But not all goals are numbers. Why not set a goal to play tag with your kids—until *they* want to stop, not you? Or to run up a flight of stairs without effort? Or to dance without missing a beat?

Rather than falling in love with one number, set as many goals as you wish. Write them down and tuck them away. Or better yet, create an I Believe box to store all of your goals, wishes, and dreams. What do *you* believe?

No matter what I weigh, I always wish I were 5 to 10 pounds lighter. I think a lot of women share this "oasis mirage" perspective on the ideal weight.

—*Amy Baxter, MD, a mom of 15- and 12-year-old sons and a 10-year-old daughter; the CEO of Buzzy4Shots.com; and the director of emergency research, Scottish Rite, of Children's Healthcare of Atlanta, in Georgia*

I'm now 44, and it seems more difficult to get back down to my college weight, which I tend to think of as my goal weight.

—*Stacey Ann Weiland, MD, a mom of a 14-year-old daughter and 9- and 7-year-old sons and an internist/gastroenterologist, in Denver, CO*

My goal was to get within a few pounds of my pre-pregnancy weight. I'd been an avid exerciser, and I knew where I felt best. I wanted to get back to that "happy place."

—*Lennox McNeary, MD, a mom of a four-year-old son, a specialist in physical medicine and rehabilitation at Carilion Clinic,*

and a cofounder of the Mommy Doctors Bakery (makers of Milkin'
Cookies), in Roanoke, VA

❧

My goal is to be in the "normal weight" category on the Body Mass Index (BMI). (Read more about BMI in "When to Call Your Doctor," below.) I want to be healthy, but not super thin.

Your BMI is based on your height and weight. You can use the calculator at http://NHLBISupport.com/bmi so you don't have to do the math.

—*Leena Shrivastava Dev, MD, a mom of 15- and 12-year-old sons and a general pediatrician and advocate for child safety, in the Baltimore, MD, area*

When to Call Your Doctor

Yes, your body has changed over time, especially if you've had children. The most obvious change is likely weight gain.

But unlike celebrities who have nannies, chefs, and personal trainers, the average woman will take longer than a few weeks to get back to her pre-pregnancy shape. In fact, it's normal and healthy for weight loss to happen gradually over several months. It's particularly important to take it slow if you're breastfeeding.

Once you're several months past giving birth, or any time in your life where your reflection in the mirror isn't quite the one you'd like to see, it might be time to look at your weight and consider whether you need to lose some of those extra pounds. One way to do that is to check your Body Mass Index (BMI). Another, easier, way is to use the BMI calculator at the National Institutes of Health website, which you'll find here: **NHL BISUPPORT.COM/BMI.** The NIH even has a BMI calculator app for your phone. Or see the chart on page 134. Or here's how to calculate it.

• Divide your weight in pounds by your height in inches, squared. (For example, if you weigh 150 pounds and you are 5 feet 7 inches tall, it would look like this: 150/4,489 = .033.)

Rather than setting a goal weight, I set a reasonable goal range of weights that are between 5 to 10 pounds apart. The actual number is meaningless; it's all about how one feels.

—*Hana R. Solomon, MD, a mom who raised four children, a grandmom of three, a board-certified pediatrician, the president of BeWell Health, LLC, and the author of* Clearing the Air One Nose at a Time: Caring for Your Personal Filter, *in Columbia, MO*

My goal weight is the weight I feel most comfortable at. It would be ideal if everyone was in the normal BMI range, but that occasionally makes weight management more daunting and unrealistic, which

• Multiply that number by 703. (For our example, it would come out to 23.5.)

If your BMI falls between 18.5 and 24.9, you're considered to have a normal weight. However, a BMI between 25 and 29.9 is considered overweight, and a BMI of 30 or higher is considered obese.

Another thing to think about is the size of your waist. That's because fat that settles around your middle might increase your risk of high blood pressure, high cholesterol, type 2 diabetes, and heart disease. Women whose waists measure 35 inches or more are advised to lose weight.

Doctors don't always address weight issues during your appointments, so you might need to be the one to start the conversation. Tell your doctor you're concerned about your weight, and ask if your weight might be related to any health conditions, such as high blood pressure or hypothyroidism, or medications you're taking. Your doctor can also give you advice about how to get started losing weight and recommend local weight loss programs or experts such as dietitians.

sometimes discourages people from starting the weight loss process in the first place. I try to find the weight where I can look in the mirror and feel confident in myself.

—Jennifer Bacani McKenney, MD, a mom of a two-year-old daughter who's expecting another baby and a family physician, in Fredonia, KS

MomMy TIME   **Make an I Believe Box**

Setting a goal or an intention is great. But committing it to paper makes it feel more concrete, real, *achievable*. An I Believe box is a special place to save your goals and dreams.

An I Believe box can be made of anything. Any sort of box or container will do. You might choose something especially meaningful to you, such as a box that looks like an antique book if you love to read. Or maybe a candy box that you saved from your first Valentine's Day with your husband.

To get started, write down as many goals and dreams as you can come up with. Some might be grand, blue sky ideas, and others might be simple, easy-to-accomplish goals. Write down both short- and long-term goals. Some might be for many years or months away, and others might be things you can do next week. Write each goal on a separate sheet of paper and tuck it into your I Believe box.

You might want to put your I Believe box in a special place. That could be somewhere you see often, to remind you to step toward your goals and follow your dreams. Or it could be somewhere more private if you wish to keep your goals and dreams close to your heart and not share them.

Every now and then, you might want to read your goals and dreams to remind yourself what you're hoping for and to see how far you've already come!

> **Setting goals is the first step in turning the invisible into the visible.**
>
> **—*Tony Robbins, an author and motivational speaker***

I have an app on my phone that I can use to set weight loss goals and track my progress. The app is called Lose It! My trainer recommended it to me. It's very easy to use, and I love it!

> —*Kristin C. Lyle, MD, FAAP, a mom of 10-, 7-, and 5-year-old daughters, the disaster medical director at Arkansas Children's Hospital, and an assistant professor of pediatrics at the University of Arkansas for Medical Sciences, both in Little Rock*

When I wanted to lose weight, I didn't set a goal weight. I didn't want to have a number in my head and risk disappointment if I didn't reach it. Instead, I used how my clothes fit as a guide. When I could fit into my pre-pregnancy clothes, I felt great. I might never get back to where I want to be in swimwear, but I'm not giving up yet!

> —*Pam D'Amato, MD, a mom of seven- and four-year-old daughters and an interventional pain management physician with University Spine Center, in Wayne, NJ*

My target used to be my pre-pregnancy weight. But I've come to the realization that I'm not going to get back to what I weighed in my twenties. I've made peace with that. Instead, I'm trying to get back to what I weighed between my two pregnancies. That's more realistic for me.

> —*Stephanie A. Wellington, MD, a mom of a 13-year-old son and an 11-year-old daughter, a hospitalist in the Level III NICU at Bellevue Hospital Center in New York City, and the medical coach and founder of PostpartumNeonatalCoaching.com*

After my kids were born, my desire to lose my pregnancy weight was a source of stress. I realized that I needed to set a realistic goal for myself. I decided I didn't need to get all the way back down to my pre-pregnancy weight. I'd be happy to get close. I adjusted my expectations, and that made it easier to achieve success.

I found that after my kids were born, my priorities really changed. I still wanted to look good, but I didn't want to put as much effort into it as I had before. With kids, so much of your energy is sucked into caring for them. Everything changes.

—*Aline T. Tanios, MD, a mom of 10- and 4-year-old daughters and an 8-year-old son and a pediatric hospitalist and assistant professor at the Washington University School of Medicine, in St. Louis, MO*

I don't set goals. Instead, I make intentions. An intention is something that you work toward, but just getting closer is success, rather than trying to meet a specific goal. Rather than setting a goal to lose 10 pounds, I made an intention to eat better and exercise more. I can't fail!

—*Jennifer Hanes, DO, a mom of a seven-year-old daughter and a four-year-old son, an emergency physician who's board certified in integrative medicine, and the author of* The Princess Plan: Shrink Your Waist, Expand Your Beauty, *in Austin, TX*

Most women intuitively know their goal weight. I was pudgy as a kid, and when I was in my twenties and thirties, I was about 15 pounds heavier than I am now. After studying obsessively what makes women feel balanced from their cells to their souls, I've concluded that a BMI of 20 to 23 is best—for me and most women. Some women prefer to be thinner, but that starts to creep into the slippery slope of the bone loss zone, or heavier, and that creeps into the you're-creating-an-inflamed-neighborhood-for-your-cells zone. Chronic inflammation is associated with many diseases.

I'm 5 feet 5 inches tall, and when I'm 125 pounds, I'm good at a

Mommy MD Guides-Recommended Product
MyFitnessPal

"I love the app MyFitnessPal," says Amy Baxter, MD, a mom of 15- and 12-year-old sons and a 10-year-old daughter; the CEO of BUZZY4SHOTS.COM; and the director of emergency research, Scottish Rite, of Children's Healthcare of Atlanta, in Georgia. "It's a free app you can use to scan barcodes, count calories, and chart the food you eat and the exercise you do. Best of all, you can connect with pals."

It's never been easier to keep a food journal and know exactly how many calories you're eating every day, thanks to food and fitness tracking apps such as MyFitnessPal. Open the app on your phone or computer every day, plug in the food you eat, and the app does the math for you. When you exercise, MyFitnessPal calculates how many calories you burned and adds it to your diary. If you choose, you can also track your weight and connect with friends who use the app.

The best part: It's free! MyFitnessPal is available across Android, iOS, Blackberry, Kindle, and Windows apps. So find the app in your phone's app store or go to **MYFITNESSPAL.COM** and set up an account.

MyFitnessPal includes a comprehensive database of more than 3,000,000 foods. You can create your own food database and add your own foods and recipes at any time and access them from anywhere with an Internet connection.

It also offers support with its discussion forums that let you learn from others, share your own tips, receive and give encouragement, and make friends.

BMI of 20.8, but I need to make sure I'm getting the minerals in my diet that I need for my bones. When I'm around 130 pounds, typically during the winter, my BMI is 21.6, which is just right. My clothes fit. I don't take radical vows of no-this and no-that every Monday. I pull on my skinny jeans and they fit, year after year, and they don't feel like sausage casing.

I set my goal weight around how I want to feel, and I want to feel at peace, generous, and celebratory. I don't want to swear off wine or sugar for the rest of my life, but I want to create the best neighborhood possible for my DNA.

—Sara Gottfried, MD, a mom of 13- and 8-year-old daughters, a board-certified gynecologist, and the author of The Hormone Cure, in Berkeley, CA

RALLIE'S TIP

The way I set a goal weight for myself has changed dramatically over time. Thank goodness! When I was young, and before I had my babies, I'd set the most ridiculous weight loss goals for myself, like "I'm going to lose seven pounds in five days!" Then I would set to work eating lettuce and cucumbers and exercising like a madwoman. Sometimes I would succeed, and sometimes I wouldn't. Either way, it was a terrible way to treat my body.

I don't do that anymore. Now that I'm older and wiser, I'm much kinder to myself, and I have far more gratitude for my good health. I don't take it for granted, and I don't want to risk losing it! When I was in my teens and early twenties, I wanted to weigh 115 pounds, like a fashion model. (Never mind that I was a tall, sturdy farm girl of 5 feet 9 inches, and I hadn't weighed 115 pounds since the sixth grade.) At that time, I wasn't really interested in having a healthy weight. I just wanted to be thin and glamorous looking. I was a member of that generation of women who equated thinness with beauty, intelligence, and self-control and all of those qualities that really have nothing whatsoever to do with how much you weigh.

Now that I have more sense and maturity about these things, and through years of trial and error, I realize that I feel healthiest, strongest, and most energetic when I weigh around 145 pounds. At 5 feet 9 inches, weighing 145 pounds gives me an acceptable BMI, so I know I'm not overloading my heart or my joints or endangering my health in other ways because of excess weight. At this weight, I can also carry enough muscle mass on my body to ride and train my horses, throw a bale of hay across a fence, or haul a couple of buckets of water to the barn if I need to. I can pick up my grandbabies and toss them into the air. I can hug my sons with gusto.

At 145 pounds, I will never be able to squeeze myself into a scrumptious pair of size 6 jeans—unless they've been mislabeled by the gods!—but I'm willing to live with that. The trade-off is that I get to feel strong, athletic, healthy, and vibrant, and I get to do all those things that I love to do every day of my life.

Getting Started

What will be the reason why you finally get serious about losing weight? It might be that it's a new year—why not become a new you? Or maybe you have an upcoming event, such as a high school reunion, for which you'd like to look more like the *old* you. Maybe your doctor urged you to lose weight—or your children or spouse did. Maybe you caught a glimpse of yourself in a mirror or a photo and thought, *Who's that?*

Whatever brought you to this moment of change is so much less important than what you do with that motivation and decision. You can make a change to be the healthiest you yet! To believe you can is everything.

❧

The first time I had a challenge with my weight was my freshman year in college. I gained the typical "freshman 15." When I felt super tired and had to buy bigger pants, I knew I needed to get motivated to lose the extra weight!

—Kay Corpus, MD, a mom of a six-year-old daughter and a two-year-old son, a family physician, and the director of Owensboro Health Integrative Medicine, in Kentucky

FitBit

You don't have to deny yourself any of your favorite foods. You just have to account for them. It's okay to eat a small serving of a sweet treat or a high-fat food every now and then. In fact, it might help keep you from going overboard and eating too much.

I gained about 50 pounds during my first few years of college. I knew I needed to get serious about losing weight when I noticed my clothes felt tight at our first college holiday break. Then I got motivated.

—*Eva Mayer, MD, a mom of a nine-year-old daughter and an eight-year-old son, an associate professor of pediatrics at Temple University, and a pediatrician with St. Luke's Pediatrics Associates, in Bethlehem, PA*

Before I was pregnant with my son, I was on the TV show *Survivor*. The show aired while I was pregnant, and it was difficult to watch myself growing thinner on the TV as I was gaining weight in real life! I looked big to myself. Plus, I was going to be on the show's live reunion episode when I was four months pregnant, and I felt pressure to look my normal weight for that. I was very motivated to get back to pre-*Survivor* weight again after my son was born.

—*Edna Ma, MD, a mom of a six-month-old son, an anesthesiologist at UCLA Olive View Medical Center, and the founder of BareEase pre-waxing numbing kit, in Los Angeles, CA*

About a year after my sons were born, I really started packing on the pounds. I think it was caused by a combination of my schedule being disrupted, falling off my regular exercise routine, and cooking—and eating—more. I realized I needed to lose weight when I moved up two dress sizes!

—*Bola Oyeyipo-Ajumobi, MD, a mom of five- and two-year-old sons, a family physician at the Veterans Health Administration, and the owner of SlimyBookWorm.com, in San Antonio, TX*

When my twins were six and my youngest turned four, I finally had the time to do a self-assessment! I think that a lot of women go through major changes when their kids begin full-day school. I took a hard look at my weight and fitness. I lost 25 pounds, and I've kept it off.

—*Katherine Dee, MD, a mom of eight-year-old twin daughters and a six-year-old son and a radiologist at the Seattle Breast Center, in Washington*

For most of my life, I didn't have a problem with my weight. I'm lucky to have inherited my father's high metabolism! But after my second child was born, getting back to exercising was very challenging. I kept expecting the added pregnancy weight to just drop off. When I finally stopped to think about my weight, I remember suddenly thinking, *I am really overweight.* That was an aha moment for me.

—*Allison Bailey, MD, a mom of a nine-year-old son and a five-year-old daughter and founder and director of Integrated Health and Fitness Associates, in Cambridge, MA*

I've had times in my life where I might have given into that three-layered chocolate cake more than once—a day. I also faced a weight gain challenge during the first year of my marriage. I had recently gotten married, started working at a new hospital, and moved to the Big Apple! Eating out at Hell's Kitchen and skipping workouts became a bad routine for me. The funny thing was the day of my wedding I was in the best shape of my life, and by my one-year anniversary I was in the worst shape of my life.

The moment I realized that perhaps I had indulged a little too frequently in the cookie jar was when I had to go to a friend's wedding. It was time to let loose and have fun celebrating, and all I could think of was how nothing fit! I had all these beautiful clothes that looked great on the rack but not on my body! It was time to undergo a lifestyle change, not a diet plan.

—*Arleen K. Lamba, MD, a mom of a three-month-old son, an anesthesiologist, the medical director of Blush Med Institute, and founder of the Blush Blends Skin Care line, in Washington, DC*

? When to Call Your Doctor

All right. You've decided it's time to lose weight. The next question is: How are you going to do it?

The answer is far from simple, considering the plethora of weight loss programs out there, some with big promises that you can lose 10 pounds the first week or that you'll have a bikini body in six weeks.

The most important thing to remember is to lose weight in a healthy way, and that typically means losing half a pound to two pounds a week (although you might lose weight faster at the beginning). When you choose a program that's more like a lifestyle plan and less like a diet, you can stick with it for many years. You'll also be more likely to achieve your goal weight and maintain that weight over the long haul. Plus, you'll be a shining example to your children of the right way to eat, exercise, and take care of yourself.

Talk to your doctor about the healthiest way for you to lose weight, given your current health. If you have diabetes or another medical condition, you'll have to take special care as you embark on a weight loss and exercise program. If you're breastfeeding, you should talk to your doctor about how cutting calories might affect your milk supply.

There might be a hospital-based weight loss program or support group in your area that your doctor can steer you toward. Or perhaps your doctor might refer you to a dietitian, who can give you further advice and recommend a weight loss program that's best for you.

If you'd rather follow a food plan online, you can talk to your doctor about using the USDA's SuperTracker, which is a place to maintain an online food diary and exercise log. There are even meal plans specifically designed for breastfeeding moms. Simply log on to CHOOSEMYPLATE.GOV/SUPERTRACKER-TOOLS/SUPERTRACKER.

I had an epiphany at the age of 39 in an unlikely place—a Madonna concert. I watched, riveted, as Madonna, 10 years older than me, sang and danced her heart out for more than two hours. I thought to myself, *That's it. I want to love my body like this woman loves her body. She is beautiful.*

Regardless of what you think about Madonna, we can probably agree that she is hot and has an incredibly lean body. From that moment on, I realized that the pain of staying the same—or lugging around the extra 15 to 20 pounds, constantly running the list of why the jeans are so tight—was worse than the pain of change.

—*Sara Gottfried, MD, a mom of 13- and 8-year-old daughters, a board-certified gynecologist, and the author of* The Hormone Cure, *in Berkeley, CA*

Before I got pregnant, I was about 5 to 10 pounds overweight. My physician told me not to diet while I was pregnant, and instead he advised me to "eat healthy." I actually lost 5 pounds in the first trimester of my first pregnancy.

But as my pregnancy went along, I had a lot of food cravings. In the Indian culture, you're supposed to give in to food cravings, so I gained quite a lot of weight. I'm a petite person, and I wasn't used to not fitting into my clothes. Being overweight took a huge toll on me emotionally. I was really looking forward to losing the weight after I had my baby.

—*Shilpa Amin-Shah, MD, a mom of a three-year-old son and a two-year-old daughter and an emergency physician and director of the recruiting team at Emergency Medical Associates, in Livingston, NJ*

I gained 40 pounds during my first pregnancy. It took me two years to lose all my baby weight from that first pregnancy. So for my second pregnancy, I was more cautious about what I ate, and I only gained 25 pounds, which was a lot easier to lose and get back to pre-baby weight.

The time of year you have your baby definitely affects your weight loss strategy. When my second daughter was born, I was really looking forward to losing the weight and getting active because she was a "summer baby." It was so much easier to get back into an exercise program during the summer than it had been with my older daughter, who was a "winter baby." I was really ready to get outside and walk off those pounds with her in her stroller.

—*Jeannette Gonzalez Simon, MD, a mom of four- and one-year-old daughters and a pediatric gastroenterologist at Staten Island Pediatrics GI, in New York*

I was amazed at how dramatically—and quickly—my body changed during pregnancy. This was hard for me.

Even after my baby was born, my body still felt so different. Before getting pregnant, I thought that after I had my baby, my body would quickly go back to its previous size. It doesn't exactly work like that.

After my baby was born, I was anxious to lose the weight. But at the same time, I wasn't going to sacrifice time with my baby to do it. I figured it could take a good 18 months to 2 years to get my weight back down to pre-pregnancy level. I wasn't going to go on a fad diet or do some super-intensive weight loss program. I was motivated to lose the weight, but to do it at my own pace. I wasn't going to push myself. I wanted to be healthy more than I wanted to be slim.

—*Christy Valentine, MD, a mom of a seven-year-old daughter, a specialist in pediatrics and internal medicine, and the founder of the Valentine Medical Center, in Gretna, LA*

I've tried all of the major weight loss programs, and they have worked for me, but only for a limited time. I think to be truly successful, you have to identify why you're overeating. For me, I discovered I was trying to distract myself with food and fulfill myself with food. I needed to find other ways to distract and fulfill myself, and then I was finally ready to be successful at losing weight.

—*Jennifer Hanes, DO, a mom of a seven-year-old daughter and a four-year-old son, an emergency physician who's board certified in integrative medicine, and the author of* The Princess Plan: Shrink Your Waist, Expand Your Beauty, *in Austin, TX*

> **The distance is nothing:**
> **It's only the first step that is difficult.**
> **—Mme. Du Deffand,**
> **a 17th-century French hostess and patron of the arts**

I've never been overweight, but I've had to work to stay that way. I ate well and exercised, but I was always "pleasantly padded."

After my first son was born, the weight came off so quickly that my husband thought there was something wrong with me! A combination of breastfeeding, walking, and getting back to my normal way of eating took the weight right off.

The weight didn't come off as easily after my second pregnancy. After my second son was born, I started to try to lose the weight by putting him into his stroller and taking him for walks when he was only a week old.

—Heather Orman-Lubell, MD, a mom of 12- and 8-year-old
sons and a pediatrician in private practice at Yardley Pediatrics of
St. Christopher's Hospital for Children, in Pennsylvania

I struggled with my weight a lot as a kid. Then, of course, it was a challenge after my pregnancies with my kids being 12 months and 2 weeks apart. I was pretty much pregnant for two years.

I tried hard during my pregnancies not to overdo it and gain a lot of weight. It's a common misconception that when you're pregnant, you're eating for two. Actually, you only need an additional 100 to 300 calories a day!

I also tried to exercise during pregnancy. During my second pregnancy, I knew I could push myself more than I had during my first. I knew I was ready to lose weight when my baby was born. I was anxious to get rid of my "soft spots."

—Antoinette Cheney, DO, a mom of a seven-year-old son and
a six-year-old daughter and a family physician with Rocky Vista
University College of Osteopathic Medicine, in Parker, CO

I never had weight problems until after my pregnancies. I gained 60 pounds. It took me a few years to get motivated, though, because I thought the weight would come off pretty much by itself. It didn't.

One day, I caught a glimpse of myself in a mirror and thought, *Maybe I need to do something about this.* That got me motivated to make a change! My weight wasn't acceptable to me anymore.

—Tiemdow Phumiruk, MD, a mom of 13-, 10-, and 7-year-old daughters, a pediatrician in the emergency department of Children's Hospital Colorado at Parker Adventist Hospital, and adjunct faculty at Rocky Vista University College of Osteopathic Medicine, in Parker, CO

MOMMY TIME: Set Up a Pinterest Account

It can feel overwhelming when you're making lifestyle changes to lose weight, and it's good to have all the information and guidance you can get. That's where Pinterest comes in. In addition to all of the advice and tips you'll get in this book, Pinterest can be a place to continue receiving support and great advice.

Pinterest is a free website that acts as an online pin board in which you share ideas with others. For weight loss, it's a great place to collect healthy recipes, workout ideas, weight loss articles, and inspiration from around the web. After you set up an account, you can "follow" other people and see the photos that they've Pinned. When you find a photo that you love, you can save it to your account. Then you can easily find a great recipe for a healthy weeknight meal whenever you need it. Or when you're in an exercise rut, look for a new treadmill or walking program. Or when you're lacking motivation, find a great quote.

Because pictures and images are at the heart of Pinterest, browsing the site feels a lot like paging through glossy magazines, which means it can feel like a guilty pleasure while it's helping you reach your weight loss goals.

In my life, I go through phases where I get really motivated to lose weight. For example, I was in Arizona recently for a meeting, and I put on my bathing suit to go swimming. But after I saw myself in the hotel mirrors, I decided to skip the good food and buffets. I just couldn't look at myself in those mirrors. Seeing myself in my bathing suit motivated me to lose some weight.

But at the same time, I think that you have to try to love yourself the way you are. It's hard to treat your body well and lose weight if you hate yourself.

I tell myself, "This is who I am, extra pounds and all." Yes, it would be nice to be a few pounds thinner, but I try to be my own best friend.

—*Judith Hellman, MD, a mom of a 15-year-old son, an associate clinical professor of dermatology at Mt. Sinai Hospital in New York City, and a dermatologist in private practice*

After my younger daughter was born, I tried to make dietary changes and exercise to lose the weight. It wasn't helping as much as it had before. The number on the scale wouldn't budge, and my clothes weren't fitting. It took me about a year to decide that I needed a new approach.

This was a turning point for me. I needed to find a way to motivate myself. So I signed up for a half marathon. Never mind I had never run more than two or three miles in the past!

I downloaded a training "recipe" to follow, and I used that to build up my stamina. I ran on my treadmill from January to March, and then in the spring I took my running outside. Then the weight finally came off.

I ran the half marathon. Meeting that goal was one of the most exhilarating moments of my life!

—*Pam D'Amato, MD, a mom of seven- and four-year-old daughters and an interventional pain management physician with University Spine Center, in Wayne, NJ*

I'm only 4 feet 8 inches tall, so gaining even five pounds is significant. After my first pregnancy, I needed to buy size 12s. Plus, because I'm short, everything needed to be hemmed. That's a pain, and it's expensive!

Because I dress in business casual for work, I needed quite a lot of clothing, and it was impacting my closet space. I felt like I was shopping all of the time. And for once in my life, I did not want to shop. It meant more time away from my precious children.

As we started to go into a new fashion season, I thought of all of those new clothes that I'd need to buy, to hem, and to store. This would take time, and I wanted to spend that time with my children, rather than at the mall. That was the straw that broke the camel's back for me. I needed to make changes to lose the weight and to get healthy for myself and for my children. Those were the things that motivated me.

A tricky thing about losing weight is that you can't put it on your to-do list until you're honestly ready to cross it off. Until you find the right time—and the right reasons—for you, you're not ready. Otherwise you'll continue to beat yourself up about needing to lose weight, but you won't be successful at it.

For me, I knew I was ready when I was confronted with the logistical challenge of having too many sizes of clothing to fit into my closet and not wanting to waste more time shopping for a new wardrobe as my waistline expanded. It was time.

—*Amy Thompson, MD, a mom of six-, four-, and two-year-old sons and an ob-gyn at the University of Cincinnati College of Medicine, in Ohio*

❧

As far back as I can remember, I have struggled with achieving a balance between what I want to weigh and what I actually do weigh. Now I firmly believe that it's all about how I feel and my health. The scale is an indication of where I am health-wise, but it's not how I define myself. At some points in my life, I've definitely been in better shape than at other times, and when life gets more complicated, controlling my weight gets harder for me.

One thing that I find very motivating is hearing success stories of other people who have lost weight. I enjoy hearing what

FitBit

Rearrange your kitchen to support your new, healthy life-style. Stock the fridge with bottled water instead of soda. Toss out the cookies and fill your cookie jar with nutritious, low-fat trail mix. Throw out the chips and cheese-twists and replace them with whole grain crackers. Keep a bowl of fresh fruit in plain sight on the kitchen counter. It's easier to make wise food choices when they're readily available.

motivated them and how they became successful at changing their lives.

As a plastic surgeon, I perform a lot of body-contouring procedures on moms who have lost their baby weight, and on men and women who have lost excess weight and have loose skin. Many patients I treat didn't have surgery to help them lose weight; they lost the weight on their own through changes in diet and exercise. More often than not, they made simple changes over long periods of time, and those small changes added up to big weight loss.

I ask every patient about the motivating factor, or the "secret," to their success. Many times, the "secret" was a defining moment—not fitting into a particular piece of clothing, seeing an unflattering photograph of themselves, or watching a family member struggle with an obesity-related illness—and then sticking with the positive changes that moment created. For example, one patient told me that she simply started eating less of everything she wanted. Another said she just started going to bed at night a little bit hungry. Most successful weight loss patients increased their activity (even just a little bit every day) and focused daily on their goals. Many of my patients come to surgery consultations with supportive family members. I think having a strong group of positive people around you makes a huge difference.

—*Michelle Spring, MD, a mom of a one-year-old son and two grown stepchildren and a board-certified plastic surgeon with Marina Plastic Surgery Associates, in Marina del Rey, CA*

RALLIE'S TIP

Starting on your weight loss journey will undoubtedly require you to make some changes—to your diet, exercise routine, and lifestyle. Change is difficult and sometimes a little scary, even if it's good change. Doing the same old thing isn't just easy—it's also comfortable and familiar.

When I'm trying to make a positive change in my life, no matter how excited I am about the intended result, I always try to remind myself to start out really small, and I've found that's the best way to succeed. For instance, if you want to start exercising, start with a goal you can master relatively easily. Rather than telling yourself that you're going to start running a mile a day on Monday morning, it's better to start out walking for 15 minutes three times a week. That's not nearly as difficult or as scary as running a mile a day, and you're much more likely to succeed without injuring your body—or your pride. Once you've mastered the trick of getting out of bed to walk for 15 minutes three mornings a week, it's far easier to take the next step of running for 15 minutes a day, and then continuing to increase your time and distance until you can run a mile with relative ease. Success generates success. When you succeed at small goals, you're motivated and confident enough to tackle the bigger ones.

It's also helpful to do all the little things that make it easier for you to succeed at making a change. Preparation is key. For instance, if you want to start eating more fresh fruits and vegetables, go to the grocery store and buy your favorites over the weekend or at the beginning of the week. Peel and cut them up and put them in single-serving containers so they'll be easy to grab when you're hungry. Buy some of your favorite veggie dip ahead of time. If you want to walk in the morning, gather up your sweatpants and walking shoes and put them where you can easily find them. Make it as easy and as painless as possible to make the change.

While you're at it, find a way to make change fun. If your new behavior is boring or painful, why in the world would you want to stick with it?

Don't listen to the negative voice in your head. We all have one, but we don't have to listen to it! When you hear the voice of resistance or doubt, drown it out with a pep talk. Remind yourself of the reasons that you're choosing to make this change, and keep your eye on the prize!

Making Time to Eat Better and Exercise More

You're a mother, wife, grocery store shopper, gift buyer, schedule organizer, laundry doer, cleaner-upper, chauffeur, errand runner, chef, dish washer, boo-boo kisser, disagreement mediator, and more. Yikes, how on earth could you have time to prepare nutritious meals and exercise too?

Actually, the more important question is: How could you *not*? To do all that you do, you need the energy of Super Mario, the strength of Popeye, and the determination of Wile E. Coyote. You need some serious fuel and energy reserves. You need to make time for *you*.

I swam in college, and I was always used to getting up first thing in the morning to work out. That's always been my routine. This works out well with kids. I get up early and get my workout done, and then I'm not interrupting them to work out.

—*Antoinette Cheney, DO, a mom of a seven-year-old son and a six-year-old daughter and a family physician with Rocky Vista University College of Osteopathic Medicine, in Parker, CO*

I set my alarm for 5 am each morning. This way I have time alone to exercise—and to get some paperwork done—before my kids are awake. This gives me more energy, so I make myself do it.

—*Eva Mayer, MD, a mom of a nine-year-old daughter and an eight-year-old son, an associate professor of pediatrics at Temple University, and a pediatrician with St. Luke's Pediatrics Associates, in Bethlehem, PA*

I typically exercise early in the afternoon before I pick up my kids from school. This schedule works for me because it's when I have time. It also gently raises my cortisol and mood.

—Sara Gottfried, MD, a mom of 13- and 8-year-old daughters, a board-certified gynecologist, and the author of The Hormone Cure, in Berkeley, CA

I have to actually make exercise a priority. I put it on my Microsoft Outlook calendar as part of my day. Sometimes, my kids and I turn on some music and have a half-hour dance party in the kitchen. That really burns calories! My husband and I take the kids to the park when the weather is nice. My kids also love practicing yoga with me. They love doing downward dogs and backbends every chance they get.

—Kay Corpus, MD, a mom of a six-year-old daughter and a two-year-old son, a family physician, and the director of Owensboro Health Integrative Medicine, in Kentucky

One of my family's time-saving tricks is for my husband to make a big pot of healthy food, such as tabbouleh, so that we can eat it through-out the week, along with other dishes. It's filled with parsley and tomatoes, it has a lot of nutrients and fiber, and it's delicious. (See the recipe on page 303.) We cook once and enjoy it all week.

—Hana R. Solomon, MD, a mom who raised four children, a grandmom of three, a board-certified pediatrician, the president of BeWell Health, LLC, and the author of Clearing the Air One Nose at a Time: Caring for Your Personal Filter, in Columbia, MO

For me, cooking is all about "semi-homemade." I want to make healthy meals, but with my schedule they have to be easy and quick. We eat a lot of salads, and to speed up the prep, I buy Dole bagged salad mixes. I also buy cleaned and prepped vegetables such as Brussels sprouts, broccoli, and green beans in the steam microwave bags. I often pick up marinated, cooked chicken breasts at Trader Joe's. They're already cooked, moist, and delicious, so I just have to make a side dish to serve alongside them, and dinner is ready for those extra busy days!

A lot of people don't realize that one of the fastest, easiest foods to cook is fish. I buy flounder, cod, or skinless salmon. I wrap it tightly in aluminum foil with a few dabs of butter and some herbs such as rosemary or dill. Then I bake it at 450 degrees for around 10 minutes.

> —*Jeannette Gonzalez Simon, MD, a mom of four- and one-year-old daughters and a pediatric gastroenterologist at Staten Island Pediatrics GI, in New York*

I try to find little time-savers throughout my day. One thing that helps save time is running errands during and making appointments for off-peak times. I shop at the mall or the grocery store on weekdays because they're a lot less crowded than on weekends.

> —*Sonali Ruder, DO, a mom of a two-month-old daughter, an emergency physician at Coral Springs Medical Center near Fort Lauderdale, FL, and a recipe developer and blogger at TheFoodiePhysician.com*

With two small children, I'm struggling more now than I have in the past to eat right and exercise. I'm so busy every day working and taking care of my kids. At the end of most days, I'm so tired I feel like there's no way I could work out. As my kids have gotten older, it's gotten even harder because I get so caught up in their activities. I've lost the time for myself.

I try hard to free up time for exercise with time-saving tactics at home. I do a lot of shopping online for clothing and household goods. Two sites I visit frequently are Diapers.com and Soap.com.

—Sigrid Payne DaVeiga, MD, a mom of a seven-year-old son and a two-year-old daughter and a pediatric allergist with the Children's Hospital of Philadelphia, in Pennsylvania

To free up some much-needed time for exercise, I always make a grocery list and organize it by sections in the grocery store. This means I do less backtracking across the store, and it helps keep me out of most of the middle aisles, which hold the processed foods. I try to shop the perimeter of the store, where the fresh ingredients are found.

Also, I have a second fridge in the garage. I love it! With three boys, we go through four gallons of skim milk a week! If I didn't have that second fridge, I would need to make two or three trips to the grocery store every week.

—Amy Thompson, MD, a mom of six-, four-, and two-year-old sons and an ob-gyn at the University of Cincinnati College of Medicine, in Ohio

Here's one of my best time-saving tips: My favorite type of clothing is leggings. If they go out of style, I'm in trouble! I wear a long sweater over a pair of leggings, with a T-shirt underneath. If I have a few spare minutes to exercise, I just pull off the sweater and voilà, I'm wearing workout clothes! They're so versatile and practical, and wearing them saves me lots of time.

If I had to spend two minutes changing clothes, it might give me time to change my mind and do something other than work out! By wearing leggings, I can drop everything at a moment's notice, and I'm ready to exercise.

—Tiemdow Phumiruk, MD, a mom of 13-, 10-, and 7-year-old daughters, a pediatrician in the emergency department of Children's Hospital Colorado at Parker Adventist Hospital, and adjunct faculty at Rocky Vista University College of Osteopathic Medicine, in Parker, CO

Life with kids and work gets so hectic. I have a dry-erase board on my refrigerator, and my husband and I note all of our activities there. We even schedule trips to the gym there. We sync our phone calendars too, but the low-tech dry-erase board is actually a better system for us.

The dry-erase board also doubles as a message center. My daughter gets a kick out of telling me, "Daddy wrote you a message."

—*Jeannette Gonzalez Simon, MD*

Mommy MD Guides-Recommended Product

KalynsKitchen.com

"After my sons were born, life was so hectic," says Amy Thompson, MD, a mom of six-, four-, and two-year-old sons and an ob-gyn at the University of Cincinnati College of Medicine, in Ohio. "My husband and I really weren't eating well.

"One day, a patient told me she had lost a lot of weight on the South Beach Diet. Resolved now to lose weight, I Googled it, and I came across a wonderful website, KALYNSKITCHEN.COM. This site offers delicious, nutritious recipes by a woman who lost 42 pounds. Many of the recipes can be used on the South Beach Diet, and many of them have a low glycemic index and are low-carb. Other diets and meal plans seemed stagnant and did not really let me cook.

"That site is so helpful. I love to cook; I find it very therapeutic. I don't like to get new recipes from cookbooks because they're static. A cookbook isn't a living thing. I needed a diet that had an infinite number of options.

"KalynsKitchen.com is ever-changing, with new recipes and ideas every day. Once I discovered it, I felt like a home chef again. I refer to the site almost daily, and I send my patients there. It's amazing!"

There's no charge for any of the recipes on KALYNSKITCHEN.COM. Visit the site to learn more.

I'm a big list maker, and it's been wonderful to see my sons develop into list-makers too! As my sons have gotten older, I'm able to delegate more tasks to them, freeing up some time for myself. We have a dry-erase board on our refrigerator, and I write to-do lists on it. My sons like to complete tasks and cross them off the list.

My sons also have regular chores that they are responsible for. My older son makes everyone's school lunches. My nine-year-old son does the laundry one day a week. My seven-year-old empties the dishwasher and puts the dishes away. (Well, the places he can reach anyway.) Even my five-year-old feeds the dogs.

—Deborah Gilboa, MD, a mom of 11-, 9-, 7-, and 5-year-old sons, a family physician with Squirrel Hill Health Center in Pittsburgh, PA, and a parenting speaker whose advice is found at AskDoctorG.com

As your kids get older, it gets so much easier to find time to exercise and eat better. During my pregnancies and the time when my kids were little, it was really hard to find time to exercise and cook. I was exhausted all of the time.

But now that my kids are older, and they're not waking up in the middle of the night, I'm not so tired, and I have more time to myself. I take a kickboxing and dance class at the gym. It's taught by a phenomenal mom of four who's in her fifties! It's a lot of fun; we dance and work out to high-energy music by Pit Bull and LMFAO.

When I don't have time to go to the gym, I do TurboFire and P90X. TurboFire is a fun combination of dance, kickboxing, and strength training, and P90X is a combination of plyometrics, strength training, and kickboxing. I must confess, I don't follow these programs exactly; I pick and choose what I want to do. These workouts are excellent for toning muscles, and they make me feel great.

—*Amy Barton, MD, a mom of an 11-year-old daughter and 8- and 5-year-old sons and a pediatrician at St. Luke's Children's Hospital, in Boise, ID*

I exercise for only 4 ½ minutes a day. No kidding! I break it down into three 90-second sessions. Right before I eat, I do 90 seconds of very strenuous exercise. For example, I might hold a plank position for a minute and a half. That might not sound like a lot, but it gets my pulse racing, and it makes me sweat. Or I might do squats, lunges, pushups, or situps for 90 seconds.

These tiny bursts of exercise are certainly better than nothing. Plus, doing them right before I eat helps stabilize my blood sugar. By exercising right before I eat, there's more blood flow to my thighs than to my gut. Consequently, I don't feel as hungry, and it's a reminder while I'm eating that I just did something great for my body.

—*Jennifer Hanes, DO, a mom of a seven-year-old daughter and a four-year-old son, an emergency physician who's board certified in integrative medicine, and the author of* The Princess Plan: Shrink Your Waist, Expand Your Beauty, *in Austin, TX*

I have a very busy medical practice, I run a skin care company, and I'm also an extremely active part of my husband's and son's lives. It's hard to find time for myself, and I feel guilty when I try. My son is an only child, and at his age he can't understand why we can't be at all of his school events and activities.

To make time to exercise, I walk everywhere, such as to and from work—unless it's minus 3 degrees outside! We also go to the gym together as a family. My son likes to walk on the treadmill and shoot baskets. He'll do pretty much anything at the gym that we'll let him do!

—*Michelle Yagoda, MD, a mom of an 11-year-old son, a facial plastic surgeon, the CEO of Opus Skincare, LLC, and cofounder of BeautyScoop, a patented and clinically proven supplement for skin, hair, and nails, in New York City*

Based on everything I knew as a psychiatrist, I spent only 20 hours a week away from my daughter for the first four years of her life. Needless to say, it was a challenge to have a career within this parameter. I worked at home a lot, and I still do.

Of course, finding time to exercise also presented a challenge.

So I exercised with my daughter. There are more ways to do this than the proverbial jogging stroller. I swam laps while she took swimming lessons. I also found a studio that offered gymnastics classes for kids while one of the moms taught a yoga class, for the adults.

—Dora Calott Wang, MD, a mom of a 10-year-old daughter, historian of the University of New Mexico School of Medicine, a unit director at Las Encinas Hospital in Pasadena, CA, and the author of The Kitchen Shrink: A Psychiatrist's Reflection on Healing in a Changing World

In addition to regular exercise, I strive to incorporate movement into everything I do. I also avoid prolonged sitting—in fact, I don't have a sit-down desk. I have a stand-up desk. So as I'm writing, reading, and talking on the phone, I'm standing. Standing burns more calories, and it facilitates movement. It takes a lot of energy to push your chair back and stand up, but if you're already standing, it's effortless to move around.

Of course, not everyone is able to have a stand-up desk in their offices! But you don't have to just sit there. Stand up and walk to the restroom, to talk to a colleague, or to get a drink. A great goal is to build 10 minutes of light activity into every hour of your day.

—Ann Kulze, MD, a mom of 24- and 17-year-old daughters and 22- and 21-year-old sons; a nationally recognized nutrition expert, motivational speaker, and physician; and the author of the best-selling, award-winning Eat Right for Life *book series, in Charleston, SC*

I'm very committed to exercising, no matter how busy I am. For most of my life I've been a fitness model, and my husband is a fitness celebrity who owns a nutrition and supplement company. Exercise is a huge part of our lives.

FitBit

If you don't have time for a 30-minute workout, exercise in three 10-minute sessions. Exercise doesn't have to be strenuous or continuous to be beneficial. Repeated short bouts of moderate-intensity activity contribute to weight loss and good health.

Even though I'm very busy, I exercise almost every day. Since my daughter was born, I've wanted to spend as much time as possible with her, so I've rearranged my schedule. Rather than exercising right after work, I exercise first thing in the morning while my baby is sleeping, or at night after she goes to sleep. I'm usually in surgery all day (which burns calories, especially with my big liposuction or mommy makeover procedures), and then I try to make dinner early, around 6 or 7 pm. I try to condense my kitchen tasks, so I'll do the dishes as I'm cooking. Right after we eat, I'll wash the remaining dishes and clean the kitchen. Then I play with my daughter until bath time at 9 pm and hug until 11 pm when she goes to bed.

The key to doing this is being very organized so I'll have that extra time to exercise. I also try to clean and put things away after I use them so that I don't have to come back to do it later. As a full-time working mom, I've become very efficient at completing tasks in a short amount of time!

—*Catherine Begovic, MD, a mom of a six-month-old daughter and a plastic surgeon at Make You Perfect, Inc., in Beverly Hills, CA*

If you want to lose weight, the most important thing you have to do is make time for yourself. Many of my patients who struggle with their weight tell me, "I don't have time to lose weight."

That might be true, but only because they're overscheduled. They're so overwhelmed with being the best wives and mothers they can be that they forget how important they themselves are.

My kids and my husband are very understanding about my need to exercise. They know that I get cranky—and a little crazy—if I don't work out regularly. If the wife and mom is happy, everyone is happy!

I don't have as much time with my kids as stay-at-home moms do, but I feel the quality of our time together is great. Part of that is because my kids allow me to do what I need to do to take care of myself and to feel good about myself. You have to schedule yourself first sometimes. Your needs are important too!

Let Hypnosis Work on Your Subconscious

How would you like a little extra motivation to make the right daily choices to lose those pounds? Hypnosis might be your ticket.

Hypnosis is about getting to a place of relaxation and concentration where you're more open to suggestion. You naturally go into that state all the time, including when you're driving, watching television, drifting off to sleep, and waking up in the morning. While you're in this relaxed state, your hypnotherapist will make suggestions for healthy behaviors that will help you get to your goal. (Unlike portrayals in the movies, hypnosis isn't about going into a deep trance where you don't have control over your movements and don't remember what you said or did.)

A few studies have found that hypnosis for weight loss might lead to an average of six pounds of weight loss. Hypnosis can also help with dealing with stress and helping you feel calm. But if you decide to try hypnotherapy, be sure to do it while exercising and making healthy changes to your diet.

A session with a hypnotherapist typically costs $75 to $125. You can find a specialist by searching the website of the American Association of Professional Hypnotherapists at **AAPH.ORG**. You can also buy hypnosis CDs or pay a fee to download pre-recorded audio sessions from hypnotherapists for as low as $3 for a short, basic session to $15 to $25 for a focused session. You can even find hypnosis apps for your phone or iPad.

—Martha Wittenberg, MD, MPH, a mom of an eight-year-old son and a six-year-old daughter and a family physician with Seal Beach Family Medicine, in California

⌒〜⌒

A major obstacle to losing weight is finding the time to do it. When I really thought about it, I realized that when I had tried to lose weight before, I had taken on too much, too fast. I had a new baby, and I had resolved to breastfeed, go back to work, and exercise. It was a recipe for disaster. I had set myself up for failure.

So I took losing weight off my to-do list, and I stopped beating myself up about it. I gave myself some time to focus on my baby, breastfeeding him and being with him. *I can't tackle my weight right now*, I thought.

After some time had passed, I took a good look at my life. I thought about all of the reasons why I had failed at losing weight in the past. Once you take stock of your failures, you can plan your success.

Next, I brainstormed ways that I could integrate healthier choices into my life, without adding any *new* tasks. I realized the two things I had to do to succeed at losing weight were to make better choices at the grocery store and at meals. *That's where I can make healthy changes without adding a lot of extra time or work*, I realized. Finally, I was ready to lose the weight.

—Amy Thompson, MD, a mom of six-, four-, and two-year-old sons and an ob-gyn at the University of Cincinnati College of Medicine, in Ohio

RALLIE'S TIP

As a mom of three sons, I spend a lot of time in the kitchen making meals and snacks and putting food on the table for my family. Over the years, I've found that the more often I cook, the more often I nibble. (After all, everything has to be taste-tested by the mom, right?) The more often I nibble, the more I end up eating, and the more weight I gain.

One of the best ways I've found to save time in the kitchen and to reduce the amount of nibbling I do is to designate one day a week as my

cooking and baking day. Sunday afternoon works best for me, and I usually try to lure my kids into the kitchen to help me out. We actually end up having fun, and my boys have learned how to make a decent meal or two in the process.

On cooking and baking Sunday, we prepare a half-dozen meals or more at once and store them all in the fridge or freezer. That way, we're not tempted to stop by a fast-food restaurant on our way home from work or school. There's already food waiting for us at home! And I'm not faced with the less than thrilling prospect of slaving over supper when I'm zapped from a long day at work. Instead, I just pop a nutritious, homemade dinner into the oven or onto the stove and steam some fresh veggies or throw together a salad to go with it.

On meal-making day, I double my recipes or plan them for maximum efficiency. If I'm browning lean ground beef for chili, it makes good sense to go ahead and prepare enough for a spaghetti dinner and some lasagna while I'm at it. When I make seven or eight meals at once, my kitchen stays cleaner throughout the week, and I end up spending far less time washing dishes and soaking pots and pans. I invest the time that I save by not cooking each evening in fitness activities, such as taking a bike ride or running on my treadmill for a half-hour.

Considering a Weight Loss Program

Turn on the TV, glance at a billboard, flip open a magazine, and you'll see plenty of weight loss programs out there. And for good reason: Some of them are very successful at what they do.

Among people who have lost weight and joined the National Weight Control Registry (NWCR), which is the largest prospective investigation of long-term successful weight loss maintenance, more than half—55 percent—used a weight loss program. The NWCR was developed to identify and investigate the characteristics of people who have succeeded at long-term weight loss. The NWCR is tracking more than 10,000 people who have lost at least 30 pounds and kept the weight off for at least a year.

In another study, researchers who analyzed data from more

than 4,000 obese people found that of those who were trying to lose weight, 40 percent saw their weight drop 5 percent or more, and another 20 percent lost 10 percent or more of their body weight by exercising and eating less fat. What worked the best? Structured weight loss programs helped the study participants be more successful.

However, like so many things in life, if a weight loss program sounds too good to be true, it probably is. The researchers found that liquid diets, weight loss pills, and diet foods and products were not helpful.

Keep in mind that humans have always eaten a natural diet of plants and animal foods. None of our ancestors flourished by eating an all-grapefruit diet; they certainly didn't inject themselves with hormones; and the ones who *didn't* get tapeworms were the ones who lived to pass on their genes!

When I was taking off my pregnancy weight, I read a book called *The Zone*. It's not so much a diet as an eating plan for life. I incorporated a lot of the principles from that book into my life. For example, I make sure to eat some protein at every meal. Protein helps you feel fuller longer.

—*Kristin C. Lyle, MD, FAAP, a mom of 10-, 7-, and 5-year-old daughters, the disaster medical director at Arkansas Children's Hospital, and an assistant professor of pediatrics at the University of Arkansas for Medical Sciences, both in Little Rock*

To lose weight, I've tried a modified 17-Day Diet program. That's a program from the book by the same name written by Michael Moreno, MD. I adjusted the program to fit my lifestyle, and I cut back on red meat and carbs and ate a lot more of other high-protein foods such as beans and lean white meat. I mostly eat all kinds of vegetables, which are packed with nutrients and low in fat and calories.

> —*Aline T. Tanios, MD, a mom of 10- and 4-year-old daughters and an 8-year-old son and a pediatric hospitalist and assistant professor at the Washington University School of Medicine, in St. Louis, MO*

When to Call Your Doctor

If you choose to try a weight loss program, it's a good idea to check with your doctor or dietitian first to make sure it's a safe and sensible choice, especially before you sign up for a commercial plan that costs hundreds of dollars.

You want to make sure that you'll be eating enough calories and a variety of foods every day. Also, you want to make sure that the program will keep your heart and bones in good health.

Your best bet is to choose a plan that's nutritious and balanced enough that you can keep it up for the long run. Diets that ban entire food groups aren't the best option for long-term success, especially if you're breastfeeding, considering getting pregnant again, or if you need to keep your energy levels up to chase after your toddler.

Your options will fall into four general categories.

Commercial plans. We've all seen the ads for Weight Watchers, Jenny Craig, Nutrisystem, eDiets, and other weight loss programs. Commercial plans range from healthy to the not-so-healthy (hint: fasting). To be sure you're going in the right direction, check with your doctor or dietitian.

Web-based programs and apps. Several online sites offer food and exercise tracking and huge databases of nutrition information for

I find it very helpful to use a free online program called FatSecret.com. For several months, I logged everything I ate, and it really helped me identify what works and what doesn't work when I'm trying to lose weight. Knowing that I'm going to log what I'll be eating makes me a lot less likely to eat to excess. The site offers a food and calorie finder that includes whole foods, restaurant foods, and packaged foods. You can find nutrition information for your recipes by plugging in the ingredients.

—*Katherine Dee, MD, a mom of eight-year-old twin daughters and a six-year-old son and a radiologist at the Seattle Breast Center, in Washington*

the foods you eat. Some even offer eating plans for low-carb, Mediterranean, or vegetarian diets and might include advice from experts. Popular sites, which might be free or charge a fee, include SparkPeople, Calorie King, MyFitnessPal, Lose It!, FitDay, SuperTracker, DietWatch, and WebMD. Again, the best choice for you will depend on your current health and fitness, so it's a good idea to check with your doctor or dietitian before jumping in.

Clinical programs. These include hospital-based programs or programs run by health care professionals in private practice. Traditionally they've been known to be very low-calorie diets, but they've evolved to become more moderate. People who sign up for these programs have the benefit of being treated by a team of medical professionals, including doctors, dietitians, exercise therapists, and psychologists. However, some programs are designed for people with a Body Mass Index (BMI) of more than 30, so you'll need to talk to your doctor about whether or not the program you're considering is right for you.

Nonprofit self-help programs. Programs such as Overeaters Anonymous and Take Off Pounds Sensibly (TOPS) offer meetings where people can get support for dealing with compulsive overeating.

When I worked in a weight loss clinic, we talked about a "therapeutic lifestyle change." That's what I've tried to do.

We worked in a comprehensive clinic that focused on total lifestyle changes. Patients met with a physician, a psychologist, a trainer, and a dietitian. I've found that I have to eat healthy foods and exercise

Mommy MD Guides–Recommended Product
Weight Watchers

"When I realized that for the first time in my life I needed to lose weight, I joined Weight Watchers," says Allison Bailey, MD, a mom of a nine-year-old son and a five-year-old daughter and founder and director of Integrated Health and Fitness Associates, in Cambridge, MA.

"I don't have time to get to meetings, so I joined their online program. It worked really well for me. I registered and created a profile. The site helped me to determine the number of Weight Watchers points I could eat each day. Each point is a simple calculation of a food's calories, fat, and fiber. The site has calculators and food charts. It uses your age, height, and current weight to help you figure out how much weight you have to lose and the appropriate number of daily points to help you reach this goal. There are even places online where you can enter your activities and get an estimate of the number of calories burned.

"I kept track of my Weight Watchers points with a smartphone app. It really helped me get back into the frame of mind of eating for one! I also set my goal weight on my phone, and the app monitored my progress toward meeting that goal."

"I am still working on my weight (although not working very hard or I would have gotten back into all of my pre-pregnancy clothes by now!)," adds Rachel S. Rohde, MD, a mom of a two-year-old daughter, an assistant professor of orthopaedic surgery at the Oakland University William Beaumont School of Medicine, and an orthopaedic upper-extremity surgeon with Michigan Orthopaedic Institute, P.C., in to maintain my weight and ideal level of fitness. But I also need to be aware of the triggers that cause me to eat (such as stress and having to do too much, and studying), and I need to find ways to keep healthy snacks on hand if I know I'm going to be triggered. I know that *if* I buy a bag of chips, I *will* eat the whole thing if I'm stressed. It's safer just

Southfield, MI. "Weight Watchers works. Joining online didn't really help me, but I and several others I know have signed up and gone to meetings. It helps to see (and hear) others who are trying to drop a few pounds as well. Many people like the 'points' system, but I like the concept of eating the 'power foods,' such as fruits, vegetables, and lean proteins. The meeting leaders' styles are *very* different, but we found one who is hilarious and full of good ideas. (She packs the room on Saturdays at 7:30 am, so you *know* she's good!) Obviously, having to step on a scale every week holds one accountable. I really just needed to get back into healthier eating habits after living by the philosophy of 'I'm pregnant and the baby wants Mexican food and chocolate ice cream all day!'"

In 2013, for the third straight year in a row, *US News & World Report* ranked Weight Watchers as the number one best weight loss diet.

Weight Watchers meetings are led by people who also lost weight with Weight Watchers. Meeting weigh-ins are completely confidential, and you don't have to "share" in meetings if you don't want to. It costs a fee to join, and a weekly fee. Weight Watchers often features special promotions, such as a chance to join for free.

Can't make meetings? Weight Watchers online might be for you. You can follow the customizable plan with your computer and/or app, using online tools to find recipes and workouts, research foods, and track your progress.

Visit **WEIGHTWATCHERS.COM** for more information.

> **The strong individual is the one**
> **who asks for help when he needs it.**
> **—Rona Barrett, columnist and businesswoman**

not to have them in the house. Ditto with a box of Girl Scout Cookies.

> —Lennox McNeary, MD, a mom of a four-year-old son, a
> specialist in physical medicine and rehabilitation at Carilion Clinic,
> and a cofounder of the Mommy Doctors Bakery (makers of Milkin'
> Cookies), in Roanoke, VA

Fad diets and diet medications don't work. Instead, I follow a simple program called the 5-2-1-0 Rule.

"5" is for eating five fruits and vegetables a day.

"2" is for two hours or less of screen time a day.

"1" is for one hour of exercise each day. This doesn't have to be intense aerobics! It can include anything that gets your heart rate up, such as walking up stairs and playing with your kids.

"0" is for no sugary drinks. I avoid sweet tea and soda. Instead I drink unsweetened tea or water flavored with lemon or frozen fruit.

> —Eva Mayer, MD, a mom of a nine-year-old daughter and
> an eight-year-old son, an associate professor of pediatrics at
> Temple University, and a pediatrician with St. Luke's Pediatrics
> Associates, in Bethlehem, PA

After my first daughter was born, I hit a wall with weight loss. I was one of those pregnant women who was anything but cute and radiant. I was like a house. I would stand in front of the refrigerator trying to figure out when it was socially acceptable to eat again. I gained so much weight that I couldn't bear to look at the scale at the doctor's office toward the end of my pregnancy.

When I gave birth to my first daughter and heaved my swollen, waistless body home, the number on the scale dropped maybe six pounds. It wasn't pretty.

I joined Jenny Craig, and it really helped me get the lid back on my disordered eating. I got back down to my pre-pregnancy weight and lost even a little more.

Ultimately, it was trial and error, the 12-step healing process, and a connection to a Higher Power that truly got me into my right-sized body, not some quickie new scheme or trick designed to fool the body.

—*Sara Gottfried, MD, a mom of 13- and 8-year-old daughters, a board-certified gynecologist, and the author of* The Hormone Cure, *in Berkeley, CA*

Mommy MD Guides–Recommended Product
Zumba

"One way I make time to exercise is by multitasking," says Aline T. Tanios, MD, a mom of 10- and 4-year-old daughters and an 8-year-old son and a pediatric hospitalist and assistant professor at the Washington University School of Medicine, in St. Louis, MO. "I got a seven-DVD Zumba set, and I did the workouts with my kids. They thought it was fun, and my weight loss results were great."

You can buy a set of three DVDs for $49.95 at **ZUMBA.COM,** or look for single DVDs at Target and Walmart for about $15 each.

You can also attend Zumba classes, which last for 45 to 60 minutes. Zumba feels more like dancing than working out!

To learn more about Zumba classes, visit **ZUMBA.COM**. To find classes near you, you can search at **ZUMBA.COM/EN-US/PARTIES/SEARCH**. The cost varies, but in general you should expect to pay about $6 per class or buy a bundle of 6 classes for $30 or 12 classes for $55.

I've learned in my life that carbohydrates are like poison to me. This makes things especially challenging around the holidays, when there are tons of carb-heavy foods such as Christmas cookies and rice pudding all over the place at work and holiday get-togethers. It's also hard when I'm under stress. I gained 10 to 20 pounds during a very stressful time in my life. It took me 10 years to lose it, but when I was faced with a choice between taking medication to control my cholesterol or losing weight, I knew what I had to do. I didn't want to take the medication. I was very motivated!

I've found that a modified Sugar Busters diet works well for me. The Sugar Busters diet is a low-carbohydrate diet that includes eating smaller portions, avoiding nighttime snacking, and limiting alcohol intake. It isn't as rigorous as the Atkins diet, which made me feel weird and gave me bowel problems. I follow a modified Sugar Busters program most of the time. I give myself some leeway about once a week and for very special occasions.

I also take my time eating. I force myself to chew slowly, and I try to spend 20 to 30 minutes at the table for each meal. When I was an intern, I learned that if you didn't eat quickly, you might not have time to eat. I had to unlearn this bad habit. Now I realize that if you eat too quickly, you don't reach a point of satiety, and you end up eating more than you need to and more than you want to.

—*Linda Brodsky, MD, a mom of a 30-year-old son and 28- and 25-year-old daughters, the president of WomenMDResources.com, a physician in private practice with Pediatric ENT Associates, and a retired professor of otolaryngology and pediatrics, in Buffalo, NY*

Staying Motivated

Getting motivated is hard enough! But staying motivated day after day, week after week, if you're losing weight, or even worse if you're not, is really the hard part. Resolutions aren't always easy to keep—even the New Year's kind. Studies show that more than half of people who make New Year's resolutions don't keep them.

The trick is doing some serious soul-searching. Why do you want to lose weight? Therein lies your best motivation. Grab onto that motivation like you might have once grabbed onto a cheesy slice of stuffed crust pizza and never, ever let go.

⌒∽⊙

I go to the gym with my husband most of the time. I find that having a workout partner helps to motivate me.

—*Sonali Ruder, DO, a mom of a two-month-old daughter, an emergency physician at Coral Springs Medical Center near Fort Lauderdale, FL, and a recipe developer and blogger at TheFoodiePhysician.com*

⌒∽⊙

While I was losing weight, there was a time when I had only one bra that fit! I really didn't want to go out and buy more bras because I knew that I wanted to lose more weight. I vowed that when my bra size got under 40 inches, I would splurge and buy more. That was very motivating!

—*Jennifer Hanes, DO, a mom of a seven-year-old daughter and a four-year-old son, an emergency physician who's board certified in integrative medicine, and the author of* The Princess Plan: Shrink Your Waist, Expand Your Beauty, *in Austin, TX*

⌒∽⊙

I remind myself that it takes a long time to put on the weight, so it will also take a long time to lose the weight. I think it's important to keep a goal weight in sight because you won't know if you're there if you don't know where you're going. I was definitely motivated by how I felt as I continued to lose weight. As you get closer to your goal weight, you feel more confident, your clothes fit better, and people tend to notice and throw out compliments, which is always fun!

—*Jennifer Bacani McKenney, MD, a mom of a two-year-old daughter who's expecting another baby and a family physician, in Fredonia, KS*

⌒∽⊙

You might not realize it, but you need a *lot* of patience when embarking on a weight loss program. To keep myself patient and motivated, I had to stop setting a time limit on things. Instead, I just took it day by day. I never put a deadline on my weight loss, such as "I must lose

> **Motivation is what gets you started.**
> **Habit is what keeps you going.**
> —*Jim Ryun, a former track athlete*
> *and a Republican member of the United States House*
> *of Representatives from Kansas*

40 pounds in one month!" It was just about getting healthy, feeling good about the choices I was making for my body, and then, yes, losing the weight. If it took a month to lose the weight, then great! But if it took longer, that was okay too.

I was on a journey to make changes in my life. I knew that those changes would lead to a lifestyle that was healthy and everlasting, and not just a short-term diet plan.

> —*Arleen K. Lamba, MD, a mom of a three-month-old son, an anesthesiologist, the medical director of Blush Med Institute, and founder of the Blush Blends Skin Care line, in Washington, DC*

One thing that's very motivating for me is the knowledge that carrying extra weight is directly linked to joint pain. I want to avoid joint pain when I'm older, so that's a great motivation for me to get to, and stay at, a healthy weight.

When I wanted to lose weight and get into shape, I signed up for a sprint triathlon! I do the same one each year. Leading up to it, I train to make sure I can go the distance in each event, biking for an hour, running for 30 to 40 minutes, and swimming for 25 minutes. Then I work my way up to combine all three events one after the other.

> —*Leena Shrivastava Dev, MD, a mom of 15- and 12-year-old sons and a general pediatrician and advocate for child safety, in the Baltimore, MD, area*

I've tried everything to lose weight, from the Atkins diet to eliminating flour and sugar to making myself earn beer. I think that when I'm really busy, anything that takes extra time or effort is a real challenge.

Having a workout buddy works best for me. I might not make time for myself, but I certainly won't stand her up. We're both competitive, so when we have weight loss bets, the contest is motivating.

—*Amy Baxter, MD, a mom of 15- and 12-year-old sons and a 10-year-old daughter; the CEO of Buzzy4Shots.com; and the director of emergency research, Scottish Rite, of Children's Healthcare of Atlanta, in Georgia*

Since having kids, I'm less critical of my body. Don't get me wrong, there are days that I step on the scale and think, *Are you kidding me?* But mentally I can bounce back more quickly from those feelings than I could when I was 20.

But the other day, my 12-year-old told me I wasn't quite "bikini ready." I have harsher critics than myself now. That's pretty motivating.

—*Heather Orman-Lubell, MD, a mom of 12- and 8-year-old sons and a pediatrician in private practice at Yardley Pediatrics of St. Christopher's Hospital for Children, in Pennsylvania*

When I was trying to lose my pregnancy weight, I found that I needed a little more motivation, so I created a deadline. I scheduled a photography session for a family portrait at my son's six-month birthday! That was a deadline—with a little bit of pressure too. I

●FitBit

Everyone is motivated by something! Take some time to think about why *you* want to lose weight. Then break that down into smaller parts so that you're motivated by many small goals, not a single far-away-feeling one. For example, do you want to drop three dress sizes? Great! But rather than trying to motivate yourself to get all the way there, focus on finding the motivation to drop one size, then another, then another.

knew that those photos would become a permanent part of my baby's history, so I wanted to look my best. I also scheduled photo sessions for my son's nine-month and one-year birthdays to keep up my motivation!

—*Edna Ma, MD, a mom of a six-month-old son, an anesthesiologist at UCLA Olive View Medical Center, and the founder of BareEase pre-waxing numbing kit, in Los Angeles, CA*

What's motivating for me is feeling fit, rather than a specific number on the scale. I feel better when I'm exercising, so knowing that I'd have more energy, sleep better, and therefore be a better mom was enough of a motivator to help me figure out how to make time for exercise.

I also know that I feel better when my diet is primarily healthy foods, and I want my son to grow up with a healthy diet, so deciding to take the extra time to prepare healthy foods also became a priority.

—*Lennox McNeary, MD, a mom of a four-year-old son, a specialist in physical medicine and rehabilitation at Carilion Clinic, and a cofounder of the Mommy Doctors Bakery (makers of Milkin' Cookies), in Roanoke, VA*

I find that going to a gym with a baby at home just doesn't work for me. It's easy to put my baby in a travel crib with a few toys and take him to the garage with me, where I can work out for however long he lets me!

We have a small home gym in our garage. (No cars in there!) It's not fancy, but we have a TV and DVD player, a treadmill, all-in-one dumbbells, a weight bench, pull-up station, medicine balls, and exercise bands. I have some DVDs that I only watch there, so it motivates me to go exercise. For example, I've watched *Food, Inc.* over and over again in 10- to 30-minute segments. When I get bored with that video, I find something new that is motivating (and that I enjoy) to help reinforce the positive things I'm doing for myself.

—*Michelle Spring, MD, a mom of a one-year-old son and two grown stepchildren and a board-certified plastic surgeon with Marina Plastic Surgery Associates, in Marina del Rey, CA*

To lose some weight, I joined a weight loss challenge program with some old friends. For that, I had to take a photo of myself when the program started and then take another photo every month.

Those photos were amazing and very motivating! It's hard to realize how far you've come without photos. I could tell that my chest

Reflect in a Personal Journal

Journaling is a proven stress-reliever. Studies in which students wrote about traumatic events for 15 minutes at a time found that when the students explored their feelings through journaling, they experienced significant emotional and physical benefits. In the long term, journaling has been shown to reduce symptoms of depression, improve mood, and boost feelings of well-being.

Whatever is happening in your life, whether you're facing a major challenge or dealing with the day-to-day stress of working, raising a family, and trying to lose weight, journaling is sure to benefit you and give you a few minutes to focus on yourself.

But how do you get started? You have a couple of options. Your first is to journal the old-fashioned way, by putting pen to paper. In this case, make a trip to a book or stationery store and buy a journal that fits your style and that will encourage you to pick it up and write. For some, this will mean a journal with lined pages. For others who like to doodle and write, a journal with blank pages might be more inviting.

Your second option is to journal on your iPad, iPod touch, or phone using a journaling app. This might be more convenient because you'll always have it with you, particularly when you unexpectedly have free time, such as when you're in the waiting room of your doctor's office, or when you're sitting in your car waiting for your children. Check out the free Maxjournal app for the iPad, I Journal for the iPhone, or any of the other dozens of paid and free apps available for journaling.

and hips got smaller in the photos. It would have been harder to spot those changes just by looking at myself in the mirror every day.

The photos are also valuable if you fall off the weight loss wagon and regain a few pounds. You can look at the photos of your thinner self and realize, "I did that once. I can do it again."

—Michelle Davis-Dash, MD, a mom of a 19-month-old son and a pediatrician in Baltimore, MD

I don't think there's ever been a time in my life that I wasn't trying to lose weight. As you get older, I think losing weight becomes not just a physical challenge, but a mental challenge as well.

When you're younger and you're trying to find someone to date, it's a huge motivation to lose weight. I remember when I was younger, I could starve myself for days to drop a few pounds to look good for a certain person or event. (Not that this is a healthy idea!)

But as we age, our reasons for wanting to lose weight change. Now when I look in the mirror, I want to like *myself*, more than I want someone else to like me. That creates a difficult situation because I can't walk away from myself if I don't like what I see in the mirror, so it's a lot less motivating than the fear of someone else's rejection of me because of my weight. Yet, although I can live with myself no matter what I weigh, I might not be totally *happy* with myself.

—Judith Hellman, MD, a mom of a 15-year-old son, an associate clinical professor of dermatology at Mt. Sinai Hospital in New York City, and a dermatologist in private practice

RALLIE'S TIP

Most of us really, really want to lose the weight we need to in order to look and feel our best. If wanting to lose weight was all we had to do to succeed, we'd all be sashaying around the house in our skinniest skinny jeans, right this very minute! Unfortunately, as we've all learned from experience, that's just not all there is to it.

Finding that spark of motivation is the very first step—and the single most important part—of your journey. From that tiny spark, you'll need to light a fire, fan the flames, and build a giant bonfire of red-hot desire. It has to be huge, and it has to be powerful. The motivation it provides has to be strong enough to carry you through the tough times, when you're feeling a little down and discouraged and your friend shows up at your house with a bottle of wine and a two-pound box of chocolates. Your motivation has to be super strong when you've promised yourself you'd go for a jog before work and it's raining cats and dogs, and you're wonderfully cozy under the covers. Or when you've been really, really good all week and the scale shows you've gained a pound, rather than lost the two you'd planned on.

To find that special spark of motivation that speaks directly to you, you have to ask yourself, Why do I want to lose weight? Then list the most powerful, meaningful reasons that come to mind. Write them down in your journal, on index cards, or in your datebook. Type them up and store them on your computer or your phone. Scribble them on your bathroom mirror in lipstick, or post them in the kitchen on your fridge. For most of us, following a diet isn't nearly fun enough to do just for the heck of it. There have to be some pretty big and powerful reasons behind it to make it worth the effort.

Without some powerful motivation, going on a diet is kind of like going to the dentist. You know you need to do it, but you're not exactly looking forward to it, and you're certainly not enthused about it. My dentist is a nice guy, but I've always had a little anxiety about people in his profession. I really don't like seeing him in his office, and I don't exactly love having him mess around in my mouth. On top of that, I have to go to lots of trouble to make it happen. I have to analyze my schedule, plan to take time off from work, and call his receptionist to make an appointment. On the day of my visit, I have to drive to his office, sit in his waiting room feeling nervous, and then sit in the exam chair feeling even more nervous. After the hygienist and my dentist are through poking around in my mouth, I have to wait for the news. Do I have a cavity? Are my teeth in danger of falling out? Do I need some scary procedure such as a root canal? The very best I can hope for is to hear, "Everything looks great! We'll see you back here in six months!"

Of course that's always great news, but it's hardly enough motivation to overcome the dread and procrastination I feel when I think about scheduling the next appointment. It's not like something really wonderful is going to happen, like my dentist is going to jump up and shout, "Oh my gosh! I just found a two-carat diamond in your right molar!" As a result, I usually only make it to my dentist's office about every 9 or 10 months, instead of every 6 months like I'm supposed to. It takes me at least 3 months to stop procrastinating. In the end, what really motivates me to go is the fear of the consequences of not going. I value my teeth, and I don't want to lose them. So I go to the dentist as regularly as I can force myself to do it.

This same kind of logic applies to dieting. If you don't have some really big and powerful and exciting reasons to lose weight, you'll have a hard time going through all the steps necessary—namely following a diet and making time to exercise—to make it happen. You'll end up procrastinating, and as you procrastinate, you're likely to gain another pound or three. So as you think about your reasons for losing weight, take your time, use your imagination, and try to generate all the excitement and positive, powerful emotions that you possibly can.

When I was much younger, the most powerful motivation of all for me was the prospect of fitting into a certain size. I would close my eyes and imagine how fabulous I would look and feel in this size, and that was all the motivation I needed.

Sadly, now that I'm older, this technique doesn't work at all for me. I don't care nearly as much about how I look as I used to. Now, I'm much more focused on how I feel and how my body performs the tasks I need it to. So when it's time to get myself fired up to lose 5 or 10 pounds, I focus completely on these things. When I look for that spark of motivation, and I ask myself why I want to lose weight, my list looks something like this:

- I'm planning to run a half-marathon in April, and I can run faster and better at my ideal weight.
- I want to take my horse to the next level in his training, and I need to be leaner and stronger to help him advance.
- I'm going skiing with my family in February, and I really want to be

as lean, strong, and as healthy as I can be so that I can keep up with my husband and my teenage boys as they whiz down the slopes. Plus, my ski pants are a bit tight, and I really don't want to buy a bigger size!

As I write my list, I visualize how I'll look and feel running the half-marathon, riding my horse, and skiing down the slopes. I generate lots of excitement, positive emotion, enthusiasm, and anticipation about these things. And I don't just do it once; I try to do it several times a day, so I'll remember what I'm working for. I keep my eye on the prize.

At the beginning of your journey, it's far more important to get yourself really worked up about why you must lose weight than how you'll manage to do it. If your why is powerful enough, the how is actually the easy part. With enough motivation, determination, and excitement, you can accomplish just about anything.

Eating Better

Life is all about choices: Paper or plastic, turn left or go right, Verizon or AT&T. Out of the gazillions of tiny decisions you make every day, what you decide to put into your mouth is one of the biggest, and it has a tremendous impact on your health.

Generally speaking, Americans aren't making wise choices with their forks. We eat too much of what we shouldn't and too little of what we should. Typically, Americans eat a little more than 1½ cups of vegetables a day, almost a full cup less than the 2½ cups recommended by the USDA. Americans also get only 1 cup of fruit a day, while the USDA recommends 2 cups. And for whole grains, Americans eat only a little more than ½ a cup a day, while the USDA recommends getting 3 cups or more.

Because Americans aren't eating enough of the healthy stuff—fruits, vegetables, whole grains, beneficial oils, and dairy—they're not getting enough fiber or nutrients such as potassium, calcium, and vitamin D. Intake levels are so low it's a public health concern, according to the 2010 Dietary Guidelines for Americans.

Eating 2½ cups or more of fruits and vegetables every day is linked to a lower risk of cancer and cardiovascular disease, including heart attack and stroke. Each meal that you eat, each bite that you take is a choice. Choose wisely.

❧

A wise friend taught me two simple tricks that help a lot: Never eat standing up. And never eat anything out of the carton or package.

—*Amy Baxter, MD, a mom of 15- and 12-year-old sons and a 10-year-old daughter; the CEO of Buzzy4Shots.com; and the director of emergency research, Scottish Rite, of Children's Healthcare of Atlanta, in Georgia*

❧

It's not always easy to eat well, and reminders are always helpful. I have a copy of the USDA Food Guide Pyramid on my refrigerator for quick reference.

—*Stephanie A. Wellington, MD, a mom of a 13-year-old son and an 11-year-old daughter, a hospitalist in the Level III NICU at Bellevue Hospital Center in New York City, and the medical coach and founder of PostpartumNeonatalCoaching.com*

❧

When I need to lose weight, I try to eat the foods that I enjoy, but I watch my portion sizes carefully. I measure portion sizes of dairy foods, such as cheese, because these foods are typically high in calories. I limit my intake of high-carb foods to one fist-size portion per meal. I also fill my plate with lean meats and veggies.

—*Bola Oyeyipo-Ajumobi, MD, a mom of five- and two-year-old sons, a family physician at the Veterans Health Administration, and the owner of SlimyBookWorm.com, in San Antonio, TX*

❧

When I was trying to lose weight, I resisted the urge to finish everything on my plate. I try to eat only until I'm no longer hungry. Satisfaction is stopping when you're no longer hungry, not eating until you're full.

—*Leena Shrivastava Dev, MD, a mom of 15- and 12-year-old sons and a general pediatrician and advocate for child safety, in the Baltimore, MD, area*

It might be cliché, but for me the most important meal of the day is breakfast. I find that if I start the day off right, the rest of the day goes well. For example, if I eat oatmeal for breakfast, I tend to eat better the whole day. But if I eat a bagel and cream cheese for breakfast, it throws the whole day off. It's too easy to fall into the mind-set of, "So much for today. I'll be better tomorrow."

—*Michelle Spring, MD, a mom of a one-year-old son and two grown stepchildren and a board-certified plastic surgeon with Marina Plastic Surgery Associates, in Marina del Rey, CA*

I recently created my own diet. I call it VEGLY. I eat as many servings of vegetables, eggs, grapefruit, lean meats or Lean Cuisines, and yogurt as I want. If I stick with that all day, I earn a treat: a glass of beer or wine or a small dessert. I've lost six pounds so far!

—*Amy Baxter, MD*

I found that setting a routine was very helpful when I was trying to lose weight. I had to have a schedule and stick to it. On days I was working, I ate the same foods for breakfast and lunch at work each day. This way, I pre-accounted for the number of calories I was eating at these meals. This made it easy for me to control what—and how much—I was eating. I was flexible about what I ate for dinner. Because dinner is our family time, I like to cook and eat with my husband and be more relaxed about eating.

>—*Arleen K. Lamba, MD, a mom of a three-month-old son, an anesthesiologist, the medical director of Blush Med Institute, and founder of the Blush Blends Skin Care line, in Washington, DC*

After my son was born, I worked with a personal trainer. He gave me a simple piece of advice that has really helped: Don't eat any carbs after 7 pm. I try not to eat at all after 7 pm, but if I do, I'll have something high in protein, such as a piece of cheese or a hard-boiled egg.

>—*Shilpa Amin-Shah, MD, a mom of a three-year-old son and a two-year-old daughter and an emergency physician and director of the recruiting team at Emergency Medical Associates, in Livingston, NJ*

My eating strategy is to stay munching all day long. I make sure to eat breakfast, and I continue eating small snacks throughout the day. If you eat every two to three hours (even if it's just a smoothie, piece of fruit, or NutriGrain bar), it keeps your metabolism going, and you burn more calories. As I go about my daily activities, I'm burning those calories off with very little effort even before I get to the gym.

A typical day might include scrambled eggs for breakfast, a NutriGrain bar for a snack, a grilled chicken salad for lunch, an orange for a snack, and a small steak (or any source of protein), rice, and vegetables for supper.

>—*Jeannette Gonzalez Simon, MD, a mom of four- and one-year-old daughters and a pediatric gastroenterologist at Staten Island Pediatrics GI, in New York*

❤FitBit

> Fruits and vegetables are low in fat and calories, but they're often served with condiments that can undermine your weight loss efforts. Use dips and dressings sparingly, because a quarter cup of some varieties contains as much as 300 calories and 40 grams of fat.

I'm an ice cream and chocolate lover, and I don't want to ever give those up. I've tried in the past without success. I can be passionate about it for about three days, and after that I feel resentful and eat an entire carton of Breyer's Mint Chocolate Chip ice cream or a package of Milano cookies. So I compromise by having dessert a couple of nights a week—instead of every night!

—*Deborah Gilboa, MD, a mom of 11-, 9-, 7-, and 5-year-old sons, a family physician with Squirrel Hill Health Center in Pittsburgh, PA, and a parenting speaker whose advice is found at AskDoctorG.com*

Everyone has one type of food that's their weakness. For me, it's sauces. I love sauces, gravies, and dressings. They can have a lot of calories. Rather than cutting them out of my diet, I searched to find flavors and brands that I like that don't have too many calories. I found Makoto Ginger Dressing, for instance, has only 80 calories in two tablespoons instead of a higher-calorie creamy dressing. You can buy it at grocery stores and stores such as Target.

Sometimes I mix a higher-calorie dressing with a lower-calorie one. For example, I'll combine Kraft Asian Toasted Sesame Light (only 50 calories per two-tablespoon serving) with a higher-calorie Asian dressing. This gives me more flavor, for fewer calories.

—*Tiemdow Phumiruk, MD, a mom of 13-, 10-, and 7-year-old daughters, a pediatrician in the emergency department of Children's Hospital Colorado at Parker Adventist Hospital, and adjunct faculty at Rocky Vista University College of Osteopathic Medicine, in Parker, CO*

I think that if people were to eat "real foods" most of the time, their weight would be fine. You just can't eat too much broccoli and other real foods!

Also I think most Americans eat too much red meat. You don't have to become a vegetarian, but I think most people could benefit by cutting back on red meat. My husband and I eat meat once or twice a week. The rest of the time, we eat chicken, fish, or vegetarian meals.

—Hana R. Solomon, MD, a mom who raised four children, a grandmom of three, a board-certified pediatrician, the president of BeWell Health, LLC, and the author of Clearing the Air One Nose at a Time: Caring for Your Personal Filter, *in Columbia, MO*

Mommy MD Guides-Recommended Product
Great Food!

So much of weight loss is knowing what you're eating and making smart choices. Thankfully, there are plenty of nutritious, convenient options at the supermarket today. Here are some to try.

Seapoint Farms Organic Edamame. These nutty soybeans come frozen in pods or shelled. They're a great choice for weight loss because they're filled with protein, which will help you feel full. Seapoint Farms offers individual packets of soybeans with Dora or SpongeBob on the bag, which might help motivate your child to eat them along with you.

One Dora-embellished pack of shelled edamame has only 59 calories. Find it in the organic freezer section of your supermarket. A bag of eight 1.5-ounce packs costs about $3.19.

Chobani Greek Yogurt. Dietitians tend to recommend Greek yogurt because it has more protein than regular yogurt, and protein helps you feel fuller. Greek yogurt also delivers calcium and live and active cultures to boot. One tip: Stir in the liquid that pools at the top of the yogurt. That's the whey, which is rich in protein.

You can find Chobani Greek Yogurt in plain nonfat (you can add

After delivering my children, I started cutting back on one thing at a time. I was—and still am—a big snacker. I cut out one snack at a time: first, the middle-of-the-night snack, next the before-dinner snack, then the after-dinner snack, and finally the mid-morning snack.

Once I was down to just three meals a day, I started reducing the number of calories I ate at these meals. For lunch I restricted myself to a serving of fruit, a granola bar, and a cup of yogurt. I also started skipping breakfast and just having coffee. Coffee is actually a great appetite suppressant. (I'm not recommending this approach as a doctor.)

—*Stacey Ann Weiland, MD, a mom of a 14-year-old daughter and 9- and 7-year-old sons and an internist/gastroenterologist, in Denver, CO*

your own fruit, honey, or agave syrup) or in several flavors, including pomegranate, blood orange, strawberry, and raspberry. One six-ounce container costs about $1.39.

Arnold Sandwich Thins Rolls. There's so much variety in breads and rolls today. It's a matter of simply taking some time to read the nutrition labels before you buy. But if you want a no-brainer, pick up Arnold Sandwich Thins Rolls. They have only 100 calories per roll, and you can use them for toast, egg sandwiches, grilled cheese, panini sandwiches, plain ol' turkey and Swiss, or burgers. They come in yummy flavors, including flax & fiber, 100 percent whole wheat, honey wheat, whole grain white, multigrain, and seedless rye. A package of eight rolls costs about $4.19.

Helen's Kitchen Burrito Bowls. When you don't have time to make lunch or dinner, throw one of these burrito bowls in the microwave, and you have a tasty vegetarian meal that's high in fiber. The bowls range in calories from 230 to 340 and come in several varieties, including Korean noodle, coconut vegetable, Baja pinto bean, and veggie fajita. One bowl costs about $4.09.

> **Nothing tastes as good as skinny feels.**
>
> **—*Anonymous***

Because I don't go to the gym, I really watch what I eat. I try to avoid foods with a lot of processed sugar and fats. Instead, I eat fruits and vegetables that I like, such as snap peas, avocados, apples, and salads. I find that crunchy foods are more satisfying than foods that you drink. Chewing takes time, and it gives me a sense of satiety.

I do allow myself to eat chocolate or ice cream if that's what I'm hungry for, but I eat some fruit first. Then if I still have the craving, I'll have the chocolate or ice cream.

I don't let myself get ravenous. Otherwise, it's too tempting to eat too much. It's like going to the grocery store hungry; it's hard to exercise any willpower.

> —*Edna Ma, MD, a mom of a six-month-old son, an anesthesiologist at UCLA Olive View Medical Center, and the founder of BareEase pre-waxing numbing kit, in Los Angeles, CA*

I have rheumatoid arthritis (RA), and it flared up immediately after my kids were born. I started to eat an anti-inflammatory diet. I avoided all processed foods and cut back on red meat. Instead I ate whole foods such as vegetables and chicken.

This diet eased my RA symptoms, and it also helped me to lose weight. It's very restrictive until you start to make adjustments to see which foods your body can tolerate and which it can't.

> —*Antoinette Cheney, DO, a mom of a seven-year-old son and a six-year-old daughter and a family physician with Rocky Vista University College of Osteopathic Medicine, in Parker, CO*

A few years ago, I switched to a gluten-free diet. I was having skin sensitivity issues and digestion problems, and I noticed that both got worse when I ate gluten.

I avoid all wheat-based pastas and breads and other foods

containing gluten. I can eat a gluten-free pasta dish if I want. I eat a lot of lean protein, fruits, and vegetables. I snack on dried fruit and trail mix. Since changing my diet, my allergy and digestive problems have gone away, and as side benefits, I feel healthier and have a lot more energy.

—Allison Bailey, MD, a mom of a nine-year-old son and a five-year-old daughter and founder and director of Integrated Health and Fitness Associates, in Cambridge, MA

⚬⁄⚬

After my pregnancies, particularly after my second, I developed food sensitivities and gastrointestinal issues. I reacted negatively to almost everything I ate! I had to watch carefully what I was eating. I went on an elimination diet. I only ate organic, whole foods, such as organic fruits, vegetables, meat, and poultry. I stopped eating gluten, dairy, corn, soy, and eggs. Eventually, my body healed. Now I can tolerate gluten, dairy, corn, soy, and eggs in small doses. I waited nearly a year before adding these foods back into my diet. I did it one at a time so I could note any reactions. For most people, it takes three to six months to add these foods back. I just felt really great eliminating them!

A side benefit to overhauling my eating was weight loss. I lost nearly 12 pounds.

—Kay Corpus, MD, a mom of a six-year-old daughter and a two-year-old son, a family physician, and the director of Owensboro Health Integrative Medicine, in Kentucky

⚬⁄⚬

At age 39, I completely, dramatically changed the way I eat. I finally practiced what I preached, and I ate seven servings of fresh fruits and vegetables, especially of the dark green variety, each day. I started to weigh my food and calibrate what really moves the needle on the scale for me. I worked with therapists, and I did a long tour through various 12-step food programs. I approached my disordered eating as an addiction.

I discovered that I do best around 125 to 130 pounds, not 145 to 150. I found out that I'm not good on grains, and I have an intolerance to both gluten and dairy. It's incredibly sad for me, but also incredibly important to realize.

Later, I found that I'm genetically programmed to perform best on a low-carb food plan, and that's what I follow. I eat carbs for breakfast, as brain fuel, but I'm a protein-and-veg girl the rest of the day. I limit alcohol, and I rarely eat sugar. That works for me. I'm still addicted, but now my addictions are toward Pema Chodron [a notable American figure in Tibetan Buddhism], running with girlfriends, and yoga.

—*Sara Gottfried, MD, a mom of 13- and 8-year-old daughters, a board-certified gynecologist, and the author of* The Hormone Cure, *in Berkeley, CA*

Mommy MD Guides-Recommended Product
Great Restaurants!

It's a real—and necessary—luxury to get together with a friend without the kids for some time to recharge, talk, laugh, and relax. It's also a perfect opportunity to work toward achieving your goals for weight loss with a healthy meal.

Make it a regular habit to get together with friends for lunch at a restaurant that offers healthy options. You'll get the nutrition you need to keep moving toward your weight loss goal and the stress relief of kicking back with good friends. And what a treat to leave behind the kid-centered fast-food chains for a day.

You can find healthy options at almost any chain restaurant, as long as you first look up the nutrition information online or on a food-tracking app. If you don't have time before you're in the restaurant, search out options on the menu that are labeled low-fat or healthy.

If you're looking for some places to get you started, try these chains.

Zoup! This chain, which is known for its soups (but also offers salads and sandwiches), has low-fat and vegetarian options, and its nutrition information is available online and in their restaurants. An eight-ounce cup of Frontier Seven-Bean Soup has only 100 calories and 1.5 grams of fat (add 190 calories for a hunk of the multigrain

It's challenging to eat well right now. My daughter is in a phase where she only wants to eat chicken nuggets and yogurt, which makes it harder for me to eat well too.

I don't want to fight with her. So to get her to eat her vegetables, I sneak them in. I shave carrots and put them into burritos. I stir a little applesauce into yogurt.

My son, on the other hand, is a more adventuresome eater. He likes to try new foods. When we visit my friend Mommy MD Guide Cheryl Wu, MD, in New York City, she prepares a lot of Asian dishes.

bread that comes with it). A half Chicken Greek Salad has only 340 calories and 12 grams of fat.

Au Bon Pain. Look up this chain's smart menu online and you'll get all the nutrition information you need to make a healthy choice, such as the Thai Peanut Chicken Wrap with 550 calories and 28 grams of protein.

Noodles & Company. This restaurant, which offers Asian-, Mediterranean-, and American-inspired dishes, has a 500-calories-or-less "cheat sheet" on its website that includes Thai Curry Soup, Chinese Chop Salad, Pad Thai, Caesar Salad, and Penne Rosa.

Corner Bakery Café. Check out the more than 100 meal combos available on the menu with fewer than 600 calories (and listed on its website), including the Uptown Turkey Sandwich and Chicken Noodle Soup, the Tomato Mozzarella Sandwich and Mixed Greens, and the Harvest Salad and Three Lentil Vegetable Soup. Keep in mind, however, that sides add more calories to the meal.

Panera Bread. You'll find the calorie info on the menu at Panera, but remember that extras will add to that number. The smoked turkey breast on country bread has only 420 calories, but you'll have to add to your calorie count if you ask for mayo.

They have tons of vegetables, and they're very healthy. My son was excited to try all of them, and he loves using chopsticks. We've adapted some of her recipes to make at home. We make big stir-fries of vegetables, a protein such as chicken, and sometimes an egg.

—*Sigrid Payne DaVeiga, MD, a mom of a seven-year-old son and a two-year-old daughter and a pediatric allergist with the Children's Hospital of Philadelphia, in Pennsylvania*

I find it helpful to keep in mind that sometimes I confuse hunger with thirst, boredom, or other "feelings." Sometimes I try to follow the advice to drink a glass of water *before eating* to make sure what I'm feeling is not thirst. Having fruit on hand is helpful, and I'll eat an apple or an orange for a snack. I think that when you go to the fridge and open it, staring into it like you're browsing at the store, you probably are something other than hungry.

—*Rachel S. Rohde, MD, a mom of a two-year-old daughter, an assistant professor of orthopaedic surgery at the Oakland University William Beaumont School of Medicine, and an orthopaedic upper-extremity surgeon with Michigan Orthopaedic Institute, P.C., in Southfield, MI*

I've always tried to watch what I eat and make healthy choices, but after my kids were born, it became even more important to me to eat well. I wanted to establish good habits for them and set a good example.

I "edited" my pantry carefully. I edited a lot of foods right out of it, such as chips, sugary snacks, and processed foods. If those foods aren't in my pantry, my family isn't going to eat them—at least not at home.

I love to cook, and I prepare most of my meals from scratch. I truly look forward to every meal! If we want to have dessert, I have a rule that we have to make it ourselves, from scratch.

—*Ayala Laufer-Cahana, MD, a mom of 17- and 15-year-old sons and a 14-year-old daughter, a pediatrician, and the founder of Herbal Water Inc., in Wynnewood, PA*

⚫FitBit

When my twins turned six years old, I vowed to lose 25 pounds. I did it with a combination of dietary changes and exercise. The important thing about changing your diet is to make sustainable changes. Otherwise, when you go back to your "normal" way of eating, the weight will come back. The key for me was to identify foods that I loved that were satisfying and filling but not high in calories. Some of these foods are yogurt and cottage cheese, nuts and nut butters, and eggs.

It's also very helpful for me to eat some protein at every meal in order to feel satiated. I like any kind of grilled meat, such as steak and chicken, and I avoid protein with fatty sauces. I buy savory baked tofu at Trader Joe's. It comes in different flavors, and it's a good way to get lots of protein with no effort. You don't even have to cook it! You can just slice it up and toss it in your salad. Kids will even eat it!

I add nuts, a bit of cheese, and a leftover high-protein food, such as steak, to salads. That combo makes me feel very full.

—*Katherine Dee, MD, a mom of eight-year-old twin daughters and a six-year-old son and a radiologist at the Seattle Breast Center, in Washington*

I learned from a nutritionist that fiber is very filling. I buy Fiber Rich crackers, which are low in calories and high in fiber. Half the calories in each cracker are indigestible. Another brand of crispbread is also an option. I have nicknamed that one "Sawdust," because that's what it tastes like straight up.

I eat those crackers with soup most of the time to counteract the sawdust factor. I strongly believe that it's not helpful to eat very tasty foods. In my case, I just want to eat more of them. It's not easy to want to overeat "sawdust."

I put a little cottage cheese or cut-up hard-boiled egg on top of the crackers. That makes them taste better too. Sometimes I eat them with ready-made organic chicken-and-vegetable soup to make a complete meal.

—Judith Hellman, MD, a mom of a 15-year-old son, an associate clinical professor of dermatology at Mt. Sinai Hospital in New York City, and a dermatologist in private practice

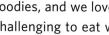

My husband and I are huge foodies, and we love to eat out and try new restaurants. It can be challenging to eat well at restaurants. I definitely splurge on special occasions and get what I want. But normally, I look at the nutrition information, which is on more and more menus these days, and this makes it easier to eat well and make healthier choices. I stay away from anything fried, and instead I order grilled food. When I order pasta, I try to avoid cream sauces, which are usually very high in fat. I also order a lot of salads and dishes with whole grains such as quinoa. I would like to say that I choose restaurants based on the nutrition information, but I can't say that I do!

I don't eat a lot of fast food, but it's encouraging that many fast-food restaurants are making an effort to have healthier options.

—Sonali Ruder, DO, a mom of a two-month-old daughter, an emergency physician at Coral Springs Medical Center near Fort Lauderdale, FL, and a recipe developer and blogger at TheFoodiePhysician.com

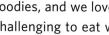

Get rid of the guilt! If you feel guilty about what you're eating, such as a slice of cake at a birthday party, your body releases the stress hormone cortisol. That actually makes your body store more fat! Instead, if you choose to have a piece of cake, enjoy it!

While we're on the subject of birthday cake, choose to eat foods that you truly enjoy. Most of the time, birthday party cake isn't even good. So why eat it? I forgo birthday party cake, and instead I'll look

Mommy MD Guides–Recommended Product
Slim-Fast Bars and Shakes

"When I'm trying to lose weight, I replace a meal with a Slim-Fast bar," says Stacey Ann Weiland, MD, a mom of a 14-year-old daughter and 9- and 7-year-old sons and an internist/gastroenterologist, in Denver, CO. "They taste good, are inexpensive, and are easy to eat when I'm on the go."

Slim-Fast bars come in four flavors: Chocolate Mint, Double-Dutch Chocolate, Peanut Butter Crunch Time, and Chocolatey Vanilla Blitz. Each bar has 100 calories. You can buy them for around $5 for a box of five at stores such as Walmart and Target and online retailers such as Amazon.com.

"I drink Slim-Fast chocolate shakes," says Stephanie A. Wellington, MD, a mom of a 13-year-old son and an 11-year-old daughter, a hospitalist in the Level III NICU at Bellevue Hospital Center in New York City, and the medical coach and founder of Postpartum-NeonatalCoaching.com. "It is my favorite way to start my day, especially when my day starts at 5 am. At 200 calories, a Slim-Fast shake is an easy way to break my hunger in the morning when I don't have the time to prepare a meal. I can even drink it at the hospital where I work. The chocolate flavor helps satisfy a chocolate craving too!"

You can buy Slim-Fast shakes in powder or premixed. They come in vanilla, chocolate, and strawberry flavors. You can buy them in stores such as Walmart and Target and at online retailers such as **AMAZON.COM**. A four-pack of 10-ounce premixed shakes costs around $6. Visit **SLIM-FAST.COM** for more information.

forward to my favorite Key lime cheesecake from a restaurant another day. Enjoy your food, and eat what you enjoy.

—*Jennifer Hanes, DO, a mom of a seven-year-old daughter and a four-year-old son, an emergency physician who's board certified in integrative medicine, and the author of* The Princess Plan: Shrink Your Waist, Expand Your Beauty, *in Austin, TX*

I've found it to be very helpful to identify a few healthy go-to meals and eat them every week. It all started when my kids were little and I tried to make it easier for my housekeeper and me to shop for and prepare meals. Most people eat the same foods over and over again, so if you make those meals healthy, it goes a long way toward promoting weight loss.

For example, we usually eat hamburgers or meat loaf and broccoli on Mondays, chicken with steamed cauliflower on Tuesdays, fish with some sort of spinach dish on Wednesdays, and pasta on Thursdays. Every day we have a fresh salad. On Fridays, we celebrate Shabbat (the Jewish Sabbath), and so we have a special meal. We start with prayers and then sit for almost two hours, often with guests, and enjoy a drawn-out meal of soup, salad, and then our main course with lots of side dishes, mostly veggies. On Friday nights we also have dessert.

When my kids were little, we'd have leftovers on weekends, and we loved to barbecue on Sunday nights. Sometimes we went out to eat, but never, ever did we take our kids out for fast food. With our dietary limitations (we eat a kosher diet and only eat vegetarian and plain fish at restaurants), it wasn't too difficult to just say, "We can't eat that." I think if more parents said that to their kids, eating habits would be much better.

—*Linda Brodsky, MD, a mom of a 30-year-old son and 28- and 25-year-old daughters, the president of WomenMDResources.com, a physician in private practice with Pediatric ENT Associates, and a retired professor of otolaryngology and pediatrics, in Buffalo, NY*

I buy as much organic food as I can, especially meat, dairy, and eggs. I think it's important to pay attention to where your food comes from. I don't eat a lot of animal products, but when I do, I buy grass-fed beef and try to shop at farmers' markets. I believe in making consumer choices that help guide our entire food industry in a healthier, more environmentally responsible direction.

I also drink a lot of vegetable juice. My family loves Columbia Gorge, Evolution, and Naked Juices vegetable juices or veggie-fruit mixes.

I make smoothies with fruits, vegetables, and ground flaxseed. These ingredients are nutrient rich and low in calories. Even my one-year-old drinks them with me! I have a Jack LaLanne juicer, and I try to make fresh juices at home, but it's a lot of work. I don't believe in any of the fad diets, such as low-carb, high-carb, or high-fat. I believe that we should eat as many colorful fruits and vegetables as we can, as well as whole grains and nuts and seeds, and that we should significantly limit our consumption of sugar, processed foods, and animal proteins.

Years ago I read a book called *The China Study* by Dr. T. Colin Campbell, which changed my outlook on food and health forever. Since then, I have done a lot of reading and research on the topic. One of my favorite experts is Dr. Joel Fuhrman for his passionate approach to superior health through diet, and my favorite movies are *Forks over Knives* and *Food, Inc.*

—*Michelle Spring, MD*

❧

I've probably lost myself—my entire body weight—four or five times. I've tried everything to lose weight. But every time I lost it, I gained it all back. Keeping the weight off has been a lifelong battle.

I was even a chubby kid. I remember as a child, my weight was treated as a negative issue. I wasn't given the same treats as other kids were. That really reinforced my negative feelings about my weight.

I've learned that I need to be vigilant about my weight all of the time. The only strategy that has worked is eating sensibly. As my grandmother used to say, "Moderation in all things." If I try to give up certain foods entirely, then I feel deprived, I rebound, and I overdo it later.

☉ Mommy MD Guides–Recommended Product
Fresco 11-Pound Electronic Kitchen Scale

If you're keeping a food journal, it's good to know you're eating all three ounces of chicken or the full one ounce of cheese you're counting. A kitchen scale can help you do that. It's as simple as turning on the scale and placing the food on the glass top.

Electronic kitchen scales are easy to find at stores such as Walmart and Bed, Bath & Beyond and aren't too expensive. A tried-and-true brand is the Fresco 11-Pound Electronic Kitchen Scale, which costs around $45 on **AMAZON.COM**.

I was a heavy teen, and when the first diet soda, Tab, came out, I went on a Tab-and-Jell-O diet. I ate nothing else for a few weeks and lost a few pounds. Then I gained them all back. Now I eat whatever I like, in moderation.

Another thing that helps is that my family keeps kosher. We can't eat out in fast-food restaurants, and that helps keep me from grabbing the high-calorie foods you find there. While keeping kosher helps me avoid the pitfalls of eating out, there are still plenty of high-calorie kosher foods available in the grocery store, so I have to be vigilant with my grocery shopping!

—*Susan Besser, MD, a mom of six grown children, ages 28, 26, 24, 22, 21, and 19, a grandmom of two, a family physician, and the medical director of Doctors Express-Memphis, in Tennessee*

Because I'm a surgeon specializing in liposuction, many of my patients ask for my advice on losing weight or avoiding weight gain after their surgery. I tell all of my patients that the key to weight loss is a combination of diet and exercise. Although both are important, I always emphasize diet and tell my patients to "watch what you put in your mouth." Exercise is great, but if you do cardio exercise, such as running or swimming, for an hour, you only burn around 300 to 400 calories. That's less than what's in a cheeseburger! You really can't use the excuse that you can eat anything you want and then work it off later.

I am extremely disciplined in what I eat, and I find that eating healthfully gives me more energy and makes me feel better overall. In general, I avoid sugars. This includes foods that have sugar in them, such as cookies, candy, sugary snacks, plus sodas and other sweet drinks. The sweet drinks are really important to look out for. Mixed coffee drinks and some energy drinks have a lot of sugar that people tend to forget about. I also don't drink alcohol at all because of the calories.

I limit my intake of carbohydrates. If I do eat them, it's at my first meal of the day, usually oatmeal for breakfast.

A typical day's eating for me is a few eggs for breakfast, a light salad with avocado for lunch, and a chicken breast and steamed broccoli for supper. I don't snack much, but if I get hungry in between meals, I'll have a pear, an apple, or another piece of fruit.

It's also important to avoid pseudo-healthy foods, such as smoothies. People think that they're nutritious, but they have a lot of sugars and a lot of calories! My best advice is to read the nutrition labels on the foods you eat, and by this I mean the quantities of calories, fat, and carbohydrates. Ignore the marketing hype that calls something "slim," "high-protein," or "low-carb" and turn the product over to see exactly what's in the food you eat.

—*Catherine Begovic, MD, a mom of a six-month-old daughter and a plastic surgeon at Make You Perfect, Inc., in Beverly Hills, CA*

⚬⁄⚬

I've been most successful at losing weight when I eliminate two elements from my diet: sugar and flour. For example, during the month of December, I swear off sugar and flour until the New Year.

It might seem like this would be especially difficult at the holidays, but actually it makes dieting easier. Around the holidays, there are so many temptations that if I had to make a decision whether or not to eat each individual treat, I would nibble continuously. But because I eliminate sugar and flour completely, it's easier to do. Studies have shown that it's easier to go cold turkey than to moderate your intake of a substance. Once you commit to a change, it takes about three or four days for that to become your new normal.

I don't avoid all carbs. For example, I eat mashed potatoes, and I put honey in my tea as a sweetener. Obviously, I avoid cookie exchanges completely!

—*Amy Baxter, MD*

I've had challenges with my weight my entire life. My weight ruined my adolescence. I remember standing in line at Walt Disney World at age 13 thinking, *I'm so fat. I want to disappear.* I was always so uncomfortable in my own skin.

I've tried so many different weight loss programs. Yet today, I weigh less than I did when I was in seventh grade. The key was finding out what works for me.

I eliminated all grains from my diet, including bread, pasta, oats, barley, and corn. Even though I tested negative for celiac disease, if I eat even a little bit of wheat, I get sick.

When you eat grains, it costs your body far more nutrients to process them than your body gets from the grains. Every time you eat a piece of bread, for example, you deplete your body's antioxidants. Your body uses up more vitamins, minerals, and nutrients to process the food than it actually gets out of the food. You're getting calories with very little nutrition. Unless you eat 5 to 10 servings of vegetables a day, your nutrient levels fall lower and lower.

It can be challenging for people to eliminate grains from their diets. I suggest people try it for a month and see how they feel. Corn is especially difficult to avoid. You have to check labels carefully for things such as corn oil and cornstarch. Even plastic is made with corn. It has completely infiltrated our lives.

It was difficult for me to control how many carbs I ate. I believe that we crave what we're allergic to. For me, that has been a huge weight revelation.

Avoiding all grains, combined with exercising at a moderate intensity, helped me to lose the weight and maintain my weight loss. Now I feel better at age 52 than I did at 32!

Instead of grains, I eat plenty of meat, vegetables, fruit, and good fats such as olive oil, coconut oil, nuts, and avocado. I think we all got fat on the low-fat diet! I especially avoid products such as light mayonnaise, which is filled with corn syrup in place of fat. I think it's far better to eat fat than all of those grains.

—*Marie Dam, MD, a mom of 24- and 20-year-old daughters and an anti-aging medicine specialist in private practice in Naples, FL, and Danbury, CT*

RALLIE'S TIP

I have a very long commute, traveling to work in several different medical clinics in rural Kentucky for one to three hours each way. Because of this, I "live" in my truck several days a week, driving to and from some rather isolated areas in the Appalachian Mountains.

Sometimes, after a hard day of working and driving, I'm almost tempted to pick up a slice of pizza and a bag of chips at a gas station on the way home, but I really don't want to get into the habit of doing that. It would be easy, and maybe even fun for a day or two, but it would be disastrous for my health and my weight.

A trick I use to eat properly on the run is what I call my "cooler diet." I put everything I want to eat for the day in a nice, roomy cooler. If it's not in the cooler, I don't get to eat it—no questions. So that means I don't get to eat the chocolate that's everywhere around me at work, or the yummy-looking cream-filled doughnuts that one of the nurses brings in from the doughnut shop for breakfast. I pack my cooler the night before work with lots and lots of whole and nutritious foods and beverages— apples, pears, oranges, and cut-up veggies with low-fat dip. A couple of bottles of water and some unsweetened tea. A container of yogurt, some string cheese, and a bag full of nutritious trail mix. A box of low-fat granola cereal.

I pack as much food as I can fit into my cooler. The only rule I have is that the food I pack must contribute to my overall good health and support a healthy weight. I might be embarrassed to admit to someone that I plan to eat this much food in a single day, unless I explain that the entire contents of the cooler have fewer calories and less fat, sodium, sugar, and cholesterol than one typical fast-food meal with a burger, fries, and a soda. I try to pack my cooler after I've eaten dinner, when my appetite is satisfied and I'm bursting with willpower and overflowing with good intentions.

I did the math once, and I calculated that I can eat four to five pounds of wholesome, nutritious food from my cooler and still end up consuming far fewer calories than if I snacked on a handful of miniature candy bars at the office and ate a couple of slices of pizza at lunch. For instance, for around 100 calories, I can spend about five minutes enjoying a nice juicy apple and feel pretty full and satisfied afterward, or for the same number of calories, I could wolf down a tiny little candy bar in three seconds flat and trigger a major, day-long chocolate binge.

Drinking Better

In our society, we often like to talk about whether your cup is half empty or half full. Maybe we should start talking more about what's actually *in* your cup. Turns out the answer might be critical for your weight loss journey.

Over the past three decades, the number of calories adults obtain from fruit drinks, sodas, gourmet coffee drinks, and other liquids has doubled, according to researchers at the University of North Carolina. This trend closely mirrors the rise in obesity in the United States.

In terms of nutrition and weight loss, what you drink is just as important as what you eat. According to the University of North Carolina researchers, most American adults consume 222 calories a day in the form of calorie-containing liquids. That's enough to produce a weight gain of 21 pounds a year!

On the flip side, one study found that drinking about 16 ounces of water before every meal helped middle-aged and older adults lose 44 percent more weight on a lower-calorie diet than people who cut calories without drinking water before meals.

～∞～

I carry a 32-ounce water bottle with me all day, everywhere I go. I try to make sure that I drink it all by the end of the day.

—*Amy Barton, MD, a mom of an 11-year-old daughter and 8- and 5-year-old sons and a pediatrician at St. Luke's Children's Hospital, in Boise, ID*

～∞～

I drink coffee in the morning, but after I drink a cup or two, I switch to plain water. I try never to drink any calories.

—*Kristin C. Lyle, MD, FAAP, a mom of 10-, 7-, and 5-year-old daughters, the disaster medical director at Arkansas Children's Hospital, and an assistant professor of pediatrics at the University of Arkansas for Medical Sciences, both in Little Rock*

～∞～

One of my favorite snacks isn't really a snack at all, but a beverage. For a quick "snack," I'll drink a box of Horizon organic milk. It's low in fat and high in calcium. The boxes hold a perfect portion. I prefer the chocolate flavor, but the vanilla is good too.

—*Jennifer Bacani McKenney, MD, a mom of a two-year-old daughter who's expecting another baby and a family physician, in Fredonia, KS*

～∞～

Before my son was born, I was a Diet Coke fiend. I drank six cans a day, straight out of the can!

But now I drink more water. Especially because I am nursing, I make an effort to drink a lot of water throughout the day. Also about

❤FitBit

Alcohol is fat free, but it's by no means calorie free. You can count on adding 100 calories for every 4-ounce glass of wine, 12-ounce bottle of light beer, or 1.5-ounce serving of hard liquor you consume. And don't forget to count the mixers!

an hour before I eat, I drink 16 ounces of water. That helps me distinguish between hunger and thirst, and it prevents me from eating too much at mealtimes.

—*Edna Ma, MD, a mom of a six-month-old son, an anesthesiologist at UCLA Olive View Medical Center, and the founder of BareEase pre-waxing numbing kit, in Los Angeles, CA*

I haven't had soda in 22 years. And I don't miss it one bit.

I also rarely drink alcohol. I don't want to drink all of those calories, plus when you're drinking, it's harder to make good food choices.

When I eat, I try not to drink too much, not even water. I've read that if you drink too much while you're eating, it dilutes your digestive enzymes.

—*Eva Ritvo, MD, a mom of 22- and 17-year-old daughters, a psychiatrist, and a coauthor of* The Beauty Prescription, *in Miami Beach, FL*

Even when I was trying to lose 25 pounds, I didn't give up alcohol. I'd limit it to one glass, especially on a "school night," but I didn't find that drinking one glass of wine at dinner was detrimental to my weight loss. Whatever pattern you adopt has to be sustainable for the long term!

—*Katherine Dee, MD, a mom of eight-year-old twin daughters and a six-year-old son and a radiologist at the Seattle Breast Center, in Washington*

I recently bought a juicer. It's a lot of work. There are actually a lot of juicing cookbooks out there; it's a juicing counterculture.

Since we bought the juicer, we buy and eat a lot more fruit. Even my son drinks the smoothies we make.

—*Michelle Davis-Dash, MD, a mom of a 19-month-old son and a pediatrician in Baltimore, MD*

I try to avoid drinking any carbonated beverages, such as soda,

Mommy MD Guides-Recommended Product
So Delicious Dairy Free Coconut Milk Creamer

Rallie's tip: I love So Delicious Dairy Free Coconut Milk Creamer. Every time I make myself a cup of coffee or tea, I check the nutrition facts panel (again!) to make sure that it really is fat free. It tastes so rich and creamy that I can't believe it doesn't have a high fat content.

I add the French Vanilla flavored creamer to my coffee every morning and to my tea in the afternoon. It makes me feel like I'm spoiling myself, having a cup of delicious gourmet coffee or tea. This creamer is dairy free, which is perfect for me because I'm a bit lactose intolerant. The company uses packaging that is BPA free, which is very important to me. And coconut milk has dozens of really important health benefits, which are always welcome!

Although coconut contains saturated fat, research shows that not all saturated fats pose a health problem, and the ones called medium chain fatty acids (MCFA), such as lauric acid and capric acid, in coconut are actually good for you. Both are known to have anti-viral and anti-microbial properties. Because they're used by the body as energy instead of being stored as fat, MCFAs help promote weight maintenance, rather than weight gain.

You can buy So Delicious Dairy Free Coconut Milk Creamers at supermarkets and health food stores for around $3.99 a pint. They're available in seven flavors. Visit **SoDeliciousDairyFree.com** for more information.

because they can contain hidden calories and carbs that add up over time and lead to weight gain. Instead I drink eight 8-ounce glasses of water each day, and this has many benefits. It supports the body's metabolism, has a purifying effect on the colon, making the absorption of nutrients much easier, and keeps your skin glowing.

—*Aline T. Tanios, MD, a mom of 10- and 4-year-old daughters and an 8-year-old son and a pediatric hospitalist and assistant professor at the Washington University School of Medicine, in St. Louis, MO*

When I was trying to lose weight, I really took a look at what I was eating and drinking. I was surprised at the amount of sugar

Mommy MD Guides–Recommended Product
Sodastream

"A gadget that helps me to drink more water is my Sodastream," says Edna Ma, MD, a mom of a six-month-old son, an anesthesiologist at UCLA Olive View Medical Center, and the founder of BareEase pre-waxing numbing kit, in Los Angeles, CA. "It adds carbonation to beverages, even water. I used to spend a lot on carbonated bottled water, but now I can make it at home. I don't feel guilty about drinking it because it's just water."

You can also make your own soft drinks with Sodastream. The company offers more than 25 regular, diet, energy, and caffeine-free flavors of syrup (sold separately). Each 500-milliliter soda mix bottle makes the equivalent of 12 liters of soda (about 33 cans). The regular soda mixes contain no high-fructose corn syrup, while the diet soda mixes contain no aspartame.

You can buy Sodastream in stores such as Target and Walmart and at online retailers such as Amazon.com. A starter kit costs around $80. Visit **SODASTREAMUSA.COM** for more information.

FitBit

The more diet sodas you drink, the greater your risk for becoming overweight. University of Texas researchers found that for every serving of diet soda a person drank daily, there was a 65 percent increase in the risk of becoming overweight, and a 41 percent increase in the risk of becoming obese. Scientists speculate that the sweet taste of diet soda interferes with the body's ability to regulate caloric intake.

and cream I was putting into my coffee! Those calories really add up. I started to measure more carefully, putting in one packet of sweetener and one teaspoon of half-and-half in place of heavy cream.

> —*Tiemdow Phumiruk, MD, a mom of 13-, 10-, and 7-year-old daughters, a pediatrician in the emergency department of Children's Hospital Colorado at Parker Adventist Hospital, and adjunct faculty at Rocky Vista University College of Osteopathic Medicine, in Parker, CO*

I find a major challenge to maintaining a healthy weight is saying no to foods and drinks that are easy to overindulge in. At the top of that list are sugary drinks! They offer only "silent" calories. When you drink them, your body doesn't "register" them as calories. You don't feel full or satisfied; in fact, you probably feel hungry! I avoid soda and juices completely.

> —*Ayala Laufer-Cahana, MD, a mom of 17- and 15-year-old sons and a 14-year-old daughter, a pediatrician, and the founder of Herbal Water Inc., in Wynnewood, PA*

I drink at least two cups of freshly brewed, unsweetened tea each day. Tea is calorie free, and it boosts energy, enhances immunity, prevents cancer, and protects against heart disease.

I also aim to drink two liters of plain clean water a day.

ᑦFitBit

Watch out for those pricey gourmet coffee drinks. They're loaded with caffeine, sugar, and fat. Many varieties have more than 300 calories and 20 grams of fat. Before you order, be sure to check the nutrition information.

To make matters worse, sugar-sweetened drinks can fatten you up, but they don't fill you up. Scientists don't fully understand the reasons our brains don't pay attention to the calories obtained from sugar-sweetened liquids. Some speculate that chewing might be important in triggering feelings of satiety and fullness.

I completely *avoid* drinking all sugary beverages, such as soda, sweet tea, fruit drinks, chocolate milk, and gourmet coffees. These beverages actually work against weight loss. They drive your blood sugar levels up and then down, too low too fast—which then makes you hungry!

—*Ann Kulze, MD, a mom of 24- and 17-year-old daughters and 22- and 21-year-old sons; a nationally recognized nutrition expert, motivational speaker, and physician; and the author of the best-selling, award-winning* Eat Right for Life *book series, in Charleston, SC*

The first thing I did to lose weight was to stop drinking calories. I'm a big hot tea drinker; tea is my thing. I used to put a lot of sugar in it, and I cut that out. I was also drinking a lot of Southern-style sweet iced tea, and I stopped that too.

The ironic thing about drinking calories is that they don't fill you up. If you ate a 300-calorie snack, you'd feel full. But if you drink a 300-calorie soda, it doesn't fill you up. You want to eat a snack with it!

I switched to putting Splenda in my tea, and I started drinking water instead of sweet tea. *I'm not going to waste calories,* I thought.

—Deborah Gilboa, MD, a mom of 11-, 9-, 7-, and 5-year-old sons, a family physician with Squirrel Hill Health Center in Pittsburgh, PA, and a parenting speaker whose advice is found at AskDoctorG.com

Dehydration is one of the big saboteurs of weight loss. Water is required to break down fat and to get it out of your body. In chemical terms, fat must be hydrolyzed in order to be excreted. So being behind on your water intake, or simply experiencing thirst, means you need to drink more.

Our bodies lose a lot of water through sweat, and also through breathing and other body functions. It's very important to drink a lot more fluids in the summertime, even if you stay indoors most of the time.

MomMy TIME — Sip a Soothing Cup of Tea

Sometimes it doesn't take much to treat yourself. One way is to take five minutes every day to make a cup of hot tea, find a comfortable place to sit, and enjoy each sip. It's soothing, it gives you a chance to slow down, and if you choose green tea, it might even help you drop the pounds.

Caffeine and catechins in green tea might help increase metabolism. Several studies have looked at whether green tea might promote weight loss, and a recent analysis of the research found that green tea appears to help people lose a small amount of weight.

But there's another reason tea might be helpful while you're losing weight: It helps keep you hydrated, and that helps keep your appetite in check. Research has shown that when people drink water before a meal, they eat fewer calories during their meal. Also, experts say that thirst might be mistaken for hunger. A cup of tea can keep you from snacking when you're thirsty—all the while giving you a few soothing minutes to recharge.

Water is usually the best way to replenish body fluid, but if you're outside a lot, alternating water with a sports drink can be beneficial. Unless you're on a fluid- or sodium-restricted diet for specific health reasons, I encourage the use of salt on food to help the body retain water and other electrolytes.

Can you be dehydrated and not be thirsty? Yes! Our thirst mechanism doesn't register until we are 3 to 5 percent dehydrated. Additionally, many prescription medications blunt this response and make the body more susceptible to the dangerous effects of heat exposure. Thus, thirst is often a poor indicator of your hydration status.

I recommend monitoring your urine to evaluate your hydration status. If you're in good health and you're well hydrated, your urine should be almost clear. If it's colored enough to make your toilet water

Mommy MD Guides-Recommended Product
Sparkletts Water Delivery

"One thing that has helped me drink more water is subscribing to a water delivery service, and having the water delivered to our home," says Edna Ma, MD, a mom of a six-month-old son, an anesthesiologist at UCLA Olive View Medical Center, and the founder of BareEase pre-waxing numbing cream, in Los Angeles, CA. "Our water delivery service is called Sparkletts.

"I've found that I drink a lot more water now because it tastes better and because I have a healthy and a tasty water option literally at my fingertips. I don't think I'm a water snob, but there are so many bottled water options that it's easy to become a more discerning water drinker. Sparkletts water comes in three- or five-gallon bottles, and the machine dispenses instant hot or cold water."

You can order it at **SPARKLETTS.COM**. They offer several different types of water: filtered water, spring water, distilled water, and fluoridated water. Sparkletts water costs about $7 for a five-gallon bottle.

> **I believe humans get a lot done, not because we're smart, but because we have thumbs so we can make coffee.**
>
> **—*Flash Rosenberg,* *a cartoonist, writer, and photographer in New York City***

appear yellow, you probably need to drink more water. (Some multivitamins can also affect the color of urine, making it almost fluorescent yellow, which is different from the yellow urine of dehydration.)

To stay properly hydrated, I recommend the following tips.

- Keep water or sports drinks on hand at all times in the hot months.
- Keep half-filled bottles in the freezer and then top off the ice with water when you're ready to leave the house. The ice keeps the water cold so you have a beverage that stays cool longer.
- Reduce your intake of caffeine and alcohol. Both of these have a diuretic effect, meaning they cause you to lose more water. It's best to limit them in the summer months.
- Keep a misting fan on hand for cooling off quickly.

  —*Jennifer Hanes, DO, a mom of a seven-year-old daughter and a four-year-old son, an emergency physician who's board certified in integrative medicine, and the author of* The Princess Plan: Shrink Your Waist, Expand Your Beauty, *in Austin, TX*

Exercising Better

The expression "no pain, no gain" has always seemed rather ironic. We're trying to lose weight, not gain it, right? Yet experts say that exercise is critical for weight loss, and especially weight maintenance.

How much exercise do you need, and maybe more importantly, how much exercise are you really getting? The average person overestimates the amount of activity she's doing by about 30 percent, and she underestimates her food intake by about 30 percent. That makes for a huge reality gap!

The U.S. Department of Health and Human Services recommends getting at least two hours and 30 minutes of moderate aerobic exercise each week, through activities such as brisk walking or dancing, plus two days a week of strength training major muscle groups, by lifting weights or doing exercises such as pushups, situps, and leg lunges.

To determine how much exercise you're really getting, you could keep a simple log, jot it down on your calendar, or use a tool such as an app. (See "Mommy MD Guides-Recommended Product: MyFitnessPal" on page 10 for a great one to try!)

I exercise every day. It's not so much that I love to exercise, but I have a belief that our bodies were built to move. I don't do anything unusual; I run or work out on my elliptical trainer.
—*Deborah Gilboa, MD, a mom of 11-, 9-, 7-, and 5-year-old sons, a family physician with Squirrel Hill Health Center in Pittsburgh, PA, and a parenting speaker whose advice is found at AskDoctorG.com*

When my kids were born, I started walking a lot. I was a huge fan of the double jogging stroller. I walked my kids everywhere. Once I was able to start running again, I did that instead. Running while pushing that stroller is twice as hard as running alone.
—*Antoinette Cheney, DO, a mom of a seven-year-old son and a six-year-old daughter and a family physician with Rocky Vista University College of Osteopathic Medicine, in Parker, CO*

One of my favorite ways to exercise is having fun in our pool with my family. We were fortunate that our home came with a pool, and we spend hours out there, just goofing around and diving underwater for pool toys. It's a fun, great workout.

We also take our kids golfing. Our kids are young, so we can't always finish 18 holes, but 12 is a good goal!
—*Amy Barton, MD, a mom of an 11-year-old daughter and*

8- and 5-year-old sons and a pediatrician at St. Luke's Children's Hospital, in Boise, ID

⌒⁄⌀

Once I got a little momentum toward weight loss with my diet alone, I started adding a workout. At first it was really simple, just some walks. Slowly I worked my way up on the workout intensity scale.

One of my favorite workouts now is hot yoga. It was tough at first, but it has become my way to relax my muscles, strengthen my soul, and get a great calorie burn.

I did Bikram yoga, which is a form of hot yoga that involves doing 26 yoga postures in a 90-minute class in a room that heats up to 104 degrees. Sound scary? To me it did, the first time I thought about trying it. But in reality, it was a big release of the stresses of the day when I completed each session. I was proud and excited as I saw my body transform and become stronger. Though it was definitely hot and strenuous, I took it slow at first and then built up to doing the classes regularly.

—*Arleen K. Lamba, MD, a mom of a three-month-old son, an anesthesiologist, the medical director of Blush Med Institute, and founder of the Blush Blends Skin Care line, in Washington, DC*

Mommy MD Guides-Recommended Product
Stairmaster

"It's well worth investing in a cardio machine to have in your home," says Lisa Campanella-Coppo, MD, a mom of a three-year-old daughter and an emergency physician with EMCARE and the Meridian Health System, in Monmouth, NJ. "When my daughter was born, my husband bought me a Stairmaster. It was the best money we've ever spent. It's much harder to find time to go to the gym than to go downstairs to exercise!"

You can buy Stairmasters for around $1,700 on up. Visit **STAIRMASTER.COM** for more information.

When I need to lose weight, I really try to ramp up the exercise. I used to go to the gym, but after my second son was born, that no longer was practical. I was paying for a gym membership I wasn't using!

Instead, I bought an elliptical trainer, and I work out on that for 10 to 20 minutes a day, usually after I put my sons to bed. I'm not a morning person, so working out at night works better for me! I set a goal for myself to exercise three or four times a week. If I know it's going to be a busy week, I try to get my workouts out of the way as early in the week as possible. I make a pact with myself, and if I don't do it, I feel like I've let myself down.

When to Call Your Doctor

It's always important to build your fitness level gradually, to warm up at the beginning of your workout (get your heart rate up by walking or taking it slow for the first 5 to 10 minutes), and to stretch after your exercise session to avoid injuring yourself. Overall, exercise should feel challenging but not painful.

If you push too hard before your body is ready, you might end up with a painful muscle strain, a sprained ankle, knee pain, or an injured back. If the injury is acute, or sudden in onset, you might feel pain during the exercise, followed by swelling, tenderness, or weakness. You might not be able to put weight on the part of your body that's injured. If your injury is chronic, or long lasting, you might notice recurrent pain when you exercise or swelling and a dull ache when you rest.

If you experience either type of pain, first, stop exercising. Don't push through it. Then decide if it's something you can treat at home or if you need to see a doctor.

Call your doctor if:

• You're experiencing severe pain, swelling, redness, or numbness.
• A joint feels unstable or looks deformed.
• You're not able to put any weight on the part of your body

—*Bola Oyeyipo-Ajumobi, MD, a mom of five- and two-year-old sons, a family physician at the Veterans Health Administration, and the owner of SlimyBookWorm.com, in San Antonio, TX*

My favorite exercise is walking. You don't need to join a gym; all you need is a good pair of walking shoes. It also helps if you have a dog. I have a lot of motivation to get out and walk my golden retriever. I live near a wildlife preserve, and it's a beautiful place to walk.

I walk outside with my dog around three days a week. I also have an elliptical trainer, and I'll work out on that for 20 minutes if the weather is bad.

that's injured, you can't walk, or you can't bend a knee.
- You heard a pop at the time of the injury, or you feel as if a bone could slide out of its socket.
- You have neck pain that extends to your arms and legs.
- The injury involved your head, especially if it's followed by changes in vision, loss of balance or coordination, vomiting, confusion or memory loss, or slurred speech.

If the injury doesn't seem severe, use the RICE method at home for the next 48 hours, which involves rest, ice, compression, and elevation.

- **Rest:** Take weight off the injured area and take it slow while you're healing.
- **Ice:** Press a cold pack or your own bag of ice wrapped in a towel to the area for 20 minutes at a time several times a day.
- **Compression:** Wrap the injured area with an elastic bandage to support it and help reduce swelling.
- **Elevation:** Keep the injured area above your heart whenever possible by placing your limb on a pillow when you're lying down.

After you've used the RICE method, call your doctor if the pain and swelling get worse over time.

I also do situps on a disk-shaped balance ball. The beauty of using a ball is that it supports my neck and it also helps me engage my core muscles. Plus, it's small enough that I can keep it in a closet.

—*Debra Luftman, MD, a mom of a 22-year-old daughter and a 19-year-old son, a board-certified dermatologist in private practice, coauthor of* The Beauty Prescription, *developer of the skincare line of products Therapeutix, and a clinical instructor of skin surgery and general dermatology at UCLA*

When I was ready to lose weight, I added Pilates to my usual routine. I didn't want to have a tummy tuck! I wanted to tone my muscles. I took a Pilates class at a local studio. I think that Pilates is a great workout for women who want to tone all of their muscle groups. When I first started doing it, I felt so sore afterward!

Mommy MD Guides–Recommended Product
Turbo Jam DVDs

"I've done the same terrific exercise program since college," says Eva Mayer, MD, a mom of a nine-year-old daughter and an eight-year-old son, an associate professor of pediatrics at Temple University, and a pediatrician with St. Luke's Pediatrics Associates, in Bethlehem, PA. "I found it at BeachBody.com: Turbo Jam DVDs. It's a high-energy workout with amazing dance music. One of the best parts is that it's easy on my joints. I used to do other dance-type workouts, and this is the only one I've found that doesn't hurt my knees."-

"I'm in the best shape I've ever been in," Dr. Mayer adds. "I do one of their workouts every day that I'm not working, so three or four days a week. I've been doing these workouts for more than 10 years, and they never get boring."

You can buy the Turbo Jam program—six workouts on two DVDs—at **BeachBody.com** for $59.85 plus shipping.

Now I take a class called CrossFit. It's a core strength condition-ing program. (Visit CrossFit.com to learn more.) The classes really help me with my strength, flexibility, endurance, and balance. You don't have to be in phenomenal shape to do it because you can scale it to your ability. The workouts are intense but a lot of fun. And it is rewarding to see yourself progress and get better. It's drawn a very loyal following.

I feel healthier and stronger than I ever have. I recently ran a half marathon and beat my personal pre-pregnancy record!

—*Martha Wittenberg, MD, MPH, a mom of an eight-year-old son and a six-year-old daughter and a family physician with Seal Beach Family Medicine, in California*

∽

When I first tried to lose weight, I jogged. That worked—until my knees started to hurt. Then I started using the elliptical trainer in our basement. That worked—until I started getting bored. Now I bike out-side on trails behind my house while my kids are in school. The fresh air and scenery keep me entertained. I really enjoy biking, and you don't have to spend a lot of money to get a decent bike.

For me, changing the type of exercise I do every so often really helps. It's important to be flexible and change your routine if it isn't working for you anymore.

—*Tiemdow Phumiruk, MD, a mom of 13-, 10-, and 7-year-old daughters, a pediatrician in the emergency department of Children's Hospital Colorado at Parker Adventist Hospital, and adjunct faculty at Rocky Vista University College of Osteopathic Medicine, in Parker, CO*

∽

I get down on myself sometimes because I don't exercise more. Before my son was born, I loved to try new activities, such as rock climbing or surfing, and I loved the mental and emotional boost that regular stren-uous activity gave me. But that's a lot harder with kids. Now I have to be more realistic. I try to get in at least 30 minutes of exercise each day. We have a dog, and I often take walks with my husband, our son, and the dog up and down the hills around our house.

> **A bear, however hard he tries,**
> **grows tubby without exercise.**
> **—*A.A. Milne*, Winnie-the-Pooh**

I've also started to bike to work. This is helpful because it kills two birds with one stone: exercise and commuting! The night before work, I pack a big backpack with my work clothes and toiletries. I also keep some clothes and shoes at work. I find if I don't pack the bag the night before, it's too easy to jump in the car and drive instead.

—*Michelle Spring, MD, a mom of a one-year-old son and two grown stepchildren and a board-certified plastic surgeon with Marina Plastic Surgery Associates, in Marina del Rey, CA*

I must confess, I don't go to the gym. Instead, I try to make everyday tasks more active. For example, when I go for walks with my husband and our baby, my husband pushes the stroller, and I carry five-pound weights. This way I can also work out my arms while I walk.

Also, I almost never take the elevator. Even when I go into work in the morning, and I'm carrying my breast pump, briefcase, and lunch, I walk up the stairs.

—*Edna Ma, MD, a mom of a six-month-old son, an anesthesiologist at UCLA Olive View Medical Center, and the founder of BareEase pre-waxing numbing kit, in Los Angeles, CA*

I set a goal for myself of exercising four times a week, for 30 minutes each time, on my stationary bike. If I meet that goal, it's awesome. We just bought an elliptical trainer. It was expensive, but I felt the money was better spent than a gym membership that we weren't able to use because of child care issues.

I also try to do more mini-exercises throughout my day. For example, I always take the stairs at work, walk to the hospital rather than taking the shuttle, and do some housework each day. It burns more calories than sitting on the couch does!

—*Aline T. Tanios, MD, a mom of 10- and 4-year-old daughters and an 8-year-old son and a pediatric hospitalist and assistant professor at the Washington University School of Medicine, in St. Louis, MO*

❧

When my son was around a year old, I found my weight creeping up. Some of my college friends are now coaches for a beach-body weight loss program, called TurboFire.

I joined their crazy challenge. It has a series of workouts that you're scheduled to do each day, such as Pilates and high-intensity interval training. I lost about 10 inches and five pounds in 90 days. I looked and felt great, and I had more energy and stamina. The only problem is that I'm not the spring chicken I used to be, so I had to stop due to a back injury. I still try to walk and do Pilates.

—*Michelle Davis-Dash, MD, a mom of a 19-month-old son and a pediatrician in Baltimore, MD*

❧

To lose and then maintain my weight, I do a combination of cardio training and weight lifting. If you do cardio training first, then weight lifting, it boosts your metabolic rate more than just doing either cardio training or weight lifting alone. Weight training helps build muscle. With better muscle tone, your clothes fit better. I like to do a lot of different types of workouts. This cross-training is important because it keeps me from getting bored, and also because different types of workouts exercise and tone different muscle groups.

I've lifted weights since college. If you want to learn how to lift weights, you can usually get a free training session or two with a personal trainer when you join a gym.

—*Katherine Dee, MD, a mom of eight-year-old twin daughters and a six-year-old son and a radiologist at the Seattle Breast Center, in Washington*

❧

In college, I gained the typical "freshman 15" pounds. All of those extra pancakes and slices of pizza really caught up with me.

To lose the weight, I started teaching aerobics and worked as a personal trainer. This might seem a little extreme, but I like knowing more about what I'm doing. Becoming a teacher is a great way to learn about a subject. I earned my Aerobics and Fitness Association of America (AFAA) certification and started teaching step aerobics. I loved working with people, and I began offering one-on-one training. I enjoy teaching people about anatomy and fitness. I also love seeing people get stronger. I pretty much became a gym rat!

It's so funny to think about it now, but it really helped me refine the skills I needed for my job today, which is promoting health and wellness.

—*Kay Corpus, MD, a mom of a six-year-old daughter and a two-year-old son, a family physician, and the director of Owensboro Health Integrative Medicine, in Kentucky*

Yoga is huge for me. But I'm not going to tell you that I do yoga three to five times a week. I set more realistic goals to have a better chance of success. I go to a yoga class just once a week.

Mommy MD Guides-Recommended Product
Billy Blanks DVDs

"For my birthday one year, my daughter bought me some Billy Blanks tapes," says Marie Dam, MD, a mom of 24- and 20-year-old daughters and an anti-aging medicine specialist in private practice in Naples, FL, and Danbury, CT. "They helped me change my shape, strengthen my core, and feel great. They helped me get an intense cardio and strength training workout at the same time, in about 40 minutes.

"I liked that I could do them at home, and I loved losing weight and feeling great. They are terrific! You get to kick and punch and really exercise your core. Doing those workouts completely changed the shape of my body."

You can buy Billy Blanks DVDs in stores such as Walmart and Target and at online retailers such as **AMAZON.COM** for around $9.99.

I find that going to a yoga class, rather than doing poses at home, is more beneficial. The ebb and flow of class helps ease stress, and the instructor helps gently guide me into the proper poses.

The overall philosophy of yoga has changed my outlook on life. It reminds me to look up and out and strive to do more—to be more.

—*Jennifer Hanes, DO, a mom of a seven-year-old daughter and a four-year-old son, an emergency physician who's board certified in integrative medicine, and the author of* The Princess Plan: Shrink Your Waist, Expand Your Beauty, *in Austin, TX*

After my son was born, I was really looking forward to losing the weight. I had a C-section, so I had to go slowly. I started with mainly cardio training, such as walking

What really jump-started my exercising was when I hired a personal trainer. People might think this is crazy expensive, but I split the cost with a friend, and we each paid $35 a session. He met with us for an hour twice a week. He exercised with us, and he also went over our eating plans. It was very helpful, motivating, and fun.

—*Shilpa Amin-Shah, MD, a mom of a three-year-old son and a two-year-old daughter and an emergency physician and director of the recruiting team at Emergency Medical Associates, in Livingston, NJ*

We have a treadmill and elliptical trainer in our basement. That's also where our TV is. TV is a destination in our house; you have to walk downstairs to watch it.

Getting to exercise with Mom and Dad is a treat in our family. If you're exercising with Mom and Dad, you get some extra screen time. I'll run on the treadmill and listen to something on my MP3 player, while one of my sons will exercise and watch cartoons.

My sons are happy to spend time one-on-one with me, and also it's a great opportunity for me to model healthy exercising behaviors for them. They see me struggling and sweating—which is better than them simply thinking, *Mommy went to the gym.*

—*Deborah Gilboa, MD*

With exercise, I'm pretty self-disciplined. I work out three or four days a week. My goal is three, but if I do four, I'm thrilled. Exercise is just part of my life.

I love to run outside on warm, sunny days. I tolerate the treadmill by recording shows that I love on the DVR. When my older son was a baby, I asked my husband to buy me a treadmill. I needed that a lot more than I needed fancy jewelry or other things. We bought a moderately priced treadmill, and it's been worth every penny. It's lasted a really long time, and it gets a lot of use.

We put the treadmill in a corner of our finished basement. This way my kids can play on one side of the room, and I can exercise and keep an eye on them at the same time.

Also, I was lucky enough to hire a personal trainer; I split the cost with a friend. It was expensive, around $35 a week, but I justified it by saying I don't get my nails done or wear expensive clothes. The cost is usually lower if you work out with the trainer at the gym, rather than having the trainer come to your home. Working out with the trainer really changed my body shape. She pushed me, but in a fun way.

—*Heather Orman-Lubell, MD, a mom of 12- and 8-year-old sons and a pediatrician in private practice at Yardley Pediatrics of St. Christopher's Hospital for Children, in Pennsylvania*

Even though I know that what I eat has a greater impact on my weight than how much I exercise, exercise is still indispensable to losing weight. I never miss a day of exercise, unless I'm sick in bed. In addition to helping me lose—or maintain—weight, exercise gives me boundless energy, alleviates stress, improves my mood, and makes me feel great. It's self-reinforcing because when I exercise, I feel great, so I want to exercise again.

A key to exercise for me is to prevent boredom. So I have a "menu" of exercise options that I enjoy from which to choose. Today, for example, I took a yoga-spin class. Yesterday I went for a walk, and tomorrow I might swim. I like to mix it up.

FitBit

When you exercise regularly, your body becomes more efficient at burning calories for energy. By working your muscle tissue with daily exercise, you can dramatically increase the number of calories your body burns daily.

I also incorporate weight and resistance training into my routine. Once you're older than 45, it's more difficult to *lose* weight unless you *lift* weight. If a 50-year-old woman has gained 20 pounds since age 20, she hasn't just gained 20 pounds. She's probably gained 20 pounds of fat, and she's probably *lost* 10 pounds of muscle.

Resistance training helps you increase your muscle mass, which burns about 70 percent of the calories you consume. It also helps prevent osteoporosis and preserve your functionality. As you age, you want to be able to do everything you want to do in life.

—Ann Kulze, MD, a mom of 24- and 17-year-old daughters and 22- and 21-year-old sons; a nationally recognized nutrition expert, motivational speaker, and physician; and the author of the best-selling, award-winning Eat Right for Life *book series, in Charleston, SC*

Having active kids helped me to stay active. When they learned to ski, I learned to ski. When they started their tennis lessons, I took up the racquet again, waiting for the day they could beat me, which came when they were about 13 years old. I found that you need to start kids exercising very early.

As much as possible, I kept my kids away from the TV and off computers, which I think are poisoning our society. Those activities encourage kids to be passive, not active. Instead, I encouraged my kids to play active games. We started asking them to help with household chores early on—picking up their own toys and cleaning their own rooms. My husband and I started swimming, biking, and

☉ Mommy MD Guides–Recommended Product
30-Day Shred

"Starting a cookie business did *not* help with the initial post-baby weight loss, and my exercise time took a backseat to family, work, and running a company," says Lennox McNeary, MD, a mom of a four-year-old son, a specialist in physical medicine and rehabilitation at Carilion Clinic, and a cofounder of the Mommy Doctors Bakery (makers of Milkin' Cookies), in Roanoke, VA. "I got up around 5 am to get ready for work and pump, back when I was still breastfeeding. Then after work, I didn't exercise because I didn't want to take any more time away from my son. For a long time, I swore that I couldn't work out late at night.

"Then I finally decided that I felt awful enough to try it," Dr. McNeary adds. "So for a week, every night after I got my son in bed, I worked out with 30-Day Shred. Within two days, I had more energy. I couldn't walk up the stairs, but I had more energy. The workouts are only about 20 minutes long, and it's really hard to make the excuse that you really can't find 20 minutes at some point during your day or night to work out. Seriously. It's 20 minutes. And it *works*.

"Once my husband decided to get back in shape, too, we bought an Arc Trainer, which we both use five or six days a week. I can catch up on watching TV, listen to podcasts or audiobooks, or just zone out to music.

Now I do about 20 to 30 minutes of cardio training (which is now my *me* time) and work my abs and lift weights, or I do the 30-Day Shred workout or another of the Jillian Michaels DVD workouts."

You can buy the 30-Day Shred DVD at stores such as Walmart and Target and at online retailers such as **AMAZON.COM** for around $10. Visit **JILLIANMICHAELS.COM** for more information, to watch sample exercise videos, check out sample fitness plans, and more.

walking with them when they were very young. Taking an after-dinner walk is good for the whole family!

As my children got older, I started going to yoga and Pilates classes, initially to spend time with my daughters, and then because I became hooked! I have a NordicTrack that's old, but it still works, so I do aerobic exercise on that, too. And I am a sucker for all sorts of exercise tapes—dance and other fun exercises.

*—Linda Brodsky, MD, a mom of a 30-year-old son
and 28- and 25-year-old daughters, the president of
WomenMDResources.com, a physician in private practice
with Pediatric ENT Associates, and a retired professor of
otolaryngology and pediatrics, in Buffalo, NY*

When I started trying to lose weight, I didn't tackle the exercise part of it. I had tried running before and had given up. Having exercised at the gym with machines that tell you how many calories you've burned, I realized that no amount of exercise was going to give me the freedom to eat indiscriminately! You just can't work out that long! You have to run a mile to burn about 30 calories. That's a joke!

But after I lost the weight by overhauling my diet, I did add exercise back into my life. My husband and I both felt it was important to set a good example for our kids. We want to show them that we're good stewards of our bodies.

We joined a gym that gives us each two hours of free child care each day. That way we could take a class and have time to shower while the kids played. Now I enjoy taking spinning classes, and I've run two half marathons! I enjoy working out at the gym, around plenty of other people. I like the social aspect of the gym and the accountability that comes with having other people around.

—Amy Thompson, MD, a mom of six-, four-, and two-year-old sons and an ob-gyn at the University of Cincinnati College of Medicine, in Ohio

Supplementing Right

In a perfect world, or maybe even in the future in this not-quite-perfect world, there would be a nutritional supplement you could take to melt the pounds away, no matter how many cheese puffs, stuffed-crust pizzas, and frosted cakes you eat. It'll no doubt be on the shelf next to the supplement that erases wrinkles and age spots and just across the aisle from the supplement that allows your IQ to increase 30 points and multitask three amazing tasks at once.

But here today, sadly none of them exist. But there are some nutritional supplements that might help you on your weight loss journey.

About a year and a half ago, I started to take chia seeds as a supplement before bed. I put them in water, and they form a jelly-like substance that I drink. When taken this way, they are not for the faint of heart. But I really love it. They have a lot of fiber and omega-3 fatty acids. Since I started taking them, I feel more energized, and I have fewer cravings for sweets because they are filling.

Mommy MD Guides-Recommended Product
Muscle Milk

"When I was really trying to lose weight, I drank Muscle Milk Lite," says Shilpa Amin-Shah, MD, a mom of a three-year-old son and a two-year-old daughter and an emergency physician and director of the recruiting team at Emergency Medical Associates, in Livingston, NJ. "It's high in protein, so it fills you up, and it tastes great. I drink it over ice, so it tastes like a milk shake. It comes in chocolate and vanilla. My favorite is the chocolate."

You can buy Muscle Milk Lite at stores such as Costco and at online retailers such as **AMAZON.COM**. A 24-pack costs around $33 dollars. Visit **MUSCLEMILK.COM** for more information.

> **A strong positive attitude will create
> more miracles than any wonder drug.**
> —*Patricia Neal, an American stage and screen actress*

—*Allison Bailey, MD, a mom of a nine-year-old son and a five-year-old daughter and founder and director of Integrated Health and Fitness Associates, in Cambridge, MA*

⌒⌒

You should see my supplement cabinet. I'm a biohacker by nature, and I was an MIT bioengineer before becoming a physician.

I take about eight supplements at a time, and I rewrite my own protocols every four to eight weeks. I struggle with PMS, sky-high cortisol (a stress hormone, which I also call the "Bad Boyfriend Hormone"), and a slow metabolism.

Daily, I take a high-potency multivitamin because it improves my thyroid function.

—*Sara Gottfried, MD, a mom of 13- and 8-year-old daughters, a board-certified gynecologist, and the author of* The Hormone Cure, *in Berkeley, CA*

RALLIE'S TIP

If there was a magic weight loss supplement that caused the pounds and inches to melt away, I feel certain that I would have found it! And if I did, I would share it with everyone I know.

I've always been fascinated by nutrition, and I love reading about and researching herbs, supplements, and nutrients. Unfortunately, I've never found that one magic weight loss supplement that we've all been searching for. Still, I do take nutritional supplements on a daily basis.

No matter how hard I try, I find it difficult to eat a perfectly balanced diet every single day, so taking a daily multivitamin and mineral supplement just makes good sense to me. I also take a combination calcium and vitamin D supplement, a vitamin C supplement, and an omega-3 fatty acid supplement. This allows me to cover most of my

⚫FitBit

Use spices such as cinnamon, cloves, ginger, nutmeg, and anise to sweeten without sugar. Sprinkling spices on a baked sweet potato or baked apple will satisfy your sweet tooth and help keep your weight loss plan on track.

nutritional bases and make sure I'm getting most of the important nutrients that I need for good health. When your body is well nourished with all the vitamins, minerals, antioxidants, and fats that you need, your immune system is better able to do its job keeping you healthy, so you're less likely to get sick. You're also more likely to have more energy, and you're better able to cope with everyday stressors. If you're not deficient in a particular nutrient, you're less likely to crave particular foods, or greater quantities of food, and it's easier to maintain control over your eating behaviors.

One supplement that I believe has helped me control my appetite more than anything is not really a supplement in the traditional sense, but rather a spice—cinnamon. Scientific studies have demonstrated that adding cinnamon to sweet foods helps reduce the spike in blood sugar that typically results afterward. The problem with having a spike in blood sugar is that when it falls to normal or slightly below normal levels (what some people call a sugar crash), it can lead to rebound hunger, which can lead to eating too much of the wrong foods, which of course can lead to weight gain. As a bonus, cinnamon has antibacterial and antifungal properties. Whenever I have a cup of coffee or tea or a bowl of oatmeal, I always sprinkle a half teaspoon of cinnamon on top. It's good for me, and it tastes great!

Here are a few of my other all-time favorite supplements.

PROBIOTICS
These are naturally occurring, friendly bacteria that dwell in the human gut. These microorganisms have several important benefits in terms of enhancing digestion, normalizing bowel function, improving immunity, and boosting overall health.

Although the human gastrointestinal tract is most commonly associated with the digestion of food and the absorption of dietary nutrients, it has another, equally vital function. The gut is a major component of the body's immune system, and it plays a critical role in defending us from disease-causing germs. Beneficial bacteria in the gastrointestinal tract protect us from colds, stomach bugs, and other infections. Because these good bacteria are constantly being turned over in the body, it's important to replenish them on a regular basis.

One of the easiest ways to boost the population of good bacteria in your gut is to add a source of probiotics to your daily diet. Probiotics can be found in dietary supplements, a cultured dairy product called kefir, and in certain brands of yogurt, including DanActive and Activia, which contain live bacterial cultures.

Studies have shown that adults who regularly consume probiotic preparations suffer significantly fewer infections of the gastrointestinal system and upper-respiratory tract. The results of several large clinical trials revealed that both children and adults taking probiotics on a daily basis experienced fewer illnesses, and they also enjoyed reduced rates of absenteeism from school and work.

If you're allergic to milk products, probiotic pills and powders are excellent choices. On the other hand, if you're merely mildly lactose intolerant, you might be able to consume dairy products containing probiotics without experiencing the slightest bit of gastrointestinal grief because the lactose is pre-digested by the friendly bacteria.

PSYLLIUM

Fiber contains no vitamins, minerals, or calories, but nonetheless, it's a key component of every woman's diet. Although adult women need at least 28 grams of fiber daily to stay healthy, most of us consume only about 15 grams a day. Needless to say, there's plenty of room for improvement. While eating a balanced, plant-based diet is one of the best ways to boost fiber consumption, that's not always easy for women on the go. If you're in search of an inexpensive and convenient fiber source, a product called psyllium is well worth considering.

Psyllium fiber is derived from the husk of a shrub-like herb that's native to parts of Asia and North Africa. In the United States, it's sold as a nutritional supplement at supermarkets and health food stores in various forms, including tablets, capsules, water-soluble crystals, and wafers. It is also the primary ingredient in several over-the-counter products, such as Metamucil and Fiberall. Although psyllium has long been used to alleviate constipation, this unique source of fiber does more than just promote regularity and good bowel health.

Clinical trials have shown that in combination with a low-fat diet, a daily dose of just 10.2 grams of psyllium can reduce the risk of heart disease by significantly lowering cholesterol levels. Among adults with diabetes, the same dose can dramatically reduce blood sugar levels.

In addition to its positive effects on cholesterol and glucose, psyllium is also beneficial in terms of weight management. The soluble fiber in psyllium and other foods, including oats, peas, and many types of fruit, helps reduce hunger and curtail overeating by contributing to a sense of fullness. Soluble fiber absorbs water like a sponge in the stomach, and it also delays gastric emptying. Both actions make you feel fuller for longer.

Adding psyllium to your diet will likely improve your health, but it's best to start with a low dose and gradually increase it. Drastic increases in fiber intake, regardless of the source, can lead to intestinal bloating, cramping, and excessive gas production, which can be uncomfortable and can also make you rather unpopular with your friends and family. Drinking plenty of water will reduce the likelihood that you'll experience any of these unpleasant side effects. If you're in search of a supplement that can lower your blood sugar and cholesterol levels, curb your hunger, or just boost your fiber intake, a daily dose of psyllium might be your best bet.

XYLITOL

Most of us get far more sugar in our diets than our bodies need. The average American consumes somewhere in the neighborhood of 150 pounds of sugar every year. Most health and nutrition experts, including those affiliated with the U.S. Department of Agriculture, recommend an intake of no more than 10 teaspoons of sugar a day. If you do the math (a pound of sugar contains 108 teaspoons), you quickly realize that the average American consumes more along the lines of 45 teaspoons of sugar each day, which undoubtedly contributes to the epidemics of obesity and diabetes in our country.

To avoid the high-calorie consequences of a sugar-laden diet, many women turn to artificial sweeteners. Although these women might temporarily avoid some of the unwanted calories, they might not be avoiding the associated weight gain. In fact, numerous studies have linked consumption of noncaloric artificial sweeteners to weight gain, rather than weight loss. Animal research suggests that calorie-free artificial sweeteners actually stimulate hunger and overeating.

While the reasons for the increased appetite are not fully understood, some experts believe that when noncaloric sweeteners are consumed, the brain responds to the sweet taste in the same way that it responds to the sweet taste of pure sugar: It alerts the pancreas to prepare for an incoming caloric load. Although there are no calories in artificial sweeteners, the brain doesn't know this. As a result, it signals the pancreas to begin pumping insulin into the bloodstream. Insulin's job is to escort sugar molecules from the bloodstream to cells in various tissues throughout the body. Because there are no sugar molecules in artificial sweeteners, the newly released insulin goes to work on sugar that is already in the bloodstream, and as a result, it can cause blood sugar levels to drop well below normal. Low blood sugar levels, in turn, are a powerful stimulus for hunger.

Because artificial sweeteners can end up causing more harm than good, you're far better off choosing a low-calorie sweetener than a no-calorie sweetener. A natural sugar substitute known as xylitol is an excellent choice, for many reasons.

Discovered in 1891 by a German chemist, the substance became popular in many European countries during World War II, when sugar was in short supply. Since the 1960s, xylitol has been used as an FDA-approved nutritive sweetener in diabetic diets. These days it can be found in a few brands of baked goods and beverages, as well as in chewing gum, mints, and toothpaste.

Xylitol isn't a true sugar but rather a naturally occurring sugar alcohol found in many plants, including some fruits and vegetables.

Although it was originally derived from birch trees, corn is now the primary source of commercially produced xylitol. In its pure form, the sweetener is a white crystalline substance that looks, tastes, and measures like sugar. Unlike table sugar, which has 15 calories per teaspoon, xylitol provides just 9.6 calories per teaspoon.

Because the human body metabolizes sugar alcohols in a unique manner, xylitol doesn't produce the rapid, dramatic spikes in blood glucose and insulin levels that commonly occur following the consumption of regular sugar. As a result, eating xylitol-sweetened foods won't leave you feeling tired, hungry, or craving sugar afterward.

While sugar is known to wreak havoc on dental health, xylitol has the opposite effect. The natural sweetener has been shown to prevent tooth decay by inhibiting the growth of Streptococcus mutans, the bacteria primarily responsible for causing dental cavities. Over the past two decades, a number of studies have shown that when volunteers chewed xylitol-sweetened gum three times daily following meals, they developed significantly fewer cavities than those chewing sugar-sweetened gum. Xylitol also has been shown to increase saliva production, help control bad breath, reduce the frequency and severity of mouth sores and ear infections, and improve oral health in individuals with periodontal disease.

Preliminary research suggests that sugar alcohol might play a role in the prevention and treatment of osteoporosis. When fed to aging rats, xylitol reduced bone loss and actually increased bone mineral density by an average of 10 percent. Scientists speculated that the sweetener might enhance bone health by boosting the body's absorption of calcium. While the optimal dose necessary to promote bone health is still unknown, a daily intake of six grams of xylitol has been shown to help prevent dental cavities and improve oral health. For best results, two pieces of gum, each containing one gram of xylitol, should be chewed three times daily following meals. In these amounts, xylitol is generally well tolerated. At doses greater than 30 grams a day, however, the sugar alcohol can have a laxative effect, which many women find to be quite beneficial.

While xylitol is perfectly safe for adults and children, dogs can't properly metabolize the sugar alcohol, so it should never be fed to your pets.

Like regular sugar, xylitol can be purchased in bulk, as well as in single-serving packages. Unlike sugar, xylitol isn't widely available in supermarkets; it's more likely to be found at stores and shops that sell natural foods and nutritional supplements. Xylitol is more expensive than regular table sugar, but if you're looking for a reduced-calorie sweetener that offers a few bonus benefits for your health, it's an excellent investment.

Finding Weight Loss Supporters

Try to get by with a little help from your friends!

A great sex life will help you lose weight! It releases endorphins, feel-good hormones that decrease stress. A great sex life also reduces cortisol levels, so you store fewer calories as fat!

> —*Jennifer Hanes, DO, a mom of a seven-year-old daughter and a four-year-old son, an emergency physician who's board certified in integrative medicine, and the author of* The Princess Plan: Shrink Your Waist, Expand Your Beauty, *in Austin, TX*

It is important to gain the support of your spouse for your weight loss efforts. It would be very hard to try to lose weight in a vacuum.

> —*Katherine Dee, MD, a mom of eight-year-old twin daughters and a six-year-old son and a radiologist at the Seattle Breast Center, in Washington*

My husband is always supportive of me. When I signed up for my first half marathon, he was very encouraging. He was already a runner, so he didn't do the training program with me, but he ran the half marathon with me. He's running a full marathon, and that's motivating and inspiring to me.

> —*Pam D'Amato, MD, a mom of seven- and four-year-old daughters and an interventional pain management physician with University Spine Center, in Wayne, NJ*

When I decided to lose weight, I started jogging. I lost 10 pounds to begin with. My youngest daughter said to me, "Wow, Mommy, you look normal." That wasn't exactly what I wanted to hear, but I understood what she meant. It was supportive and encouraging to me.

—*Tiemdow Phumiruk, MD, a mom of 13-, 10-, and 7-year-old daughters, a pediatrician in the emergency department of Children's Hospital Colorado at Parker Adventist Hospital, and adjunct faculty at Rocky Vista University College of Osteopathic Medicine, in Parker, CO*

∽⌒∾

A major obstacle to weight loss can be an unsupportive partner or spouse. If your spouse is eating fattening food, it makes it a lot more tempting to cheat on your diet.

I'm fortunate that my husband is always on the same page as me with diet and exercise so that our family has a healthy lifestyle. I would encourage any women who are trying to get in shape to ask their partners to do it with them. The extra support makes it fun and much easier to do.

—*Catherine Begovic, MD, a mom of a six-month-old daughter and a plastic surgeon at Make You Perfect, Inc., in Beverly Hills, CA*

∽⌒∾

I think a major challenge to weight loss—and good health in general—is the naysayers. You can't lose weight if you're surrounded by people telling you that you can't! It's also hard to lose weight when you're surrounded by people who are focused on their own failures.

I seek out people who inspire me. If you see people who are successful at something, you want to glom onto them! I found a terrific running partner who supports me and inspires me to do my best.

My husband is also very supportive of me. Even before he was trying to lose weight himself, he was very encouraging to me.

—*Amy Thompson, MD, a mom of six-, four-, and two-year-old sons and an ob-gyn at the University of Cincinnati College of Medicine, in Ohio*

∽⌒∾

When my family knows I'm making a change, such as eliminating sugar and flour from my diet, they buy into it. This gives me accountability.

> **Don't wait for someone to take you under their wing.**
> **Find a good wing and climb up underneath it.**
>
> *—Frank C. Bucaro,*
> *a motivational speaker and business ethics expert*

My children inherited my husband's family's genetics: They're all thin. They're all old enough to understand now that I'm concerned about my weight even though they don't have the same concerns. Two of them are very sweet about it, such as saying, "Mom, *I* don't think you're fat, but weren't you going to not eat that?" My 12-year-old will mischievously say, "Oh, I thought you didn't like your 'squishy,'" and poke my too-big tummy.

—Amy Baxter, MD, a mom of 15- and 12-year-old sons and a 10-year-old daughter; the CEO of Buzzy4Shots.com; and the director of emergency research, Scottish Rite, of Children's Healthcare of Atlanta, in Georgia

I read the book *The Five Love Languages of Children* to help me better understand the types of support and love that my son needs. An unanticipated benefit was that it also helped me learn what my husband and I need.

Once you figure out someone's "love language," you can share and receive support on any journey more easily. For example, my love language is "acts of service." When someone does things for me that lighten my "to-do" list, it relieves my stress and makes me a happier, healthier person. Knowing someone's love language enables you to support him or her in a way that is well received and nourishing. Buy the book! It's the best $10 you'll ever spend.

—Michelle Yagoda, MD, a mom of an 11-year-old son, a facial plastic surgeon, the CEO of Opus Skincare, LLC, and cofounder of BeautyScoop, a patented and clinically proven supplement for skin, hair, and nails, in New York City

After my daughter was born, it was hard to find time to exercise. I made a plan to meet a few friends who also are moms to exercise in the mornings before work. We encouraged and supported each other. Initially we just worked out together, but then we joined a ladies-only boot camp–style weight loss program. I liked the fact that the group was for women only because I could go there and not care a bit about how I looked.

My daughter's father was very supportive of this. He watched our daughter while I went to work out.

—*Christy Valentine, MD, a mom of a seven-year-old daughter, a specialist in pediatrics and internal medicine, and the founder of the Valentine Medical Center, in Gretna, LA*

Ironically, my coworkers present my toughest weight loss challenge, by ordering pizza for lunch and by bringing cakes into the office, but they can also be my biggest supporters. Whenever one of us is trying to lose weight, the others rally behind her. For example, one of my coworkers was going on a cruise and wanted to lose weight. On her

Start Your Own Support Group

If you're trying to lose weight and someone else close to you, such as your spouse, friend, sister, or mom, is too, why not start your own informal support group? You could share ideas and recipes, meet to *work* out instead of to *eat* out, brainstorm solutions to challenges facing you and, most important, celebrate your successes.

It's not for everyone, but some people might find a little competition motivating! You could challenge your workout buddy to a bet, such as whoever loses 10 percent of her body weight first wins a gift card for her favorite clothing store. Or whoever loses the first 10 pounds wins a gift certificate for a massage. Put your money where your mouth is, which incidentally is where the junk food *won't* be!

breaks, she'd walk up and down the stairs at the hospital, and three or four of us would join her!

Each year as winter turns to spring, most of us start to think about our weight. We all watch what we eat and encourage each other. It's a wonderful place to work. I feel very supported by my friends and coworkers.

—Stephanie A. Wellington, MD, a mom of a 13-year-old son and an 11-year-old daughter, a hospitalist in the Level III NICU at Bellevue Hospital Center in New York City, and the medical coach and founder of PostpartumNeonatalCoaching.com

RALLIE'S TIP

Making yourself accountable to someone else is an excellent way to overcome the mental resistance to change. If you want to start exercising but fear that you'll let yourself down, ask a friend to accompany you on your morning walks.

You might not be motivated to drag yourself out of bed for your own sake, but you'll probably have a hard time breaking your word to a friend. Especially if she's waiting for you in front of your house in the predawn hours!

Monitoring Your Weight

One of your most powerful weight loss tools—next to your fork!—is your scale. In a study of people in the National Weight Control Registry, who have all lost at least 30 pounds and kept them off for at least a year, scientists found that more than one-third of them weighed themselves at least once a day. The researchers discovered that when people stopped weighing themselves daily, their weight was more likely to creep back up. But when they went back to daily weigh-ins, their weight came back down.

The scientists think that weighing yourself each day helps you to catch weight gains before they really get going and to adjust your eating accordingly.

&FitBit

Don't let anyone feed you something you wouldn't allow them to feed your dog. Would you let your coworker feed your dog a doughnut? Would you let your mom give your dog an extra serving of mashed potatoes and gravy?

Stepping on the scale might not be your favorite thing to do, but it could prove to be a critical step in your weight loss journey.

∽⌒

The best way for me to monitor my weight is also the easiest: How do my pants feel?

—*Sonali Ruder, DO, a mom of a two-month-old daughter, an emergency physician at Coral Springs Medical Center near Fort Lauderdale, FL, and a recipe developer and blogger at TheFoodiePhysician.com*

∽⌒

I don't weigh myself. In fact, I hate going to the doctor because I hate being weighed! I track my weight by how my clothes fit. If a skirt starts to feel tight, I know it's time to exercise more and be more mindful of what I'm eating.

—*Amy Barton, MD, a mom of an 11-year-old daughter and 8- and 5-year-old sons and a pediatrician at St. Luke's Children's Hospital, in Boise, ID*

∽⌒

Having a "weigh in" day has helped me maintain my weight. I try to do this once a week. Usually, I aim to weigh in at the same time on the same day of the week. So for me that day is Tuesday, and I weigh myself as soon as I wake up, right before I hit the shower. I picked Tuesday because it allows me a day to "normalize" my weight after a weekend of fun and food!

—*Arleen K. Lamba, MD, a mom of a three-month-old son, an anesthesiologist, the medical director of Blush Med Institute, and founder of the Blush Blends Skin Care line, in Washington, DC*

I try to make myself get on the scale a few times a week, but I try not to get too caught up in the number on the scale. It hurts too much when it doesn't go down. Instead, I try to pay attention to how I feel and to how my clothes fit.

—Kristin C. Lyle, MD, FAAP, a mom of 10-, 7-, and 5-year-old daughters, the disaster medical director at Arkansas Children's Hospital, and an assistant professor of pediatrics at the University of Arkansas for Medical Sciences, both in Little Rock

When to Call Your Doctor

Making healthy choices offer benefits that can be measured by your doctor, especially if health issues prompted your weight loss efforts to begin with.

When you first talk to your doctor about embarking on a weight loss program, ask about setting up a follow-up appointment to track your progress. At your next appointment, your doctor might look at the following factors to measure the positive effects that weight loss is having on your health.

- Blood pressure. Losing just 10 pounds can lower your blood pressure, which is a good sign that dropping weight is improving your heart health.
- Cholesterol level. Losing 5 to 10 percent of your weight can also improve your cholesterol numbers.
- Blood sugar. With every single pound you lose, you lower your risk of developing diabetes. The Diabetes Prevention Program, a study of more than 3,000 people, found that a weight loss of 5 to 7 percent of total weight slowed the development of type 2 diabetes.

Having something other than the scale to confirm you're getting healthier can help motivate you to keep going. If you give yourself three months before going back to your physician for a follow-up appointment, you'll have enough time to lose about 10 pounds and see positive results.

Facebook

Facebook doesn't only have to be for looking up pictures of old high school friends. Use the site to your advantage by starting a virtual weight loss support group and inviting friends who are also working on dropping pounds. You'll be able to trade tips, celebrate each person's successes, and keep your motivation high for months.

I used to check my weight each day on a scale at home. It turned out that wasn't helpful. If my weight hadn't gone down—or worse yet, had gone up—it affected my mood and motivation the rest of the day!

So I got rid of that scale, and now I check my weight once a week on the scale at the gym.

—*Leena Shrivastava Dev, MD, a mom of 15- and 12-year-old sons and a general pediatrician and advocate for child safety, in the Baltimore, MD, area*

As you age, losing weight and maintaining your weight get harder. You burn fewer calories as you age, and so if you eat at age 40 the same way you ate at age 20, you're going to gain weight.

The really tricky thing is that this type of weight gain is insidious. Just burning 80 to 100 fewer calories each day can add several pounds to your body in a year. You don't feel the weight piling on, but at the end of the year, you've gained a few pounds. If you don't reverse the trend, in a few years, you'll find that somehow you're carrying a lot of extra weight.

To monitor my weight, I notice how my clothes fit. If they seem tight, I cut my chocolate allowance. (Chocolate is my daily indulgence; I treat myself to some every day.) I weigh myself infrequently, but at my annual checkup with my gynecologist I make sure that I'm the same weight that I was the year before.

—*Ayala Laufer-Cahana, MD, a mom of 17- and 15-year-old sons and a 14-year-old daughter, a pediatrician, and the founder of Herbal Water Inc., in Wynnewood, PA*

RALLIE'S TIP

Clothing—especially warm winter clothing—gives us plenty of opportunities to hide under bulky sweaters, long pants, and fluffy coats. It's easy to become less aware of weight gain, and we can become less motivated to keep our bodies in good shape by eating properly and exercising regularly.

To combat this, when I step out of the shower, I take a look at my body in the mirror, sans clothing. It's hard to ignore those extra pounds and inches when you're naked! I find this to be a more accurate—and more motivating—assessment of my weight than the scale. Numbers on the scale aren't nearly as powerful to me as a visual image of my body.

Most of us expect—and accept—that we'll gain a little weight as we age. We might tell ourselves that we'll get around to losing it, but that doesn't always happen. And unfortunately, that extra weight seems to get harder and harder to lose the older we get. While a weight gain of less than two pounds isn't necessarily a cause for alarm, the fact that most folks never shed the extra weight year after year is more worrisome. In spite of all those New Year's resolutions to slim down, the majority of Americans tend to gain—and keep—at least one additional pound each year throughout adulthood.

I find that I'm far more likely to gain weight in the winter than in the summer, spring, or fall. To combat this, I pay attention when my jeans start getting tighter, and I keep an eye on my winter weight by weighing myself more often during the winter months. When my weight gets into the "danger zone" (five pounds over my summer weight), I know that it's time for me to get busy and start eating better and exercising more.

Facing Challenges and Overcoming Obstacles

On the road to weight loss success, there are many parking places. And fast-food chains, all-you-can-eat buffets, and late-night-pizza-delivery places.

Yes, you'll face many challenges on your journey, and you'll have to overcome obstacles.

For example, there are twice as many fast-food restaurants today compared to 40 years ago. Studies have found that the more fast-food joints in your neighborhood, the higher your community's collective BMI.

Plus, we literally have more food at our fingertips. Between 1970 and 2008, the amount of food available went up by 600 calories per person per day in the United States. Our life today is like a 24/7 buffet. We can buy—and eat—food around the clock.

Portion sizes are getting bigger and bigger. Restaurant meals in particular have gotten larger—with an emphasis on getting more for your money. Signs in fast-food restaurants scream "Value Meals, Biggie Sizes!" Also, ready-to-eat, convenience food portion sizes are growing. Studies show that portion sizes of these foods began increasing in the 1970s and have continued to do so. Today, most of these serving sizes exceed federal serving size standards. Scientists compared portion sizes for a few key foods: salty snacks, desserts, soft drinks, fruit drinks, French fries, burgers, pizza, and Mexican food. The study found that between the late 1970s and late 1990s, portion sizes increased for all of the categories, except pizza.

Research shows that the more food is put in front of you, the more calories you're likely to consume. One study found that people ate 30 percent more calories of macaroni and cheese when offered the largest of four portions, compared with the smallest!

But if you make a point of serving yourself less or seeking out restaurants with smaller portions, you're more likely to lose weight.

Also, paying attention to why you're eating is also helpful. In a survey by the Consumer Reports National Research Center, psychologists said taking note of emotional eating and working on the emotional issues that might have led to gaining weight help people succeed at weight loss.

⌒⌒

Going out to eat is a challenge. The portions are huge! When we go to a restaurant, I eat only half of what they give me, and I take the rest home.

—*Tiemdow Phumiruk, MD, a mom of 13-, 10-, and 7-year-old daughters, a pediatrician in the emergency department of Children's Hospital Colorado at Parker Adventist Hospital, and adjunct faculty at Rocky Vista University College of Osteopathic Medicine, in Parker, CO*

A challenge to my weight loss is when I'm sick, or when my kids are sick. I try to exercise anyway because it makes me feel better and gives me energy. When my kids are sick, when I'm sick, or if I've had a crazy day, I give myself a break and do a quicker, 20-minute, workout.

—*Eva Mayer, MD, a mom of a nine-year-old daughter and an eight-year-old son, an associate professor of pediatrics at Temple University, and a pediatrician with St. Luke's Pediatrics Associates, in Bethlehem, PA*

When I was trying to lose weight after my babies were born, I had such a difficult time. I became so frustrated. I remember thinking, *It used to be so easy to lose weight. Is this what getting older is like? Is it always going to be this hard?*

At the same time, I was also very tired. I had some blood work done, and it turned out my thyroid hormone levels were low. My doctor prescribed some medication, and the weight started to come off.

—*Martha Wittenberg, MD, MPH, a mom of an eight-year-old son and a six-year-old daughter and a family physician with Seal Beach Family Medicine, in California*

FitBit

Weight loss is one measure of success. Find other ways to gauge your progress. Did you try a new fruit or vegetable today? Did you resist the temptation to eat junk food? Did you exercise a little longer or harder? Give yourself credit and a big pat on the back for every step you take in the right direction.

> **The elevator to success is out of order.**
> **You'll have to use the stairs—one step at a time.**
>
> *—Joe Girard, an American salesman*
> *who was recognized by the* **Guinness Book**
> **of World Records** *as the world's greatest*
> *salesman for 12 consecutive years*

My job presents a weight loss challenge. On days that I'm doing surgery in the operating room, I only have very short breaks to eat between cases. It's tempting to grab something quick that's not good for me. I bring along healthy snacks, such as bananas, oranges, or yogurt, so that I'm not tempted by the treats at the nurses' station or in the vending machines!

> *—Edna Ma, MD, a mom of a six-month-old son, an*
> *anesthesiologist at UCLA Olive View Medical Center, and the*
> *founder of BareEase pre-waxing numbing kit, in Los Angeles, CA*

The biggest challenge to my weight is when I'm working a lot. As an emergency physician working very busy shifts, it's not easy to eat well at work. The food options at the hospital cafeteria aren't the best. The hospital I used to work at had a McDonald's in the lobby instead of a cafeteria!

I often pack food instead. I pack a sandwich and some snacks, such as fruit, granola, and nuts. With healthy options at my fingertips, I can work a 12-hour shift without being tempted by the vending machine.

> *—Sonali Ruder, DO, a mom of a two-month-old daughter,*
> *an emergency physician at Coral Springs Medical Center near*
> *Fort Lauderdale, FL, and a recipe developer and blogger at*
> *TheFoodiePhysician.com*

At my job, we work long shifts and unusual hours. To keep our morale high, we take any opportunity to celebrate, and those celebrations usually include food. We celebrate everything—even simply

"It's Friday!"—by ordering pizza or sandwiches or bringing in dessert.

Because these celebrations are about being part of the team, I want to be a part of them, but they make it difficult to eat properly. I try to compensate by eating small portions, such as half a slice of pizza. Or I'll take the cheese off and eat only that. Sometimes I'll be a part of the celebration, but I say "no thanks" and walk away when they break out the food.

—*Stephanie A. Wellington, MD, a mom of a 13-year-old son and an 11-year-old daughter, a hospitalist in the Level III NICU at Bellevue Hospital Center in New York City, and the medical coach and founder of PostpartumNeonatalCoaching.com*

◦✓◦

At the end of a long day, I come home and want something to eat. If I grab something fattening, such as a container of nuts, I'll eat and read and lose track of how many I've eaten.

To combat this, I count out a reasonable serving of nuts and put them into a small bowl. Also I try to limit my downtime after work to only about an hour. I read and relax, and then I get up and get moving.

—*Debra Luftman, MD, a mom of a 22-year-old daughter and a 19-year-old son, a board-certified dermatologist in private practice, coauthor of* The Beauty Prescription, *developer of the skincare line of products Therapeutix, and a clinical instructor of skin surgery and general dermatology at UCLA*

◦✓◦

I didn't gain that much weight during my pregnancy, and I lost it quickly after my son was born. My challenge began after my son started eating table food. Suddenly, I started to nibble on Goldfish crackers, Teddy Grahams, and other "little kid" foods!

My grandmother always told me, "Never eat after your kids, off of their plates."

Now I throw his leftovers in the trash or put them in the fridge. And we don't share plates!

—*Michelle Davis-Dash, MD, a mom of a 19-month-old son and a pediatrician in Baltimore, MD*

FitBit

One of the pitfalls for me was finishing my daughter's food. All those mini waffles, cheese sticks, and Goldfish crackers add up. I started reminding myself that I could always give my daughter more food if she was still hungry, rather than giving her too much and then eating the "leftovers" so as not to waste them!

It helps me stay on track if I choose healthier snacks, such as an apple, and try not to keep too many indulgent desserts around. I'm a sucker for anything chocolate!

—*Rachel S. Rohde, MD, a mom of a two-year-old daughter, an assistant professor of orthopaedic surgery at the Oakland University William Beaumont School of Medicine, and an orthopaedic upper-extremity surgeon with Michigan Orthopaedic Institute, P.C., in Southfield, MI*

Snacking can be challenging. I try to adopt the same strategy I use for my kids. I might allow myself to have a less-than-healthy snack, but only after I've eaten a healthy one.

For example, I might eat some cut-up apples or carrots, and then I might eat a few chips or a cookie.

—*Leena Shrivastava Dev, MD, a mom of 15- and 12-year-old sons and a general pediatrician and advocate for child safety, in the Baltimore, MD, area*

A major challenge to losing weight is tempting snacks. My solution is simple: Don't bring them into your house. If I don't buy soda, chips, and sugary cereals, I don't eat them.

—*Jeannette Gonzalez Simon, MD, a mom of four- and one-year-old daughters and a pediatric gastroenterologist at Staten Island Pediatrics GI, in New York*

⌒⌀

Keeping snacks on the table next to the TV can really sabotage my weight loss efforts. Watching TV encourages mindless eating, and if there are snacks within reach, I'll be tempted to eat them.

I rarely watch TV, but when I do, the only snacks within my reach are fruits and vegetables, such as apple slices and carrots!

—*Ayala Laufer-Cahana, MD, a mom of 17- and 15-year-old sons and a 14-year-old daughter, a pediatrician, and the founder of Herbal Water Inc., in Wynnewood, PA*

⌒⌀

A challenge that a lot of women face is nighttime snacking. I'm not a big snacker, and so I've never gotten into the habit of snacking at night. Snacking can simply be something you do out of habit.

Instead of snacking at night, I keep myself busy by playing with my daughter. After she goes to bed, I work on my computer and get caught up on paperwork.

—*Catherine Begovic, MD, a mom of a six-month-old daughter and a plastic surgeon at Make You Perfect, Inc., in Beverly Hills, CA*

⌒⌀

It's helpful to identify nutritious snacks that fill you up. When I get hungry in the afternoon around 4 pm, I eat a small handful of almonds with a container of Greek yogurt. They taste delicious, and the protein really fills me up.

I do allow myself to eat some sweets in moderation. I'll have a small handful of peanut M&M's, a container of sugar-free chocolate pudding, or frozen fat-free Cool Whip. When you freeze it, it tastes like ice cream.

—*Eva Mayer, MD*

⌒⌀

When I'm trying to lose weight, grocery shopping with my kids is a challenge. When I bring them along to the grocery store, they have

> **If you find a path with no obstacles,**
> **it probably doesn't lead anywhere.**
> **—*Unknown***

lots of requests for foods that they want. My grocery budget could quickly be used up with all of their requests!

I have to remember to buy some healthy foods that I like too, even if my kids don't like them, such as cottage cheese, blackberries, and asparagus.

> —*Sigrid Payne DaVeiga, MD, a mom of a seven-year-old son and a two-year-old daughter and a pediatric allergist with the Children's Hospital of Philadelphia, in Pennsylvania*

A challenge to my weight is that I'm a chocoholic. This is especially difficult during the holidays, when chocolate is *everywhere*.

I enjoy five or six Hershey's Kisses every day, spread out over the day. I don't chew them up and gobble them down! I let them slowly dissolve in my mouth. That handles my chocolate craving.

> —*Susan Besser, MD, a mom of six grown children, ages 28, 26, 24, 22, 21, and 19, a grandmom of two, a family physician, and the medical director of Doctors Express-Memphis, in Tennessee*

My babies were very big, between 9 and 10 pounds each, and I'm not quite 5 feet 2 inches tall. Pregnancy was very hard on my muscles. My rectus abdominis muscle, the one that runs down your midsection, split open. I had no waistline! I had plastic surgery to repair the muscle. It's very important to have those muscles repaired because otherwise you can't have a strong core. This can lead to aches, pains, and strains.

Also, after three years of breastfeeding, my breasts didn't go back to their pre-pregnancy size. I felt they were disproportionate to my height and frame. It was causing me to have back pain. I had breast reduction surgery. Since having the surgery, my back pain is gone.

These procedures have helped also my weight loss journey and my self-esteem.

—Kristin C. Lyle, MD, FAAP, a mom of 10-, 7-, and 5-year-old daughters, the disaster medical director at Arkansas Children's Hospital, and an assistant professor of pediatrics at the University of Arkansas for Medical Sciences, both in Little Rock

Stress poses a major challenge to my weight loss efforts. Some people eat less when they're stressed. Not me.

Also, when you're stressed, your cortisol level spikes, and that promotes fat storage around your waist and upper back. That's what happened to me.

A few years ago, I went through a period of intense stress. Even though I was eating right and exercising, I wasn't losing weight. Because I was doing Zumba and eating well, my body was fit and toned—except for my waistline.

I understood that stress was working against me, and I was able to keep up my healthy habits. And when the stress level went down, my weight did too. Looking back, if I hadn't continued my healthy habits, my weight gain during that time probably would have doubled.

—Aline T. Tanios, MD, a mom of 10- and 4-year-old daughters and an 8-year-old son and a pediatric hospitalist and assistant professor at the Washington University School of Medicine, in St. Louis, MO

For me, one challenge to losing weight is lunchtime at work. It's easy to just grab something quick—and unhealthy.

To combat that, I plan my meals ahead, even writing down what I plan to eat. Then I take my lunch with me to work. Usually I bring a salad or soup and some high-fiber crackers. I try to take a break for lunch when I'm hungry because if I let myself get too hungry, I'll order whatever comes to mind and eat something I wasn't planning on.

—Judith Hellman, MD, a mom of a 15-year-old son, an associate clinical professor of dermatology at Mt. Sinai Hospital in New York City, and a dermatologist in private practice

When I wanted to lose weight, I spent some time thinking about why I was eating. I found that sometimes I was eating simply because it was on my to-do list, not necessarily because I was hungry! I'd eat breakfast—check! Lunch—check! Supper—check! Instead, I started to pay attention to my hunger, and I now eat when I'm hungry, not just because it's something I'm supposed to do.

Also, I found that I was eating to distract myself. I really thought about what makes me happy, and what I enjoy doing. I changed jobs, and I started writing. I found that when I write, I completely lose track of time and don't think about eating. For me, activities like that are "gold star" activities.

—Jennifer Hanes, DO, a mom of a seven-year-old daughter and a four-year-old son, an emergency physician who's board certified in integrative medicine, and the author of The Princess Plan: Shrink Your Waist, Expand Your Beauty, *in Austin, TX*

Mommy MD Guides–Recommended Product
Belly Bandit

"A challenge for me after my son was born was getting my tummy 'situated' back in place, " says Arleen K. Lamba, MD, a mom of a three-month-old son, an anesthesiologist, the medical director of Blush Med Institute, and founder of the Blush Blends Skin Care line, in Washington, DC. "One thing that helped was my Belly Bandit. Carrying the extra weight sometimes left my back sore. My Belly Bandit helped my posture and gave more support to my back."

Belly Bandit is an adjustable band you wear around your midsection. The elastic is latex free, and it can be adjusted to fit around the belly, waist, and hips. It's designed to help a new mom go back to her pre-pregnancy shape.

You can buy Belly Bandit at **BELLYBANDIT.COM** for $49.95.

🍎FitBit

Avoid TV dining. It's easy to overeat when you're watching television, because when you're tuned in to your favorite show, you're more likely to tune out your internal signals of hunger and satiety.

Instead, make what you eat a treat, use real silverware, even light a candle.

I think one of the keys to losing weight and maintaining your weight is to know yourself and what makes you cheat on your diet.

I'm very impulsive, especially when I'm sleep deprived. To combat this, I have completely cut out snacking after working a shift at the hospital. At that time, I have no willpower, and I will inhale any food that's left over. Most of the time, I'm not even hungry. Now instead of eating, I just go to bed.

—Amy Baxter, MD, a mom of 15- and 12-year-old sons and a 10-year-old daughter; the CEO of Buzzy4Shots.com; and the director of emergency research, Scottish Rite, of Children's Healthcare of Atlanta, in Georgia

Having a C-section made it difficult for me to lose weight. I had to wait for six very long weeks before I could exercise. It was difficult to see my body this way. I remember asking my doctor, "Where did my six-pack go?"

Because I'm a "do-er" and a "fixer"—meaning instead of sitting around complaining or disliking something, I do something about it to fix the problem—being forced to do nothing was extremely challenging for me. I knew better than to disobey my doctor, because I didn't want to get a hernia or have complications after my surgery. Being a surgeon, I always stress to my patients to follow all instructions and allow their bodies to heal, but it was hard for me to take my own advice when I was on the other side of the knife! I was literally counting down the days until I could get back into the gym and was so thankful to go back after the six weeks passed.

—Catherine Begovic, MD

I believe that a huge red flag for what might be impeding weight loss is this test: Can you sit in the bathtub, alone with your thoughts, for 10 minutes? If not, that's a really big clue that you have a lot of internal turmoil. That might be a good reason to consider counseling to deal with those issues before tackling your weight.

On my own weight loss journey, spending time with my thoughts meant quelling the army of critics in my head that had taken root long ago in childhood. I started by telling myself positive statements while looking in the mirror each day. I also try to look at myself objectively and ask, "Would you allow somebody to speak to the mother of your children that way?" At first, I could be more loving as the mother of my children than simply "loving myself."

—*Jennifer Hanes, DO*

Having to eat my breakfast on the go and my lunch at work has always been a challenge to my weight loss success. When I was trying to lose weight, my husband bought a bunch of Tupperware for me to use, and I made a bit of fun of him. But actually it's helpful. I double the recipe that I cook from KalynsKitchen.com for supper and take the leftovers with me to work for lunch the next day.

I usually eat my breakfast in the car. I found a great recipe for an egg casserole I can eat while driving. I also like making egg

MomMy TIME **Start Tweeting**

Sometimes you need to keep your hands busy to avoid opening the fridge. Enter Twitter. You can follow your favorite celebrities, keep up with trending topics, join a weight loss group, keep a food journal, set your meal plans, read jokes, and—best of all—share your pounds lost with your followers. As a bonus: You can avoid snacking on ice cream while watching television and instead follow live tweets about shows such as *Survivor* to make it more fun to watch.

🍎FitBit

muffins, which are a good source of protein. Eating protein early in the morning helps suppress my appetite. (See the Egg Muffins recipe on page 188.)

Or I might just drink a glass of fat-free milk in the car and eat Greek yogurt midmorning at work.

—*Amy Thompson, MD, a mom of six-, four-, and two-year-old sons and an ob-gyn at the University of Cincinnati College of Medicine, in Ohio*

RALLIE'S TIP

I wish I had learned sooner that my health is far more valuable to me than the appearance of my house. My Stairmaster is not a very attractive piece of exercise equipment, and I've had it hidden away in my basement for the past two years since we moved into this house. Even though I know it's there, waiting patiently for me, I find it really hard to make myself go downstairs to use it. One reason is that I've never been all that crazy about basements. They seem dark, damp, and depressing to me.

The other reason is that I feel that I'm isolated from my family when I'm downstairs exercising in the basement. I can't see or hear what's going on upstairs, and I guess I'm afraid I'll miss something. All of my favorite people and pets and rooms are upstairs! It takes a major act of willpower to make myself go downstairs to exercise. It's almost like driving to the gym: I've got to get all my ducks in a row before I leave life in the main part of the house and make the trek down the stairs.

When I do manage to go downstairs to work out, I feel like I need to stay there for at least an hour to make it worth my while. If I don't have an entire hour to exercise, I find that I won't even bother going downstairs. With all of these mental obstacles, I wasn't using my Stairmaster nearly as much as I wanted to.

About a month ago, I asked my husband and my teenage sons to help me bring my Stairmaster upstairs to our bedroom, and we put it right in front of the big window overlooking my farm where I can see the land and the horses and the sunshine. My husband didn't completely understand my reasons for this. He thought that because we have a perfectly good exercise room downstairs in the basement, why not leave it there? But he was very kind to support me in my decision. And we've both been very happy with the results!

Since we moved the Stairmaster upstairs to our bedroom, I've exercised nearly every single day, even if it's just for 15 minutes, something I never did when I had to go down to the basement. I think I might have already lost a pound or two, and I definitely feel a lot healthier and more energetic.

A bonus benefit is that now my husband exercises more too. Now that the Stairmaster is in our bedroom, he'll hop on it for 20 to 30 minutes two or three times a week and listen to the news and weather on the radio.

I'm pretty sure that most interior designers would be appalled that we have this huge hunk of metal and rubber exercise equipment in our bedroom, because it really does nothing to enhance the room décor. But it's made a huge difference in how my husband and I feel and in our overall health. That's really the most important thing.

Coping with Setbacks

"When things go wrong, as they sometimes will,
When the road you're trudging seems all uphill,
When the funds are low and the debts are high,
And you want to smile, but you have to sigh,
When care is pressing you down a bit,
Rest, if you must, but don't you quit."

No one knows who authored these famous lines. It's often called the "Don't Quit" poem. When your motivation is low and your weight is high, rest if you must, but don't you quit!

⚬✀⚬

I love to snack. When I find that I'm gaining weight, I try to cut back on the snacks. If I am really doing poorly, I start eating more salads and less bread and other high-carb foods at dinner.

—Stacey Ann Weiland, MD, a mom of a 14-year-old daughter and 9- and 7-year-old sons and an internist/gastroenterologist, in Denver, CO

⚬✀⚬

A big weight loss challenge for me is coming home late at night, tired and hungry. It's hard not to eat whatever I want and blow my diet completely.

When that does happen, I avoid the scale the next morning. I tell myself, "I screwed up. But today is a new day."

I try to tell myself the same kinds of supportive things I would tell other people. We should treat ourselves with the same kindness that we show other people.

—*Judith Hellman, MD, a mom of a 15-year-old son, an associate clinical professor of dermatology at Mt. Sinai Hospital in New York City, and a dermatologist in private practice*

The most important thing to remember is to never give up. Everyone has bad days when the weight goes up, not down. Sometimes I step on the scale and feel horrible.

Tomorrow is another day, I think to myself. I try to shake it off and renew my commitment to the strategies that work for me, such as eating in moderation and logging what I eat.

—*Susan Besser, MD, a mom of six grown children, ages 28, 26, 24, 22, 21, and 19, a grandmom of two, a family physician, and the medical director of Doctors Express-Memphis, in Tennessee*

I've experienced all of the overuse injuries that occur when taking care of an infant or toddler, and that makes it challenging for me to lose weight. I feel like I didn't get the memo that said: While caring for your child, your lower back will hurt and one of your knees might feel lousy for a while.

I always carried my kids on the left side of my body because I am so dominantly right-handed, I needed my right hand free to do things. Because of this, my right knee became strained when my daughter turned two years old. The hardest part of having this kind of injury is understanding that you really do have to rest and take some time to recuperate for it to get better. It was hard for me to sit still and not work out, and I gained several pounds over a few months. Then one day, my knee felt better, and I began the process of disciplining myself to go slow so that I wouldn't reinjure myself.

—*Sigrid Payne DaVeiga, MD, a mom of a seven-year-old son and a two-year-old daughter and a pediatric allergist with the Children's Hospital of Philadelphia, in Pennsylvania*

RALLIE'S TIP

Stress can derail any diet, and everyone knows that moms face plenty of stress on a daily basis.

Regular exposure to stress increases our propensity to gain—and to regain—weight. That's because a primary stress hormone, known as cortisol, is secreted by the adrenal glands of the body. High cortisol levels have been shown to increase appetite, especially for sweet foods. They also promote weight gain, especially around the midsection of the body. Elevated cortisol levels are known to promote obesity and diabetes.

In addition to the very real stress-induced physiological changes that promote weight gain, many women (including me!) also engage in "stress-eating" behavior. When we feel anxious, eating often calms us down. Many of us gravitate toward comfort foods, such as chocolate, chips, bread, and pasta. These foods are typically high in calories and fat, and eating too much of them can easily promote weight gain.

When I'm feeling so stressed out that I could gnaw the handles off my refrigerator, I try to stop myself before I engage in some heavy-duty emotional eating. I remind myself that eating a carton of ice cream and a giant bag of chips won't alleviate my stress. It will only make it worse! Instead, I try to calm myself down with activities that have nothing to do with food. If I'm stressed and I feel physically tired, I give myself a time-out, and I allow myself to sit down in a comfy spot and relax with my dogs and cats and a good book. If I'm really exhausted, I might even curl up and take a 20-minute nap to "erase my brain."

If I'm stressed and feeling physically wound up, I try to burn off some steam and energy by going for a walk or a run, attacking my kitchen floor with a scrub brush on my hands and knees, or mowing the grass with a push mower. I've found that just about any activity that occupies my hands, mind, and body—besides eating, of course—is usually an excellent stress reliever.

Losing the Last 10 Pounds

Many people get frustrated and discouraged when they're trying and trying to lose those last 10 pounds. But actually, they should

> **I have not failed.**
> **I've just found 10,000 ways that won't work.**
> **—*Thomas Edison***

be celebrating! Maybe they've lost sight of the fact that they've succeeded in losing so much weight already, and they only have 10 pounds to go!

If you find yourself in this fortunate place, take a moment to celebrate! You did it! Now think about how you came to this happy place, and there you'll find the secrets to losing the last 10. You can do it!

Want to "lose" 10 pounds in an instant? Sit up straight, pull your shoulders down and back, and arch your back to get "cheerleader butt." By pulling your shoulders down, your neck looks thinner, and with a C-curve in your lower back, your thighs and tummy look thinner. Voilà, you'll look 10 pounds slimmer.

—*Jennifer Hanes, DO, a mom of a seven-year-old daughter and a four-year-old son, an emergency physician who's board certified in integrative medicine, and the author of* The Princess Plan: Shrink Your Waist, Expand Your Beauty, *in Austin, TX*

I've been having a hard time losing the last five pounds. My weight seems to be "stuck." It doesn't go down, and oddly enough it doesn't go up either. Sometimes I think that I could eat cheesecake for every meal, and the number still wouldn't change. I've tried to just give up on the number on the scale.

—*Kristin C. Lyle, MD, FAAP, a mom of 10-, 7-, and 5-year-old daughters, the disaster medical director at Arkansas Children's Hospital, and an assistant professor of pediatrics at the University of Arkansas for Medical Sciences, both in Little Rock*

I struggled losing the last 5 to 10 pounds of baby weight, despite the

FitBit

The more sweets you eat, the more you want. When you eat foods made of simple sugars, such as cookies, candy, cakes, and chips, your blood sugar level rises quickly, triggering a similar rise in insulin. Researchers at Yale University found that people are hungriest and prefer sweet tastes more when their insulin levels are high.

fact that I was doing everything I thought I needed to do to lose the weight. I was breastfeeding, walking each day with my baby, drinking plenty of water, and eating well.

I realized that the difficulty I had losing this "baby" weight was likely due to chronic lack of sleep and the excess cortisol production that results, making weight loss challenging. This was particularly difficult for me as a mother of a baby who didn't sleep through the night until he was 24 months old!

Once I started sleeping through the night, I had more energy—and probably more stable cortisol production!—so I was able to increase my activity and lose most of the weight. My son is now three years old, and I still have a few stubborn pounds left to lose, but despite this, I feel good about my weight.

—*Jennifer A. Gardner, MD, a mom of a three-year-old son, a pediatrician, and the founder of an online child wellness and weight management company, HealthyKidsCompany.com, in Washington, DC*

RALLIE'S TIP

I've had many women tell me that they struggle the most to lose those last 10 pounds. Me too! After really looking at my diet and exercise, I realized there's one thing that might be holding me back: my propensity to eat at odd times.

Shuffling kids back and forth to school functions and sports practice, working late, and attending social events make it hard for me to eat dinner on time. I often end up eating late at night. The results of a new study suggest that when it comes to losing weight, the timing of your meals and snacks may be just as important as the number of calories you consume. Published in the medical journal Obesity, the study provides the first concrete evidence linking meal timing and weight gain.

Until recently, most scientists believed that weight loss was a matter of simple mathematics: To lose a pound of body weight by dieting alone, you must consume approximately 3,500 fewer calories than your body needs to support itself at your current weight and activity level. Researchers at Northwestern University challenged this theory. Using laboratory animals, they demonstrated that eating during normal sleeping hours promotes more weight gain than would be predicted by caloric intake alone.

Translated to human terms, this means that eating a slice of leftover pizza as a late-evening snack could cause you to gain significantly more weight than if you ate the same slice of pizza in the afternoon. (The scientists' interest in the connection between late-night eating and weight gain arose after noting that nightshift workers, whose schedules force them to eat at times that are in conflict with natural body rhythms, tend to be more overweight than their dayshift counterparts.)

Based on the results of their research, the Northwestern University scientists speculate that nighttime eating in humans might disrupt the body's biological clock, known as the circadian rhythm, which governs daily cycles of feeding, activity, and sleep. Eating at inappropriate times appears to trigger a chain reaction of hormonal and metabolic events in the body that ultimately leads to excess weight gain.

When I stopped eating at crazy hours and got back on a normal schedule, I found that it was a lot easier to finally lose those last 10 pounds.

Where you start is not as important as where you finish.
—Zig Ziglar, a salesman, motivational speaker,
and author of See You at the Top

Bonus!

Take Five!
The Mommy MD Guide Program
for Maximum Weight Loss Success

If you're carrying a few extra pounds, you're in very good company. Nearly 70 percent of Americans are currently overweight or obese, and this percentage is expected to continue to rise. Although we often tend to think of excess weight as a cosmetic issue, in reality, it's a tremendous threat to our health. Obesity contributes to dozens of life-threatening diseases, including type 2 diabetes, heart disease, and cancer, and it's responsible for more than 300,000 preventable deaths in the United States each year.

In addition to causing physical harm, obesity inflicts a substantial measure of emotional suffering. It's important to remember that your weight is not—by any stretch of the imagination—a measure of your worth. Talented, attractive, and successful people come in all shapes and sizes. Although your weight is not a reflection of your character, it is a reasonably good predictor of your current and future health, and even your longevity. Being overweight just isn't good for you.

What's Your Weight Status?

Most of us don't need a diagnostic tool to know whether we're overweight. A hard look in the mirror is usually all it takes. Still, it's helpful to use a tool called the Body Mass Index (BMI) to assess your weight status. The BMI graph plots your weight against your height to determine if you are of normal weight, overweight, or obese. For the vast majority of us, this simple tool is sufficient to determine if excess weight is putting our health at risk.

Determining Your Body Mass Index (BMI)

To determine your BMI, find your height in the left-hand column of the chart below, and then move across the row to find your weight. Your BMI is listed in the top row above the point where these two numbers intersect.

BMI	19	20	21	22	23	24	25	26	27	28	29	30	31	32	33	34	35
58	91	96	100	105	110	115	119	124	129	134	138	143	148	153	158	162	167
59	94	99	104	109	114	119	124	128	133	138	143	148	153	158	163	168	173
60	97	102	107	112	118	123	128	133	138	143	148	153	158	163	168	174	179
61	100	106	111	116	122	127	132	137	143	148	153	158	164	169	174	180	185
62	104	109	115	120	126	131	136	142	147	153	158	164	169	175	180	186	191
63	107	113	118	124	130	135	141	146	152	158	163	169	175	180	186	191	197
64	110	116	122	128	134	140	145	151	157	163	169	174	180	186	192	197	204
65	114	120	126	132	138	144	150	156	162	168	174	180	186	192	198	204	210
66	118	124	130	136	142	148	155	161	167	173	179	186	192	198	204	210	216
67	121	127	134	140	146	153	159	166	172	178	185	191	198	204	211	217	223
68	125	131	138	144	151	158	164	171	177	184	190	197	203	210	216	223	230
69	128	135	142	149	155	162	169	176	182	189	196	203	209	216	223	230	236
70	132	139	146	153	160	167	174	181	188	195	202	209	216	222	229	236	243
71	136	143	150	157	165	172	179	186	193	200	208	215	222	229	236	243	250
72	140	147	154	162	169	177	184	191	199	206	213	221	228	265	242	250	258
73	144	151	159	166	174	182	189	197	204	212	219	227	235	242	250	257	265
74	148	155	163	171	179	186	194	202	210	218	225	233	241	249	256	264	272
75	152	160	168	176	184	192	200	208	216	224	232	240	248	256	264	272	279
76	156	164	172	180	189	197	205	213	221	230	238	246	254	263	271	279	287

IF YOUR BMI IS:	YOUR WEIGHT STATUS IS:
18.5 to 24.9	Normal
25 to 29.9	Overweight
30 or greater	Obese

By current standards, optimal BMI falls in the range of 19 to 21, but in general, a BMI of 24 or lower is consistent with good health as it relates to weight. A BMI of 27 or higher is associated with a greater risk of developing dozens of debilitating conditions, including type 2 diabetes, heart disease, stroke, some types of cancer, and even death.

Your Body Shape: Apple or Pear?

Excess body fat is undoubtedly a health hazard, but the location of the fat might be the best predictor of future health risks. The larger your waist is, the greater your risk for developing a number of deadly diseases. Folks who store excess fat around their waists are said to have apple-shaped bodies, because like the fruit, they are largest around their middles. Those who tend to deposit fat around their hips, buttocks, and thighs, on the other hand, are said to have pear-shaped bodies, because like pears, they are widest at the bottom.

Which fruit do you resemble? The answer lies in a measurement called the waist-to-hip ratio (WHR). To determine your WHR, all you need is a tape measure and a calculator. Standing erect, measure your waist at a point about one inch above your belly button. Next, measure your hips by placing the tape measure around your buttocks at the widest point. To determine your WHR, divide your waist measurement by your hip measurement. If your WHR is 0.80 or less, your body can be classified as pear-shaped. If your WHR is higher than 0.80, your body shape falls into the apple category.

There's a great deal of scientific evidence to support a strong link between an apple-shaped body and type 2 diabetes, stroke, and heart disease. Individuals with pear-shaped bodies are less prone to these diseases, but there is some evidence to suggest that they're at greater risk of developing osteoporosis. Regardless of your body shape, the risk of developing serious health problems increases with every inch you add to your midsection. Conversely, losing just two inches from your waist has been shown to lower total cholesterol levels and blood pressure, and to significantly reduce the risk of heart disease and diabetes. Keeping your waist circumference below 35 inches (below 40 inches for men) is an excellent way to increase your chances of living a long and healthy life.

Losing excess weight and inches can be challenging, but it is absolutely achievable if you're willing to make a few simple changes in your eating habits and activity level. Nutrition has a dramatic impact on your weight, and also on your health, energy levels, moods, and the way you look and feel. Because you can consume only a finite number of calories each day, it's essential to make every calorie count. As you're making decisions about what foods to eat to optimize your health, it's a good idea to take a closer look at some of the foods you normally choose. Before you dig in, ask yourself if the food you've chosen is merely a filler—a food that might taste good but contains only empty calories—or if it is truly a source of high-quality fuel, chock-full of beneficial nutrients.

The Three Key Nutrients

No matter what foods you eat, your diet undoubtedly contains varying amounts of three nutrients: carbohydrates, proteins, and fats. Although each is necessary for good health, it's the *balance* of these nutrients that is most important. By getting the proper proportions of carbohydrates, proteins, and fats in your daily diet, you'll immediately notice that your hunger is suppressed, your food cravings are quieted, and your metabolic rate is maximized. You'll find it far easier to achieve and maintain your goal weight than you ever imagined.

Carbohydrates

Carbohydrates are an essential part of a healthy diet. Their primary role in the diet is to provide a readily available, easily accessible form of energy for the brain and body. Getting adequate amounts of carbohydrates in your diet is important, but it's even more important to choose the right kinds. There are two types: simple carbohydrates and complex carbohydrates.

SIMPLE CARBOHYDRATES

Both simple and complex carbohydrates are made up of smaller building blocks, which are sugar molecules, linked together by chemical bonds. Simple carbohydrates consist of either monosaccharides, which are one-sugar units, or disaccharides, which are two-sugar units. Because of their small structure, they are quickly and easily broken down in the digestive tract. They're rapidly converted to single-sugar molecules in the stomach and almost instantly released into the bloodstream.

When you eat a food made of simple carbohydrates, such as a sugar cookie, it practically melts in your mouth. There's a good reason for this: The digestion of simple carbohydrates begins the instant they enter your mouth. In the presence of amylase and other enzymes in your saliva and your stomach, the bonds holding the individual sugar molecules together rapidly disintegrate. Free of their bonds, these sugar molecules make a beeline for your bloodstream. The result is a rapid spike in your blood sugar level and an immediate, intense surge of energy.

Unfortunately, the energy rush is short-lived. In response to the sugar overload in your bloodstream, your pancreas releases insulin, which is the hormone responsible for regulating blood sugar levels. Insulin ushers sugar molecules from the bloodstream to various cells and tissues in the body, where they are used as energy to fuel thousands of life-sustaining processes.

When you consume a sizeable load of simple carbohydrates in a short period of time, as you would if you ate two or three sugar cookies, you create several problems for your body. Spurred into action by a hefty dose of sugar, your pancreas might overshoot the mark and release too much insulin. The excess insulin clears your bloodstream of more blood sugar than necessary, resulting in a below-normal blood sugar level. This, in turn, can leave you feeling weak, shaky, and irritable. In the presence of low blood sugar levels, your brain attempts to restore normalcy by activating the hunger signal, sending you in search of another sugary snack. This destructive cycle can repeat itself dozens of times every day.

A suboptimal blood sugar level stimulates hunger and also creates a strong preference for sweet-tasting foods. The more simple-carbohydrate foods you eat, the more you'll want. In addition, elevated insulin levels have a profound influence on the storage of body fat. The longer and more frequently blood insulin levels remain high, the more likely you are to accumulate excess body fat. Because simple-carbohydrate food can wreak havoc with your blood sugar and insulin levels and make it difficult to lose weight, it's important to choose them with great care.

Sources of simple carbohydrates: Simple carbohydrates are abundant in most products that fall into the category of junk food. Any food that tastes delightfully sweet or seems to melt in your mouth is likely a simple-carbohydrate food, including cookies, candies, sodas, pastries, and potato chips. White and brown sugar, molasses, corn syrup, and maple syrup also make the list of simple carbohydrates.

Empty calories: While they're typically packed with sugar and calories, most simple-carbohydrate junk foods are virtually devoid of anything that's even remotely good for you, including fiber, vitamins, and minerals. Because they contain very few substances that contribute to your good health, calories from these foods are appropriately referred to as "empty" calories. You'll be doing yourself a huge favor if you eliminate these foods from your diet completely.

Some simple-carbohydrate foods are a little harder to recognize because they don't fall into the traditional junk food category. White rice and pastas, breads, and cereals made from refined grains are composed of simple carbohydrates. Although these foods might seem far superior to chips or cookies, their basic structures are similar, and they can have a similar effect on blood sugar and insulin, as well as on energy levels and mood. For this reason, these carbohydrate-rich foods should be eaten in moderation, if at all. Whenever possible, it's best to substitute whole grain products, such as oat cereal, brown rice, and whole grain varieties of bread and pasta.

Not all simple-carbohydrate foods are bad for you. In fact, many of them are necessary for good health. Some examples are many varieties of fruit, which contain the sugar fructose, and dairy products, which contain the sugar lactose.

COMPLEX CARBOHYDRATES

As their name suggests, complex carbohydrates have a more complex chemical structure. Similiar to simple carbohydrates, they're made up of individual sugar molecules, but instead of consisting of just one or two sugar molecules (monosaccharides or disaccharides), complex-carbohydrate foods are made up of polysaccharides, which contain hundreds or thousands of sugar molecules.

Time-released energy: Because they're so large, the polysaccharides in complex-carbohydrate foods are broken down slowly in the digestive tract, and the individual sugar molecules that form them are very gradually released into the bloodstream. This slow, steady release of sugar doesn't create a spike in blood sugar levels, and as a result, it doesn't trigger a dramatic insulin response from the pancreas.

As the individual sugar molecules enter the bloodstream in a leisurely fashion over a period of one to four hours, insulin levels rise slowly and gently. The overall effect is a gradual, sustained rise in blood sugar level, which is reflected in your mood and energy levels. Because they fuel your body and your brain for hours after you eat them, you can think of complex carbohydrates as time-released energy foods.

COMPLEX CARBOHYDRATES	SIMPLE CARBOHYDRATES
Whole grains: brown rice, cracked or whole wheat, rye, barley, whole grain breads and pasta	Refined, processed foods: white rice, white breads, refined cereals, refined pasta, chips, crackers, cookies, candy, cakes, pastries, pies
Legumes: lentils, chickpeas, navy beans, kidney beans, pinto beans, dry beans, peas	Sugars: table sugar, brown sugar, high-fructose corn syrup, maple syrup, honey
Cereals: bran, wheat, oatmeal	Soft drinks: sodas, sports drinks, punch, flavored sweet teas, sugar-sweetened beverages
—	Fruit drinks: 100% fruit juices, fruit "-ades," and fruit "cocktails"

Mood food: Complex carbohydrates play another vital role in your diet. They stimulate your body's production of a hormone norepinephrine and the neurotransmitter called serotonin. Norepinephrine, which is structurally similar to adrenaline, boosts energy levels and revs up the metabolic rate so that you burn more calories, even while you're at rest.

The brain chemical serotonin is an important appetite regulator and mood stabilizer: It exerts a calming effect and helps ward off depression. If you've ever found yourself eating in response to anxiety, depression, or stress, you might have noticed that the foods you crave are rich in carbohydrates. This is your body's built-in mechanism to increase serotonin levels in your brain. A diet rich in complex carbohydrates makes you feel good physically, and it also helps satisfy your hunger and enhances your sense of emotional well-being.

Sources of complex carbohydrates: Complex carbohydrates are found in whole grain foods, such as brown rice and whole grain breads, pastas, and cereals. Legumes, including dry beans and peas, are also good sources. Some fruits, including prunes, apples, and grapefruit, contain complex carbohydrates, as do some vegetables, such as okra, celery, corn, and spinach. Most complex-carbohydrate foods are relatively low in calories and rich in vitamins, minerals, and fiber.

Carbohydrate requirements: Calories from carbohydrate foods—both simple and complex—should make up roughly 40 to 50 percent of your daily caloric intake. This means if your body requires 1,600 calories a day, approximately 640 to 800 of these calories should come from carbohydrate foods. Ideally, the bulk of your carbohydrate calories will come from fruits, vegetables, whole grain foods, and legumes. Both simple and complex carbohydrates have four calories per gram, so when you eat 640 to 800 carbohydrate calories a day as part of a 1,600-calorie-per-day diet, you'll get a total of 160 to 200 grams of carbohydrates, the majority of which should be complex carbohydrates.

Protein

An adequate amount of high-quality protein in your diet is essential to your good health. Minus the water in your body, about three-quarters of your weight is protein. Most of it makes up your muscle tissue, but it's also an important component of your bones, teeth, cartilage, skin, organs, and even blood and body fluids. The components of your immune system are made up of proteins, and it depends on replacement proteins from the foods in your diet to effectively fend off minor infections and major illnesses.

Proteins serve as the catalysts for countless life-sustaining biochemical reactions and physiological processes that occur throughout your body each and every day. Your body naturally loses millions of protein-containing cells daily. They're used up, worn out, and even rubbed off your body. To replace these and repair others, you need a steady source of protein from your diet.

Dietary protein performs an important maintenance role in the body, and it also serves as a long-lasting source of energy. Eating protein-rich foods doesn't lead to dramatic spikes in blood sugar and insulin levels, and it won't wreak havoc with your energy levels and moods. When you eat a mixture of proteins and complex carbohydrates, such as grilled chicken breast on whole grain bread, your blood sugar tends to rise very gradually and remain steady for as long as three to four hours.

Sources of protein: If you're an avid meat eater, getting enough protein in your diet probably isn't a problem for you, because meat is especially rich in the nutrient. If you don't consider yourself to be an enthusiastic carnivore, however, you might have to work a little harder to meet your body's protein requirements.

Almost all foods have some protein. Fruits and vegetables have relatively little: A half-cup serving typically provides just a gram or two of protein. Meats, nuts, and beans are protein-rich, with many types providing 15 to 30 grams of protein per serving.

Because many high-protein animal products are also high-fat, high-cholesterol foods, it's important to choose them wisely, with an emphasis on low-fat dairy products, skinless poultry, fish, and lean meats that are trimmed of all visible fat. In the produce department, nuts, dried beans, peas, and other legumes are excellent sources. Smaller amounts of protein also can be found in corn, brown rice, and whole wheat pasta.

Protein requirements: As part of a nutritious and well-balanced diet, calories from protein foods should make up about 30 percent of your daily intake. If, for example, your body requires 1,600 calories a day, roughly 480 of those calories should come from protein-rich foods. Similar to carbohydrates, proteins have four calories per gram, so a well-balanced diet consisting of 1,600 calories a day includes about 120 grams of protein.

Fats

The typical American diet is notoriously high in fat, and it's taking a tremendous toll on our health. High-fat diets contribute to obesity, high cholesterol levels, heart disease, and various cancers. Although too much dietary fat is bad, having some fat in the diet is beneficial. In fact, it's absolutely essential. Fat is an important source of stored energy, and it's found in every cell in the body. It helps keep your skin soft and supple while it cushions, supports, and protects your internal organs. It aids in the body's absorption and circulation of the fat-soluble vitamins, A, D, E, and K. Fat enhances the taste and improves the texture of foods, contributing to feelings of fullness and satiety after eating.

With this said, not all fats are created equal. Unsaturated fats, including monounsaturated and polyunsaturated fats, are beneficial when consumed in moderation. Polyunsaturated fats are found in oils made from plants, including soybeans, corn, and sunflower seeds. They're especially abundant in fatty fish, including tuna and salmon, as well as nuts and seeds. Sources of monounsaturated fats include olive oil, peanut oil, canola oil, and avocados.

Saturated fat, trans fat, and dietary cholesterol are commonly referred to as "bad" fats because they're known to raise levels of LDL (low-density lipoprotein) cholesterol in the blood and contribute to heart disease. Saturated fat and cholesterol are found primarily in foods from animal sources, including fatty beef, veal, pork, and poultry with skin.

Dairy products made from whole milk also tend to be high in saturated fat and cholesterol. A few plant foods that are rich in saturated fat include cocoa butter and the tropical oils, specifically coconut oil, palm oil, and palm kernel oil.

The most dangerous type of fat is trans fat, which elevates LDL cholesterol levels and actually reduces levels of heart-healthy HDL (high-density lipoprotein), dramatically increasing the risk of heart disease. In addition, consumption of excess quantities of trans fat is linked to elevated triglyceride levels and an increased risk of developing diabetes. Trans fat turns up in many types of margarine and vegetable shortenings, deep-fried fast foods and snack foods, and many commercially baked goods such as pies, cookies, and crackers.

Fat requirements: Getting enough dietary fat isn't a problem for most folks. American adults routinely consume twice the amount their bodies need. As part of a nutritious and well-balanced diet, calories from fat should make up roughly 20 to 30 percent of your daily intake. For people consuming a diet of 1,600 calories a day, fat should contribute around 320 to 480 calories. Unlike carbohydrates and proteins, which have just four calories per gram, fat has a whopping nine calories per gram, and that's precisely what makes it so fattening. If you consume 320 to 480 calories of fat each day, you'll be getting around 36 to 53 grams of fat.

While you're watching your fat intake, be sure to pay attention to the types of fats that are working their way into your diet. Strive to consume mostly monounsaturated and polyunsaturated fats, while limiting your intake of dietary cholesterol, saturated fat, and trans fat.

Fiber

Fiber is a type of carbohydrate, but it isn't considered a true nutrient because it can't be digested or absorbed by the body. Still, fiber is a critical component of a well-balanced diet. Also known as roughage or bulk, fiber forms the structural framework of all food plants, including fruits, vegetables, grains, legumes, and nuts. Because humans lack the enzymes necessary to fully digest it, fiber travels through the gastrointestinal tract relatively unchanged, and that's exactly what makes it so beneficial.

High-Fiber Diets Promote Weight Loss

You probably know from experience that eating a bowl of bran cereal or a serving of beans can fill you up pretty fast. High-fiber foods are bulky and filling. Ounce for ounce, they're typically far lower in calories than fiber-free foods.

Because high-fiber foods require some serious chewing, they take longer to eat, and this property dramatically increases their ability to satisfy your hunger. Time spent chewing slows the pace at which you eat, giving your brain a chance to notice when your stomach is full and you're no longer hungry.

As a result, eating high-fiber foods makes it much more difficult to overeat. Numerous studies have shown that people who consume high-fiber diets tend to be thinner and healthier than those whose diets are lacking in roughage.

There's no doubt that the sheer bulk of high-fiber foods helps make you feel full, but there's another important reason for their ability to satisfy. Foods that are rich in fiber trigger the release of a specific hormone in the bloodstream called cholecystokinin, or CCK for short. This hormone is known to produce feelings of fullness and satiety.

Sources of fiber: Fiber is mainly found in plant foods. Only traces of roughage are found in heavily refined or processed foods, including white rice, white bread, refined breakfast cereals, and most types of cookies, crackers, and white pasta. With every phase of processing that occurs during the manufacture of food, fiber content is diminished. Rich sources of roughage include bran and multigrain cereals, whole grain bread products, oatmeal, and dried beans and other legumes. Fiber-rich fruits include apples, berries, figs, pears, and prunes, while fiber-rich vegetables include broccoli, Brussels sprouts, carrots, and cauliflower.

Fiber requirements: If you aren't getting enough fiber each day, you can boost your intake by taking fiber supplements and eating a wider variety of plant foods. Eating the typical American diet, most adults get only about 11 to 15 grams of fiber per day, less than half the recommended amount. For optimum health, adults should aim for an intake of at least 28 grams of fiber daily.

When you increase the fiber in your diet, be sure to start slowly and work your way up gradually. It's a good idea to drink plenty of water, because fiber absorbs water in the digestive tract. If you switch abruptly from a low-fiber diet to one rich in roughage, you might suffer a bit of gastrointestinal distress in the form of bloating, cramping, and excessive gas production. These symptoms will resolve as your body adjusts, but adding fiber to your diet slowly will allow you to avoid them altogether.

Water

Although water isn't nutritious in the true sense of the word, it is vital to life, second only in importance to oxygen. In terms of body composition, water makes up the vast majority of the human brain, organs, tissues, and fluids. Because water is the primary ingredient of our very beings, it's easy to see why drinking it is so critical. A loss of 5 percent of body water results in weakness, irritability, and impaired concentration. A loss of 15 to 20 percent can be fatal.

You need to drink plenty of water throughout the day to keep your immune system functioning optimally. Water also helps lubricate your joints, cushion your internal organs, moisten your eyes, and keep your skin soft and supple. It carries food through your digestive tract, delivering nutrients to the bloodstream and removing waste from cells and tissues.

Drinking water can help with weight control and improve energy levels. Many people feel hungry when, in reality, they're thirsty. Drinking a glass of water between meals helps fill your stomach and reduces the likelihood of overeating. Because one of the signs of mild dehydration is fatigue, increasing your fluid intake might give you a boost of energy and help you avoid turning to food for a quick pick-me-up.

Water requirements: If you don't consume enough liquid, your body will remind you to drink up by signaling you that you're thirsty. Unfortunately, your built-in sensation of thirst isn't a very reliable indicator of your body's state of hydration, and you might not feel thirsty until your body is considerably dehydrated. Because thirst isn't an ideal indicator of your body's hydration status, you shouldn't count on it exclusively to regulate your fluid intake. Most healthy adults require about a quart of water a day for every 50 pounds of body weight. When you're active, your water requirements will be greater. In general, you should drink at least eight 8-ounce glasses of water each day.

Caloric Requirements

Now that you understand the importance of carbohydrates, proteins, and fats in your diet, you're ready for some solid numbers. The first number you'll need is the total number of calories you should consume daily to achieve and maintain your goal weight. The exact number varies from person to person depending on level of activity, body composition, metabolism, age, and gender, but most moderately active women require around 11 calories to support each pound of body weight on a daily basis, while most moderately active men need around 13 calories per pound of body weight.

If, for example, you're a 150-pound woman, you'll need to eat about 1,650 calories every day to maintain that weight (150 x 11 = 1,650). What if your goal weight is 150 pounds, but you currently weigh 200 pounds? If you weigh 200 pounds right now, it's likely that your current daily diet consists of around 2,200 calories (200 x 11 = 2,200), because it takes about 2,200 calories a day to support and maintain 200 pounds of body weight for a moderately active woman.

The good news is that if you feed only 150 pounds of your body, the extra, unwanted 50 pounds will eventually get lost. By feeding your 200-pound body 1,650 calories a day instead of 2,200 calories a day, you'll be cutting your daily intake by 550 calories, enough to net you a weight loss of a little more than a pound a week. As you continue to slim down, the rate at which you lose weight will gradually slow, but ultimately, you'll reach your goal weight of 150 pounds.

It sounds too simple to be true, but it works. All you have to do is start eating like the person you want to become, and you'll eventually become that person. If you want to lose your excess weight and keep it off forever, you have to permanently change your eating habits. You have to begin eating the way you *must* eat for the rest of your life to maintain your desired body weight.

Determining your personal nutrient needs for a balanced diet is as easy as performing some simple calculations and filling in the blanks on the following pages, so grab your calculator and let's get started!

One Program, Five Numbers

After you complete the worksheet on pages 150 and 151, the only numbers you'll need to remember are the numbers of grams you should consume for carbohydrates, protein, fat, and fiber, plus the number of glasses of water you should drink (You'll calculate these numbers on the worksheet on pages 150-151.) If you choose foods and beverages that allow you to approximate these numbers on a daily basis, everything else will take care of itself. You'll be

Nutrition Facts

Serving Size 1 cup (228g)
Serving Per Container 2

Amount Per Serving

Calories 250   Calories from Fat 110

% Daily Value*

Total Fat 12g	18%
Saturated Fat 3g	15%
Trans Fat 3g	
Cholesterol 30mg	10%
Sodium 470mg	20%
Total Carbohydrate 31g	10%
Dietary Fiber 0g	0%
Sugars 5g	
Protein 5g	

Vitamin A	4%
Viatmin C	2%
Calcium	20%
Iron	4%

*Percent Daily Values are bsed on a 2,000 calorie diet. Your Daily Values may be higher of lower depending on your calorie needs.

		Calories	2,000	2,500
Total Fat	Less than		55g	80g
Sat Fat	Less than		20g	25g
Cholesterol	Less than		300mg	300mg
Sodium	Less than		2,400mg	2,400mg
Total Carbohydrate			300g	375g
Dietary Fiber			25g	30mg

eating a nutritious, well-balanced diet, and you'll find that your energy levels soar. Because you'll be maximizing your metabolic rate in the process, losing weight or maintaining your current weight will be easier than you ever imagined!

In order to meet your daily nutrient requirements, you'll need to know the nutrient contents of various foods. Fortunately, nearly every packaged food in the United States comes with a handy Nutrition Facts panel attached. If you look at the sample nutrition label at left, you'll find all the information you need. The first thing you'll want to know is the suggested serving size. According to the sample label, a single-serving size of the food inside the package is one cup. Next, you'll need to know how many grams of carbohydrates, protein, fat, and fiber a serving of this food contains. As you can see, one cup contains 31 grams of carbohydrates, 5 grams of protein, and 12 grams of fat.

Determining the nutrient content of the food that you eat is no great feat when it comes packaged with a Nutrition Facts panel. It's not quite as simple to figure out the nutrient content of the foods that you prepare from scratch, or those that are served to you in restaurants. For those items, you can use a reference book, website, or app that features the nutrient content of many popular foods. You won't have to consult a reference book every time you open your mouth for a morsel of food, but it is very important to do it initially, while you're still learning. It's also important to record your daily caloric intake each day and to make sure that your *actual* daily totals for carbohydrates, proteins, fat, fiber, and water match your *intended* totals. Before long, you'll get a feel for the nutrient values of your favorite foods, and eating a nutritious, well-balanced diet will become second nature. You'll find a 3 weeks' worth of log pages in this book, beginning on page 163.

Take Five! Daily Menu Planning

After completing your worksheet, you might learn, for example, that your balanced diet consists of 188 grams of carbohydrates, 112 grams of protein, 33 grams of fat, 28 grams of fiber, and eight 8-ounce glasses of water. You'll use these five numbers to design a balanced menu each day, like the one on page 152.

Write your numbers here:

_____ GRAMS CARBOHYDRATE

_____ GRAMS PROTEIN

_____ GRAMS FAT

_____ FIBER

_____ GLASSES OF WATER

TAKE FIVE! WORKSHEET

Daily Caloric Needs

Women: GOAL WEIGHT **=** _____ POUNDS

x   **11** calories per pound

= _____ CALORIES (*Daily Caloric Intake*)

Men: GOAL WEIGHT **=** _____ POUNDS

x   **13** calories per pound

= _____ CALORIES (*Daily Caloric Intake*)

Your *Daily Caloric Intake* is the number of calories your body needs to support itself at your goal weight.

Daily Nutrient Needs

A nutritious, well-balanced diet consists of 40 to 50 percent carbohydrates, 30 percent protein, and 20 to 30 percent fat for a total of 100 percent. For this worksheet, we'll balance the diet with 50 percent carbohydrates, 30 percent protein, and 20 percent fat.*

Carbohydrates

Because 50 percent of your daily calories will come from carbohydrate foods, multiply your Daily Caloric Intake by .50 to determine the total number of carbohydrate calories you should eat every day.

There are 4 calories in each gram of carbohydrate, so divide this number by 4 to get the total number of carbohydrate grams you should eat every day.

_____ **x .50 =** _____ **÷ 4 =** _____
DAILY   CARBOHYDRATE   CARBOHYDRATE
CALORIC   CALORIES YOU   GRAMS YOU
INTAKE   SHOULD EAT   SHOULD EAT
                   EACH DAY   EACH DAY

Proteins

Proteins make up 30 percent of the Take Five! plan. Multiply your Daily Caloric Intake by .30 to determine the number of protein calories you should eat every day.

Because there are 4 calories in each gram of protein, divide this number by 4 to get the total number of protein grams you should eat every day.

_____ x .30 = _____ ÷ 4 = _____
| DAILY CALORIC INTAKE | PROTEIN CALORIES YOU SHOULD EAT EACH DAY | PROTEIN GRAMS YOU SHOULD EAT EACH DAY |

Fats

Because 20 percent of your daily calories will come from fat, multiply your Daily Caloric Intake by .20 to determine the number of fat calories you should eat every day.

Each gram of fat has 9 calories, so divide this number by 9 to get the number of fat grams you should eat every day.

_____ x .20 = _____ ÷ 9 = _____
| DAILY CALORIC INTAKE | FAT CALORIES YOU SHOULD EAT EACH DAY | FAT GRAMS YOU SHOULD EAT EACH DAY |

Some individuals might prefer to opt for a diet consisting of 40 percent carbohydrates, 30 percent protein, and 30 percent fat, which is a balance of nutrients that also supports good health and weight loss. As you balance your diet, remember that the percentages of carbohydrates, proteins, and fats should add up to a total of 100 percent.

TAKE FIVE! SAMPLE MENU

FOOD	AMOUNT	CALORIES	CARBS (G)	PROTEIN (G)	FAT (G)	FIBER (G)	WATER (8 OZ)
BREAKFAST							
Oatmeal	1 cup	140	24	6	2	4	
Fruit yogurt	6 oz.	90	16	5	0	0	
Fresh blueberries	1 cup	93	20	1	1	2	
Water							1
SNACK							
Strawberries	1 cup	45	10	1	0	4	
Whole grain raisin toast	2 slices	165	28	4	4	2	
Almonds, dry-roasted	8	145	4	5	11	1	
Water							1
Water							1
LUNCH							
Low-calorie frozen meal	60g	210	14	30	4	6	
Tangerine	1 medium	37	8	1	0	1	
Green salad	2 cups	50	8	3	0	4	
Water							1
SNACK							
Broccoli, raw	1 cup	40	8	2	0	2	
Carrots, raw	1 cup	80	18	1	0	1	
Chicken, baked	1.5 oz.	70	0	13	2	0	
Water							1
Water							1

FOOD	AMOUNT	CALORIES	CARBS (G)	PROTEIN (G)	FAT (G)	FIBER (G)	WATER
DINNER							
Turkey breast, baked	6 oz.	240	0	36	6	0	
Sweet potato, baked	1 (2.5 oz.)	84	20	1	Trace	2	
Eggplant, grilled	4 slices (7 oz)	38	7	2	0	1	
Zucchini, grilled	1 cup	28	4	2	0	2	
Water							1
Water							1
Totals	—	1,555	189	113	30	32	8

The Physiology of Weight Loss

Although weight loss might often seem elusive, there's nothing really magical about it. It all boils down to the simple, irrefutable principles of mathematics. In order to lose weight, you must consume fewer calories than your body needs to support itself at your current weight. Like your bank account, your body weight is a reflection of the deposits and withdrawals that you make. When you deposit excess cash into your bank account, it swells. As you withdraw funds, it shrinks. The same is true of your body: Whenever you deposit excess calories, your weight increases, and when you make withdrawals, your weight decreases.

A pound of body weight represents around 3,500 calories. When you consume 3,500 calories more than your body needs to support itself at your current weight, you gain a pound. When you consume 3,500 fewer calories than your body needs to support itself at your current weight, or when you expend 3,500 additional calories through activity, you lose a pound. To determine approximately how long it will take for you to lose your excess body weight, use the worksheet on pages 156-157.

Get Up, Get Moving, and Slim Down

One of the best ways to slim down and tone up is to work out. Regular activity helps you lose weight by burning calories while you're exercising, but it also increases your metabolic rate, allowing your body to use more calories, even at rest. In addition to helping you achieve weight loss success, putting your body in motion helps boost your mood and energy levels, reduce your appetite, and promote more restful sleep. For maximum weight loss success, you'll want to incorporate both aerobic exercise and strength training into your weekly routine.

Aerobic Exercise

Aerobic exercise is any extended activity that involves moving the large muscle groups of your body at a pace sufficient to increase your heart rate and breathing. Brisk walking, jogging, cycling, swimming, and rowing are all excellent aerobic activities. Aerobic exercise strengthens the muscles of your arms and legs, and it also strengthens the heart muscle itself, improving your cardiovascular fitness and stamina. Other health benefits of regular aerobic activity include reduction in blood pressure, blood sugar, and cholesterol levels, and a lower risk of heart disease, type 2 diabetes, and many types of cancer.

Knowing Your Target Heart Rate Zone

To make sure you're getting the most from the time you invest in your aerobic workout, it's important to move your body fast enough to elevate your heart rate. How high you strive to raise your heart rate depends primarily on your age. The average adult has a resting heart rate, or pulse, of about 60 to 80 beats per minute. As a general rule, the better your physical condition, the lower your resting heart rate.

In general, your maximum heart rate can be determined by subtracting your age from 220. If you're 40 years old, for example, you'll subtract 40 from 220, which equals 180. But don't worry; you don't have to get your heart beating to the tune of 180 beats

DAY 01

FOOD FOR THOUGHT

The way to get stated is to quit talking and begin doing.
—Walt Disney

DAILY FOOD LOG/DATE:

MY TAKE FIVE! NUMBERS: ____(G) CARBS ____(G) PROTEIN ____(G) FAT____(G) FIBER ____(GLASSES) WATER

	FOOD	AMOUNT	CARBS (GRAMS)	PROTEIN (GRAMS)	FAT (GRAMS)	FIBER (GRAMS)	WATER (GLASSES)	SUPPLEMENTS
BREAKFAST								
SNACK								
LUNCH								
SNACK								
DINNER								
SNACK								
DAILY TOTALS			(GRAMS)	(GRAMS)	(GRAMS)	(GRAMS)	(GLASSES)	

DAILY EXERCISE LOG:

ACTIVITY_____ DURATION_____ COMMENTS_____

TAKE FIVE! WEIGHT LOSS WORKSHEET

If you're moderately active:

Multiply your current body weight by 11 (for women) or 13 (for men) to determine the approximate number of calories you're *currently* consuming daily, and write that **(A)**.

Next, decide on the number of calories you plan to consume each day. *(Multiply your goal weight by 11. Keep in mind that it's never wise to consume fewer than 1,000 calories a day without a physician's supervision.)* Write that **(B)**.

Subtract the number on line B from the number on line A to determine your daily caloric deficit, and write that **(C)**.

If you plan to create an even greater caloric deficit by exercising, write the number of calories you plan to expend exercising each day here **(D)**.

Add the numbers on lines **C** and **D** to get your total daily caloric deficit created by dietary changes and physical activity. Write this number **(E)**.

To determine your total weekly caloric deficit, multiply the number on line **E** by 7, and write the number **(F)**.

To determine how many pounds you can lose in one week, divide the number on line **F** by 3,500, and write that number **(G)**.

If this number is more than two pounds per week, you might want to increase your daily caloric consumption. If you plan to engage in rapid weight loss of more than two pounds a week, be sure to consult your doctor. On the other hand, if the number you wrote on line F is less than 3,500, you wouldn't even lose one pound per week. You can adjust the amount of weight you lose by adding more exercise or by consuming fewer calories per day, as long as you don't go under 1,000 calories. Plus, the closer you get to your goal weight, the longer it takes to lose a pound. That's why the scales often get stuck and why the last 10 pounds are the hardest to lose!

To determine how long it will likely take you to lose your total excess weight, simply subtract your goal weight from your current weight, and write that number **(H)**.

Now divide **H** by **G**, and you'll have the approximate number of weeks it will take you to achieve your goal weight.

If losing your excess weight will take longer than you'd like, don't be discouraged. With every pound you lose, you'll feel better and stronger, both physically and emotionally, and your self-confidence will grow by leaps and bounds. And remember, losing just one pound per week adds up to a weight loss of 52 pounds per year!

   _____ **=** Your Weight

x   11 (13 for men)

= _____ **(A) =** Calories Currently Consumed Daily

− _____ **(B) =** Calories Planned to Consume Daily

= _____ **(C) =** Daily Caloric Deficit

+ _____ **(D) =** Calories Expended by Exercising

= _____ **(E) =** Total Daily Caloric Deficit

x   7

= _____ **(F) =** Weekly Caloric Deficit

÷   3500

= _____ **(G) =** # Pounds Lost in 1 Week ·····

   _____ **=** Current Weight

− _____ **=** Goal Weight

= _____ **(H) =** Total Excess Weight

÷ _____ **(G) =** # Pounds Lost in 1 Week ◄··

= _____ **=** # of Weeks to Achieve Goal Weight

TARGET HEART RATE ZONE FOR HEALTHY ADULTS

AGE	TARGET HEART RATE ZONE
20	100–150
30	95–143
40	90–135
50	85–128
60	80–120

per minute to get a good cardiovascular workout. You just need to step up your pulse to a number that falls between 50 to 75 percent of your maximum heart rate. This range of numbers is known as your target heart rate zone.

Strength Training

Strength training, or weight training, is one of the most beneficial types of exercise you can perform, but unfortunately, it's one that is often neglected. If you can fit just two 20- to 30-minute weight training sessions into your weekly schedule, you'll see dramatic results in a short period of time. Within just a few weeks, you'll notice that you're stronger and more energetic. In a month or two, the muscles of your arms, legs, chest, and back will be more toned and defined, and your abdomen will be flatter and firmer.

If weight loss is your goal, strength training can help. Like moderate-intensity aerobic workouts, weight training exercises can burn up to seven to eight calories a minute. In addition to the calories burned during your workout, weight training creates an "after burn" effect. It causes your body to continue to burn calories at a higher rate for hours after the workout. Studies have shown that after a half-hour weight lifting session, the metabolic rate remains elevated for up to 15 hours, making this type of exercise an excellent investment of your time.

FitBit

In addition to aiding weight loss, strength training also helps you develop strong bones, boost stamina, and sharpen focus.

As you continue to engage in strength training, your body composition gradually changes, so that your percentage of body fat declines as your percentage of body muscle increases. Pound for pound, muscle tissue burns far more calories than fat does, even when you're resting. The more muscle tissue you have, the more calories your body burns each day, making weight loss even easier.

The Ever-Declining Metabolic Rate

For many people, maintaining a desirable body weight becomes increasingly challenging with each passing year. There's a good reason for this phenomenon: Research shows that with age, the metabolic rate begins a slow, steady decline. Scientists once believed that a sluggish metabolism was an inevitable part of aging, but that theory isn't entirely correct. As it turns out, the primary determinant of your metabolic rate is the amount of lean muscle tissue your body is sporting.

Because most people become less active with age, their muscle mass gradually dwindles. This process starts sooner than you might think. Muscle loss begins in the mid-twenties, and by age 30, the average sedentary person can expect to lose muscle tissue at the disturbing rate of about 2 percent per year. As more muscle tissue is lost, the metabolic rate continues to fall, along with the number of the fewer calories the body requires to support itself.

Mature, sedentary adults might require 200 to 400 fewer calories each day than they did when they were fit, active teenagers. Individuals who don't fine-tune their eating habits and make time for exercise can expect to gain about three to five pounds each decade after the age of 35.

CALORIES BURNED WITH EXERCISE
(30-MINUTE SESSION)

ACTIVITY (MODERATE INTENSITY)	130 POUNDS	155 POUNDS	190 POUNDS
Aerobics	177	211	259
Basketball	236	282	345
Bicycling (12 to 14 mph)	236	282	345
Bicycling, stationary	207	247	302
Calisthenics	133	159	194
Dancing	133	159	194
Frisbee playing	89	106	130
Gardening	148	176	216
Golf (carrying clubs)	163	194	237
Hiking	207	247	302
House cleaning	74	88	108
Mowing lawn	163	194	237
Racquetball	207	247	302
Raking lawn	118	141	173
Rowing (stationary)	251	299	367
Running	236	282	345
Shoveling snow	177	211	259
Skiing (downhill)	177	211	259
Soccer	207	247	302
Softball	148	176	216
Sweeping	118	141	173
Swimming	236	282	345
Tennis	207	247	302
Volleyball	89	106	130
Walking (3 mph)	104	123	151
Weight lifting	177	211	259

The Stress-Weight Connection

Eating right and exercising regularly can be especially challenging in the face of stress. When you're feeling stressed out, you might find yourself eating more—and more often—because you're tired or anxious or simply because you're seeking an energy boost or emotional comfort. Overeating definitely contributes to weight gain, but weight gain during periods of excessive stress also might be at least partly due to the effect of cortisol.

The hormone cortisol is secreted by the adrenal glands, and it plays an important role in regulating energy for the body. It is responsible for stimulating the metabolism of fat and carbohydrates, as well as the release of insulin and the maintenance of blood sugar levels. During periods of excessive stress, the adrenal glands often secrete more cortisol than they normally would. Several studies have demonstrated that high cortisol levels promote weight gain, especially in the abdominal region. High cortisol levels have been linked to increased appetite and cravings for foods that are high in sugar and fat. Over time, high levels of cortisol can increase the risk for developing high blood pressure, high cholesterol levels, type 2 diabetes, cardiovascular disease, and, of course, obesity.

Losing weight is by no means the easiest task you'll undertake, but it's certainly possible for virtually every individual who is willing to make the necessary changes. Following the Take Five! program, you *can* achieve your desired weight and comfortably maintain that weight for the rest of your life. Even better, you can feel confident knowing that while you're losing weight, you'll be gaining greater health and happiness in the process.

Are you ready to get started? Now that you have the tools you need, it's time to experience a Take Five! Best wishes for weight loss success!

TAKE FIVE! SUCCESS TRACKER

INITIAL GOAL WEIGHT: _____

INTERMEDIATE GOAL WEIGHT: _____

ULTIMATE GOAL WEIGHT: _____

Use the following table to record your measurements:

	DAY 1	DAY 30	DAY 60	DAY 90
WEIGHT				
BODY MASS INDEX				
WAIST CIRCUMFERENCE				
CHEST/BUST				
HIPS				
NECK				
RIGHT ARM				
LEFT ARM				
RIGHT THIGH				
LEFT THIGH				
RIGHT CALF				
LEFT CALF				

DAY 01

FitBit

Wholesome, nutritious food does more than contribute to good health and weight control. It helps you avoid cravings for foods high in sugar and fat and helps ensure your success at the next meal or snack—or even the next day!

DAILY FOOD LOG/DATE:

MY TAKE FIVE! NUMBERS: _____(G) CARBS _____(G) PROTEIN _____(G) FAT_____(G) FIBER _____(GLASSES) WATER

	FOOD	AMOUNT	CARBS (GRAMS)	PROTEIN (GRAMS)	FAT (GRAMS)	FIBER (GRAMS)	WATER (GLASSES)	SUPPLEMENTS
BREAKFAST								
SNACK								
LUNCH								
SNACK								
DINNER								
SNACK								
DAILY TOTALS		(GRAMS)	(GRAMS)	(GRAMS)	(GRAMS)	(GLASSES)		

DAILY EXERCISE LOG:

ACTIVITY_____ DURATION_____ COMMENTS_____

FOOD FOR THOUGHT
Motivation is what gets you started.
Habit is what keeps you going.
—Jim Rohn, an American entrepreneur and motivational speaker

DAILY FOOD LOG/DATE:

MY TAKE FIVE! NUMBERS: _____(G) CARBS _____(G) PROTEIN _____(G) FAT_____(G) FIBER _____(GLASSES) WATER

	FOOD	AMOUNT	CARBS (GRAMS)	PROTEIN (GRAMS)	FAT (GRAMS)	FIBER (GRAMS)	WATER (GLASSES)	SUPPLEMENTS
BREAKFAST								
SNACK								
LUNCH								
SNACK								
DINNER								
SNACK								
DAILY TOTALS		(GRAMS)	(GRAMS)	(GRAMS)	(GRAMS)	(GLASSES)	

DAILY EXERCISE LOG:

ACTIVITY_____ DURATION_____ COMMENTS_____

DAY 03

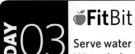 **Fit**Bit

Serve water with every meal, even if you drink another beverage. Water helps fill you and keeps you from overeating.

DAILY FOOD LOG/DATE:

MY TAKE FIVE! NUMBERS: _____(G) CARBS _____(G) PROTEIN _____(G) FAT_____(G) FIBER _____(GLASSES) WATER

	FOOD	AMOUNT	CARBS (GRAMS)	PROTEIN (GRAMS)	FAT (GRAMS)	FIBER (GRAMS)	WATER (GLASSES)	SUPPLEMENTS
BREAKFAST								
SNACK								
LUNCH								
SNACK								
DINNER								
SNACK								
DAILY TOTALS			(GRAMS)	(GRAMS)	(GRAMS)	(GRAMS)	(GLASSES)	

DAILY EXERCISE LOG:

ACTIVITY_____ **DURATION**_____ **COMMENTS**_____

DAY 04

FOOD FOR THOUGHT
Success is the sum of small efforts,
repeated day in and day out.
—Robert J. Collier, an American publisher

DAILY FOOD LOG/DATE:

MY TAKE FIVE! NUMBERS: ____(G) CARBS ____(G) PROTEIN ____(G) FAT____(G) FIBER ____(GLASSES) WATER

	FOOD	AMOUNT	CARBS (GRAMS)	PROTEIN (GRAMS)	FAT (GRAMS)	FIBER (GRAMS)	WATER (GLASSES)	SUPPLEMENTS
BREAKFAST								
SNACK								
LUNCH								
SNACK								
DINNER								
SNACK								
DAILY TOTALS			(GRAMS)	(GRAMS)	(GRAMS)	(GRAMS)	(GLASSES)	

DAILY EXERCISE LOG:

ACTIVITY_____ DURATION_____ COMMENTS_____

DAY 05

ぁFitBit

When you have a choice, always opt for fresh fruit rather than fruit juice. Fruit juice is high in sugar, and it's easy to down an entire serving in mere seconds. Eating a piece of fruit, on the other hand, requires chewing, which increases satiety.

DAILY FOOD LOG/DATE:

MY TAKE FIVE! NUMBERS: _____(G) CARBS _____(G) PROTEIN _____(G) FAT_____(G) FIBER _____(GLASSES) WATER

	FOOD	AMOUNT	CARBS (GRAMS)	PROTEIN (GRAMS)	FAT (GRAMS)	FIBER (GRAMS)	WATER (GLASSES)	SUPPLEMENTS
BREAKFAST								
SNACK								
LUNCH								
SNACK								
DINNER								
SNACK								
DAILY TOTALS		(GRAMS)	(GRAMS)	(GRAMS)	(GRAMS)	(GLASSES)		

DAILY EXERCISE LOG:

ACTIVITY_____ **DURATION**_____ **COMMENTS**_____

FOOD FOR THOUGHT
Just go out there and do what you've got to do.
—Martina Navratilova

DAILY FOOD LOG/DATE:

MY TAKE FIVE! NUMBERS: _____(G) CARBS _____(G) PROTEIN _____(G) FAT_____(G) FIBER _____(GLASSES) WATER

	FOOD	AMOUNT	CARBS (GRAMS)	PROTEIN (GRAMS)	FAT (GRAMS)	FIBER (GRAMS)	WATER (GLASSES)	SUPPLEMENTS
BREAKFAST								
SNACK								
LUNCH								
SNACK								
DINNER								
SNACK								
DAILY TOTALS			(GRAMS)	(GRAMS)	(GRAMS)	(GRAMS)	(GLASSES)	

DAILY EXERCISE LOG:

ACTIVITY_____ DURATION_____ COMMENTS_____

DAY 07

FitBit

Studies show that most people clean their plates, so if you're using an 11- or 12-inch plate, imagine how many more calories you could be eating. Slash calories by switching to a salad plate.

DAILY FOOD LOG/DATE:

MY TAKE FIVE! NUMBERS: _____(G) CARBS _____(G) PROTEIN _____(G) FAT_____(G) FIBER _____(GLASSES) WATER

	FOOD	AMOUNT	CARBS (GRAMS)	PROTEIN (GRAMS)	FAT (GRAMS)	FIBER (GRAMS)	WATER (GLASSES)	SUPPLEMENTS
BREAKFAST								
SNACK								
LUNCH								
SNACK								
DINNER								
SNACK								
DAILY TOTALS		(GRAMS)	(GRAMS)	(GRAMS)	(GRAMS)	(GLASSES)	

DAILY EXERCISE LOG:

ACTIVITY_____ DURATION_____ COMMENTS_____

DAY 08

FOOD FOR THOUGHT
Clear your mind of "can't."
—Samuel Johnson, 18th Century English writer

DAILY FOOD LOG/DATE:

MY TAKE FIVE! NUMBERS: ____(G) CARBS ____(G) PROTEIN ____(G) FAT____(G) FIBER ____(GLASSES) WATER

	FOOD	AMOUNT	CARBS (GRAMS)	PROTEIN (GRAMS)	FAT (GRAMS)	FIBER (GRAMS)	WATER (GLASSES)	SUPPLEMENTS
BREAKFAST								
SNACK								
LUNCH								
SNACK								
DINNER								
SNACK								
DAILY TOTALS			(GRAMS)	(GRAMS)	(GRAMS)	(GRAMS)	(GLASSES)	

DAILY EXERCISE LOG:

ACTIVITY_____ DURATION_____ COMMENTS_____

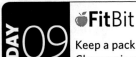

DAY 09

🍎FitBit

Keep a pack of gum in the kitchen to avoid nibbling while preparing meals. Chew a piece while you cook and keep it in your mouth until it's time to eat.

DAILY FOOD LOG/DATE:

MY TAKE FIVE! NUMBERS: _____(G) CARBS _____(G) PROTEIN _____(G) FAT_____(G) FIBER _____(GLASSES) WATER

	FOOD	AMOUNT	CARBS (GRAMS)	PROTEIN (GRAMS)	FAT (GRAMS)	FIBER (GRAMS)	WATER (GLASSES)	SUPPLEMENTS
BREAKFAST								
SNACK								
LUNCH								
SNACK								
DINNER								
SNACK								
DAILY TOTALS			(GRAMS)	(GRAMS)	(GRAMS)	(GRAMS)	(GLASSES)	

DAILY EXERCISE LOG:

ACTIVITY_____ DURATION_____ COMMENTS_____

DAY 10

FOOD FOR THOUGHT
To every problem there is already a solution, whether you know it or not.
—Grenville Kleiser, North American author

DAILY FOOD LOG/DATE:

MY TAKE FIVE! NUMBERS: _____(G) CARBS _____(G) PROTEIN _____(G) FAT_____(G) FIBER _____(GLASSES) WATER

	FOOD	AMOUNT	CARBS (GRAMS)	PROTEIN (GRAMS)	FAT (GRAMS)	FIBER (GRAMS)	WATER (GLASSES)	SUPPLEMENTS
BREAKFAST								
SNACK								
LUNCH								
SNACK								
DINNER								
SNACK								
DAILY TOTALS			(GRAMS)	(GRAMS)	(GRAMS)	(GRAMS)	(GLASSES)	

DAILY EXERCISE LOG:

ACTIVITY_____ DURATION_____ COMMENTS_____

DAY 11

⚫FitBit
Aim to eat two or three half-cup servings of fruits or vegetables at every meal. They'll help fill you up for few calories. Plus, diets rich in fruits and vegetables can also improve your health by reducing the risk for disease.

DAILY FOOD LOG/DATE:

MY TAKE FIVE! NUMBERS: _____(G) CARBS _____(G) PROTEIN _____(G) FAT_____(G) FIBER _____(GLASSES) WATER

	FOOD	AMOUNT	CARBS (GRAMS)	PROTEIN (GRAMS)	FAT (GRAMS)	FIBER (GRAMS)	WATER (GLASSES)	SUPPLEMENTS
BREAKFAST								
SNACK								
LUNCH								
SNACK								
DINNER								
SNACK								
DAILY TOTALS			(GRAMS)	(GRAMS)	(GRAMS)	(GRAMS)	(GLASSES)	

DAILY EXERCISE LOG:

ACTIVITY_____ **DURATION**_____ **COMMENTS**_____

DAY 12

FOOD FOR THOUGHT
Nothing diminishes anxiety faster than action.
—Walter Anderson, 20th Century American painter

DAILY FOOD LOG/DATE:

MY TAKE FIVE! NUMBERS: _____(G) CARBS _____(G) PROTEIN _____(G) FAT_____(G) FIBER _____(GLASSES) WATER

	FOOD	AMOUNT	CARBS (GRAMS)	PROTEIN (GRAMS)	FAT (GRAMS)	FIBER (GRAMS)	WATER (GLASSES)	SUPPLEMENTS
BREAKFAST								
BREAKFAST								
BREAKFAST								
SNACK								
SNACK								
LUNCH								
LUNCH								
LUNCH								
SNACK								
SNACK								
DINNER								
DINNER								
DINNER								
SNACK								
SNACK								
DAILY TOTALS			(GRAMS)	(GRAMS)	(GRAMS)	(GRAMS)	(GLASSES)	

DAILY EXERCISE LOG:

ACTIVITY_____ DURATION_____ COMMENTS_____

FitBit

Never go grocery shopping without a list, and never go when you're hungry. Avoid aisles where the processed foods lurk and concentrate on the perimeter of the store where you'll find produce, dairy, meat, and whole grains.

DAILY FOOD LOG/DATE:

MY TAKE FIVE! NUMBERS: _____(G) CARBS _____(G) PROTEIN _____(G) FAT_____(G) FIBER _____(GLASSES) WATER

	FOOD	AMOUNT	CARBS (GRAMS)	PROTEIN (GRAMS)	FAT (GRAMS)	FIBER (GRAMS)	WATER (GLASSES)	SUPPLEMENTS
BREAKFAST								
SNACK								
LUNCH								
SNACK								
DINNER								
SNACK								
DAILY TOTALS			(GRAMS)	(GRAMS)	(GRAMS)	(GRAMS)	(GLASSES)	

DAILY EXERCISE LOG:

ACTIVITY_____ DURATION_____ COMMENTS_____

FOOD FOR THOUGHT
*The delay of our dreams does not mean
that they have been denied.*
—Sarah Ban Breathnatch, author of *Simple Abundance* and other books about

DAILY FOOD LOG/DATE:

MY TAKE FIVE! NUMBERS: _____(G) CARBS _____(G) PROTEIN _____(G) FAT_____(G) FIBER _____(GLASSES) WATER

	FOOD	AMOUNT	CARBS (GRAMS)	PROTEIN (GRAMS)	FAT (GRAMS)	FIBER (GRAMS)	WATER (GLASSES)	SUPPLEMENTS
BREAKFAST								
SNACK								
LUNCH								
SNACK								
DINNER								
SNACK								
DAILY TOTALS			(GRAMS)	(GRAMS)	(GRAMS)	(GRAMS)	(GLASSES)	

DAILY EXERCISE LOG:

ACTIVITY_____ **DURATION**_____ **COMMENTS**_____

DAY 15

▸FitBit

When you eat a food very high in fat, you set yourself up for fat cravings at the next meal because consuming large quantities of fat triggers hormone changes that make you crave more.

DAILY FOOD LOG/DATE:

MY TAKE FIVE! NUMBERS: _____(G) CARBS _____(G) PROTEIN _____(G) FAT_____(G) FIBER _____(GLASSES) WATER

	FOOD	AMOUNT	CARBS (GRAMS)	PROTEIN (GRAMS)	FAT (GRAMS)	FIBER (GRAMS)	WATER (GLASSES)	SUPPLEMENTS
BREAKFAST								
SNACK								
LUNCH								
SNACK								
DINNER								
SNACK								
DAILY TOTALS			(GRAMS)	(GRAMS)	(GRAMS)	(GRAMS)	(GLASSES)	

DAILY EXERCISE LOG:

ACTIVITY_____ DURATION_____ COMMENTS_____

DAY 16

FOOD FOR THOUGHT
I've never been afraid to fail.
—Michael Jordan

DAILY FOOD LOG/DATE:

MY TAKE FIVE! NUMBERS: _____ (G) CARBS _____ (G) PROTEIN _____ (G) FAT _____ (G) FIBER _____ (GLASSES) WATER

	FOOD	AMOUNT	CARBS (GRAMS)	PROTEIN (GRAMS)	FAT (GRAMS)	FIBER (GRAMS)	WATER (GLASSES)	SUPPLEMENTS
BREAKFAST								
BREAKFAST								
BREAKFAST								
BREAKFAST								
SNACK								
SNACK								
SNACK								
LUNCH								
LUNCH								
LUNCH								
LUNCH								
SNACK								
SNACK								
SNACK								
DINNER								
DINNER								
DINNER								
DINNER								
SNACK								
SNACK								
SNACK								
DAILY TOTALS			(GRAMS)	(GRAMS)	(GRAMS)	(GRAMS)	(GLASSES)	

DAILY EXERCISE LOG:

ACTIVITY_____ DURATION_____ COMMENTS_____

DAY 17

🍎 **Fit**Bit

Choose protein wisely. Six ounces of broiled beef ribs has 36 grams of protein but 800 calories and about 70 grams of fat. Six ounces of baked salmon, on the other hand, has 44 grams of protein, 310 calories, and about 22 grams of fat.

DAILY FOOD LOG/DATE:

MY TAKE FIVE! NUMBERS: _____ (G) CARBS _____ (G) PROTEIN _____ (G) FAT _____ (G) FIBER _____ (GLASSES) WATER

	FOOD	AMOUNT	CARBS (GRAMS)	PROTEIN (GRAMS)	FAT (GRAMS)	FIBER (GRAMS)	WATER (GLASSES)	SUPPLEMENTS
BREAKFAST								
SNACK								
LUNCH								
SNACK								
DINNER								
SNACK								
DAILY TOTALS			(GRAMS)	(GRAMS)	(GRAMS)	(GRAMS)	(GLASSES)	

DAILY EXERCISE LOG:

ACTIVITY_____ DURATION_____ COMMENTS_____

FOOD FOR THOUGHT
Optimism is the faith that leads to achievement.
Nothing can be done without hope and confidence.
—Helen Keller

DAILY FOOD LOG/DATE:

MY TAKE FIVE! NUMBERS: _____(G) CARBS _____(G) PROTEIN _____(G) FAT_____(G) FIBER _____(GLASSES) WATER

	FOOD	AMOUNT	CARBS (GRAMS)	PROTEIN (GRAMS)	FAT (GRAMS)	FIBER (GRAMS)	WATER (GLASSES)	SUPPLEMENTS
BREAKFAST								
SNACK								
LUNCH								
SNACK								
DINNER								
SNACK								
DAILY TOTALS			(GRAMS)	(GRAMS)	(GRAMS)	(GRAMS)	(GLASSES)	

DAILY EXERCISE LOG:

ACTIVITY_____ DURATION_____ COMMENTS_____

DAY 19

FitBit

Plan your weekends and days off around fitness fun. Go for a bike ride, take a hike, go roller-skating, or work in your garden. No gym required. Just step outside and start moving!

DAILY FOOD LOG/DATE:

MY TAKE FIVE! NUMBERS: _____ (G) CARBS _____ (G) PROTEIN _____ (G) FAT _____ (G) FIBER _____ (GLASSES) WATER

	FOOD	AMOUNT	CARBS (GRAMS)	PROTEIN (GRAMS)	FAT (GRAMS)	FIBER (GRAMS)	WATER (GLASSES)	SUPPLEMENTS
BREAKFAST								
SNACK								
LUNCH								
SNACK								
DINNER								
SNACK								
DAILY TOTALS			(GRAMS)	(GRAMS)	(GRAMS)	(GRAMS)	(GLASSES)	

DAILY EXERCISE LOG:

ACTIVITY_____ **DURATION**_____ **COMMENTS**_____

DAY 20

FOOD FOR THOUGHT
Continuous effort—not strength or intelligence—
is the key to unlocking our potential.
—Winston Churchill

DAILY FOOD LOG/DATE:

MY TAKE FIVE! NUMBERS: _____(G) CARBS _____(G) PROTEIN _____(G) FAT_____(G) FIBER _____(GLASSES) WATER

	FOOD	AMOUNT	CARBS (GRAMS)	PROTEIN (GRAMS)	FAT (GRAMS)	FIBER (GRAMS)	WATER (GLASSES)	SUPPLEMENTS
BREAKFAST								
SNACK								
LUNCH								
SNACK								
DINNER								
SNACK								
DAILY TOTALS			(GRAMS)	(GRAMS)	(GRAMS)	(GRAMS)	(GLASSES)	

DAILY EXERCISE LOG:

ACTIVITY_____ DURATION_____ COMMENTS_____

DAY 21

🍎**Fit**Bit

Achieving your goal weight is a process, not an event. You'll begin reaping rewards the minute you begin making positive change in your eating and exercising habits. The journey is every bit as fun and exciting as the destination.

DAILY FOOD LOG/DATE:

MY TAKE FIVE! NUMBERS: _____(G) CARBS _____(G) PROTEIN _____(G) FAT_____(G) FIBER _____(GLASSES) WATER

	FOOD	AMOUNT	CARBS (GRAMS)	PROTEIN (GRAMS)	FAT (GRAMS)	FIBER (GRAMS)	WATER (GLASSES)	SUPPLEMENTS
BREAKFAST								
SNACK								
LUNCH								
SNACK								
DINNER								
SNACK								
DAILY TOTALS			(GRAMS)	(GRAMS)	(GRAMS)	(GRAMS)	(GLASSES)	

DAILY EXERCISE LOG:

ACTIVITY_____ DURATION_____ COMMENTS_____

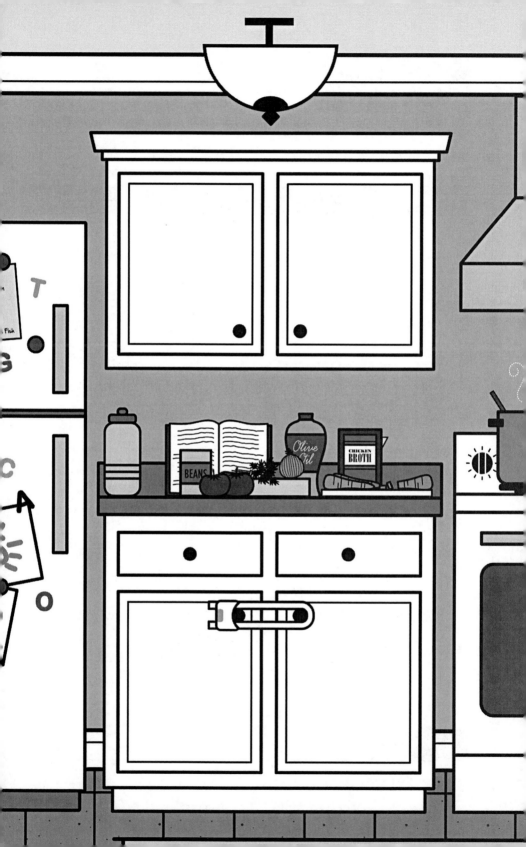

Chapter 2

Recipes for Losing Weight

Isn't it wonderful to have a recipe that's delicious, nutritious, and a family favorite? You probably prepare that recipe again and again, both for special occasions and on days you need to get something tried-and-true on the table—fast!

We asked our Mommy MD Guides for their family favorites, and here are our top picks that will help you to lose weight. These recipes are lower in fat and calories, and they're all chock-full of healthy nutrients.

You can use any of these recipes with our Take Five! program with ease. We've included the carbohydrates, protein, fat, and fiber counts for each.

We tested each of these recipes in our Mommy MD Guides kitchen—with delicious, nutritious results!

Enjoy!

> **The discovery of a new dish does more for the happiness of mankind than the discovery of a star.**
> —*Anthelme Brillat-Savarin,*
> *a 19th-century French lawyer and politician*

Dr. C's Green Smoothies

Contributed by Kay Corpus, MD. "I recommend using organic ingredients for this smoothie whenever possible. Sometimes I switch out mangoes for the pears. The first five ingredients can be blended together for a simpler version that's quite delicious!"

2 pears, cored and roughly chopped
2 Granny Smith apples, cored and roughly chopped
1 piece (½ to 1 inch) peeled fresh ginger, roughly chopped
2 cups torn kale leaves (ribs removed)
1 cup spinach
1 stalk celery, roughly chopped
½ cucumber, roughly chopped
½ avocado
Juice of ¼ lemon
1 large sprig parsley, or more to taste, roughly chopped
2 cups filtered water

In a high-powered blender, process the pears, apples, ginger, kale, spinach, celery, cucumber, avocado, lemon juice, parsley, and water until smooth.

Makes 4 servings
Per serving: 139 calories, 30 g carbohydrates,
3 g protein, 3 g fat, 7 g fiber

🍽️ RightBites

If apples have a regular place in your fruit bowl, there's good news. Eating apples regularly has been found to lower the risk of illnesses such as the common cold and even cardiovascular disease and cancer, thanks to the antioxidants found in these sweet treats.

Breakfast Pita

Contributed by Rallie McAllister, MD, MPH. "These pitas are rich in protein to power you through your busy day."

2 egg whites

¼ cup fresh or frozen vegetables of choice, chopped

¼ cup diced cooked lean ham, turkey, or tofu

1 ounce (¼ cup) grated low-fat Cheddar cheese or other cheese of choice

1 tablespoon prepared salsa

1 whole wheat pita, halved

Spray a microwave-safe bowl with cooking spray, then add the egg whites. Lightly scramble the eggs with a fork, cover the cup with waxed paper or plastic wrap, and microwave on medium power for 30 seconds. Stir the eggs, cover again, and microwave on medium power for 30 to 60 seconds, just until set. Set aside.

Place the vegetables; ham, turkey, or tofu; cheese; and salsa in a microwave-safe bowl. Microwave on high power for about 2 minutes, or until the vegetables are heated through and the cheese is melted. Add the vegetable mixture to the eggs, and stir to combine. Place into the pita halves.

Makes 1 serving

Per serving: **339 calories, 44 g carbohydrates, 30 g protein, 6 g fat, 7 g fiber**

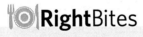 **Right**Bites

The delicious vegetables in salsa make for a nutrient-rich sauce. Tomatoes, onion, and garlic are low in calories and healthy for your heart, and tomatoes are a major source of the beneficial antioxidant lycopene.

Egg Muffins

Contributed by Amy Thompson, MD. "This recipe is from KalynsKitchen.com. These little 'muffins,' made of egg, vegetables, and cheese, are a perfect grab-and-go breakfast. You can personalize them by using more egg whites and fewer egg yolks, adding favorite veggies, or replacing some of the cheese with a choice of meat."

12 to 15 eggs (12 eggs for metal muffin tins or individual silicone cups or 15 eggs for silicone muffin pans)

1 to 2 teaspoons Spike Seasoning, or any seasoning blend that tastes good with eggs (optional)

4 to 8 ounces (1 to 2 cups) grated low-fat cheese, such as sharp Cheddar or Cheddar Jack cheese

3 scallions, thinly sliced

4 ounces chopped vegetables, such as blanched broccoli, red pepper, zucchini, or mushrooms (optional)

8 ounces diced Canadian bacon, lean ham, or crumbled cooked turkey sausage (optional)

Preheat the oven to 375°F.

If using a silicone muffin pan or individual silicone muffin cups, spray with cooking spray. If using a metal muffin pan, put 2 paper liners into each tin, then spray the liners with cooking spray.

In a large measuring bowl with a pour spout, combine the eggs and Spike Seasoning, if using, and beat well.

In the bottom of the muffin cups, layer the cheese, scallions, vegetables, if using, and meat, if using. (Fill the muffin cups about two-thirds full, with just enough room to pour a little egg around the other ingredients.)

Pour the egg mixture into each muffin cup until three-quarters full. Stir slightly with a fork. Set the muffin trays or cups on a baking sheet. Bake for 25 to 35 minutes, until the muffins have risen and are slightly browned and set.

The muffins will keep for 1 week in the refrigerator. Microwave on high for 1 to 2 minutes to reheat.

Makes 12 muffins
Per muffin: 89 calories, 1 g carbohydrates, 9 g protein, 6 g fat, 0 g fiber

RightBites

You might be Mom Strong, but are your bones strong? Women younger than 50 need 1,000 milligrams of calcium a day to keep their bones strong, and researchers have found that getting this important mineral from food is better than getting it from a supplement. In a study of 183 postmenopausal women, researchers found that those whose calcium intake came mainly from food had greater bone density than women who got most of their calcium from a supplement.

One way to reach your calcium goal is with cheese. An ounce and a half of part-skim mozzarella cheese has 333 milligrams of calcium, while the same amount of Cheddar provides you 307 milligrams. Even cottage cheese will give you a calcium bump, with 138 milligrams in a cup.

Adding cheese to your diet along with other calcium-rich foods such as low-fat yogurt, nonfat milk, kale, Chinese cabbage, tofu, and calcium-fortified foods such as cereal means you'll be well on your way to getting the recommended amount of calcium each day.

Busy Morning Oatmeal

Contributed by Lennox McNeary, MD. "I don't like instant oatmeal for several reasons. First, it takes at least 2 packets to fill me up, and that gets expensive. Second, it doesn't keep me full for long. I make my own healthier, less expensive version. On Sunday evening, I fill several small glass bowls with the dry ingredients so I can just grab a bowl on my way out to work and fix it once I get settled at my desk a little later. Sometimes I add dried cherries or blueberries and cut back on the sugar. Now you have a warm, yummy, healthy breakfast."

1 cup old-fashioned rolled oats (do not use instant oats)
1 tablespoon brown sugar
$\frac{1}{2}$ to 1 teaspoon ground cinnamon
$\frac{1}{4}$ cup chopped almonds (optional)

In a small bowl, combine the oats, brown sugar, cinnamon, and almonds, if using. Add hot water just to cover the oatmeal. Microwave on high for 30 seconds, or until the oatmeal is at the desired consistency. (If you like it mushier, add a little more water and microwave a little longer.)

Makes 1 serving
Per serving: 376 calories, 69 g carbohydrates, 14 g protein, 5 g fat, 9 g fiber

🍴🍽 RightBites

Researchers are looking into cinnamon's role in helping control type 2 diabetes, but so far studies haven't been definitive. However, cinnamon has been used as a folk remedy for everything from gastrointestinal problems to bronchitis. Here's one sure benefit of cinnamon: It adds flavor to dishes without adding calories.

Healthy Buffalo Chicken Dip

Contributed by Sonali Ruder, DO. "Traditional buffalo chicken dip
is very high in calories and fat because of the cream cheese, bottled
ranch or blue cheese dressing, and loads of shredded cheese. I decided
to perform a recipe resuscitation on this crowd-pleasing dish to shave
some calories and fat without sacrificing flavor. Serve the dip with baked
pita chips or celery and carrot sticks."

8 ounces Neufchâtel cheese, softened
1 cup plain 0% Greek yogurt
8 ounces shredded cooked chicken breast (about 2 cups)
½ cup sliced scallions, plus extra for garnish
⅓ cup Frank's Red Hot Cayenne Pepper Sauce,
    plus more to taste
½ teaspoon garlic powder
½ teaspoon onion powder
¼ teaspoon black pepper
1 ounce (¼ cup) grated reduced-fat Cheddar cheese or crumbled
    reduced-fat blue cheese (optional)

Preheat the oven to 400°F. Lightly coat a 2-quart baking dish with
cooking spray.

In a large bowl, mix together the Neufchâtel cheese and yogurt. Stir
in the chicken, scallions, hot sauce, garlic powder, onion powder, and
pepper. Top with the Cheddar cheese, if using. (If using blue cheese,
sprinkle it on top as soon as you remove the dip from the oven.)

Pour the dip into the prepared baking dish and bake for 15 to
20 minutes, or until bubbly. Garnish with the sliced scallions. Store the
remaining dip, covered, in the refrigerator, for up to 3 days.

Makes 16 (¼-cup) servings
Per serving: **70 calories, 2 g carbohydrates,
7 g protein, 4 g fat, 0 g fiber**

Quinoa Salad with Spinach, Strawberries, and Goat Cheese

Contributed by Sonali Ruder, DO. "This salad uses quinoa, which is a popular whole grain that's packed with protein and fiber as well as several vitamins and minerals. The quinoa is tossed with nutrient-packed spinach, luscious strawberries, fresh basil, and tangy goat cheese. Toasted, sliced almonds add a delightful, earthy crunch. The entire salad is tossed in a simple, homemade balsamic dressing that infuses the ingredients with bright, fresh flavor. The salad is delicious on its own, but it's also great topped with grilled chicken breast. Eating healthy never tasted so good."

1 cup quinoa, rinsed
2 cups water
$1/4$ teaspoon kosher salt
2 cups baby spinach leaves
$2/3$ cup sliced strawberries
1 ounce goat cheese, crumbled
2 tablespoons chiffonaded fresh basil
$1^1/2$ tablespoons sliced almonds, toasted

For the balsamic dressing:
2 tablespoons balsamic vinegar
1 teaspoon Dijon mustard
$1/2$ teaspoon honey or agave nectar
2 tablespoons extra-virgin olive oil
Salt
Black pepper

In a medium saucepan, combine the quinoa, water, and salt. Bring to a boil over medium-high heat, then cover and reduce the heat to low. Simmer the quinoa for about 15 minutes, or until tender and translucent. Remove the lid and cook for another 2 to 3 minutes, or until all the water has evaporated. Remove from the heat and fluff with a fork. Let the quinoa cool to room temperature.

Meanwhile, make the balsamic dressing. In a small bowl, whisk together the vinegar, mustard, and honey or agave nectar. Slowly pour in the oil while you continue to whisk. Season the dressing with salt and pepper to taste.

Place the quinoa in a salad bowl along with the spinach, strawberries, goat cheese, basil, and almonds. Add the dressing and toss to combine all ingredients.

Serve with additional goat cheese, if desired.

 Makes 2 servings
Per serving: **567 calories, 71 g carbohydrates, 17 g protein, 26 g fat, 7 g fiber**

🍴 **Right**Bites

When you eat spinach, you're getting a healthy dose of all of the benefits leafy greens have to offer. The folate and potassium help keep your heart healthy and normalize blood pressure. Spinach is also rich in vitamin K, which is important for normal blood clotting, and beta-carotene, an antioxidant that helps your body make vitamin A, which is essential for healthy vision, skin, bones, and strong immunity. Washing spinach and microwaving it is the healthiest way to cook it because it keeps almost all of its nutrients.

Spinach is available year round, and there are different varieties, including savoy, semi-savoy, smooth-leaf, and baby.

Quick Salmon Salad

Contributed by Ann Kulze, MD. "*Canned salmon is an inexpensive, convenient, and delicious way to take advantage of the awesome nutrients in oily fish. I love this salmon salad with a side of whole grain tortilla chips. You can also have it on a sandwich with 100 percent whole grain bread.*"

1 can (6 ounces) sockeye salmon, drained and broken apart
¼ cup finely chopped fresh parsley
3 tablespoons finely chopped red onion
2 tablespoons plain Greek yogurt
½ tablespoon canola oil mayonnaise or olive oil mayonnaise
½ tablespoon country-style Dijon mustard
Juice of ½ lemon
Salt
Black pepper

In a medium bowl, gently combine the salmon, parsley, onion, yogurt, mayonnaise, mustard, and lemon juice. Stir until thoroughly blended, then season with salt and pepper to taste. Store any remaining salad in an airtight container in the refrigerator for up to 3 days.

Makes 2 servings
Per serving: **177 calories, 4 g carbohydrates, 18 g protein, 9 g fat, 1 g fiber**

Lentil Soup

Contributed by Eva Mayer, MD. "This is a favorite recipe of my family. Brown and red lentils cook quicker. Green and black take longer. You can make this soup thicker by pureeing part of it to the desired consistency.

6 slices bacon, chopped
1 onion, finely chopped
2 stalks celery, finely chopped
2 medium carrots, finely chopped
1 clove garlic, minced
1 bag (16 ounces) brown lentils, rinsed
1 chicken–flavored bouillon cube
Salt
Black pepper

In a stockpot over medium heat, cook the bacon until it begins to render some of its fat, about 2 minutes. Add the onion, celery, carrots, and garlic and cook, stirring occasionally, until the vegetables are tender, about 8 minutes. Add the lentils and enough water to cover plus about 1 inch more. Bring to a boil. Add the bouillon cube, and season with salt and pepper to taste. Turn the heat down to medium-low and simmer, partially covered, for about 30 minutes, or until the lentils are tender.

 Makes 6 servings
Per serving: **391 calories, 50 g carbohydrates, 23 g protein, 11 g fat, 24 g fiber**

🍴 **Right**Bites

Like lentils? Great! A study of more than 90,000 women showed that women who regularly ate lentils and other beans had a significantly lower risk of breast cancer compared with women who rarely ate them.

French Onion Soup

Contributed by Sonali Ruder, DO. "*My French onion soup is a classic recipe that will warm you up and earn you accolades from your family. Besides being a crowd pleaser, it's also inexpensive to make. (It doesn't get much cheaper than onions!) It's delicious served alone or topped with a crusty piece of French bread and gooey, melted Gruyère cheese.*"

1 tablespoon olive oil
2¼ pounds sweet yellow onions (about 3 large onions),
    thinly sliced (about 8 cups)
½ teaspoon kosher salt
½ teaspoon sugar
2 cloves garlic, minced
2 or 3 sprigs fresh thyme
1 bay leaf
1 tablespoon flour
1 cup dry white wine or sherry or a mixture of the two
¼ cup cognac or brandy
8 cups low-sodium beef broth, chicken broth, or vegetable broth
Black pepper
6 slices (1 ounce each) French baguette
2 ounces (½ cup) Gruyère cheese, grated

In a large pot or Dutch oven, heat the oil over medium heat and add the onions. Stir to coat the onions with the oil.

Cook, stirring occasionally, for 15 minutes, or until the onions start to soften. Add the salt and sugar and stir to combine. Continue to cook the onions, stirring occasionally, until they are a rich golden brown, about 45 minutes. (Take your time with this step, because this provides the rich flavor of your soup. If the onions start to burn or catch on the bottom, you can add a small amount of water to deglaze the pan.)

Once the onions are caramelized, add the garlic, thyme, and bay leaf. Cook for another minute or two and then stir in the flour. Cook, stirring, for another 2 to 3 minutes, until the raw flour is completely absorbed by the onions. Turn the heat up to high and add the wine or sherry and cognac or brandy. Cook until reduced by half. Add the broth. Bring to a boil and then reduce the heat to medium-low. Simmer the soup, partially covered, for 20 to 30 minutes. Season to taste with salt and pepper.

Top the bread with equal amounts of grated cheese. Toast the bread in a toaster oven or under the broiler for 1 to 2 minutes, or until the cheese melts and the bread is crisp. Ladle the soup into bowls and top each one with a slice of cheesy toast. Serve hot.

Makes 6 servings
Per serving: 331 calories, 39 g carbohydrates,
15 g protein, 8 g fat, 4 g fiber

🍽️ **Right**Bites

Onions are a nutritious addition to your meals for several reasons. They're a rich source of flavonoids, including quercetin, which give them their red or yellow color. Flavonoids help reduce the risk of atherosclerosis and cardiovascular disease.

Onions also contain alkenyl cysteine sulphoxides, which give onions their distinctive taste and smell. Onion compounds have been found to help reduce the risk for cancer and asthma.

Butternut Squash Soup

Contributed by Ann Kulze, MD. "I am totally in love with butternut squash. It's a comfort food that is as good for you as it is delicious!"

3 tablespoons extra-virgin olive oil
1 large onion, chopped
3 cloves garlic, minced
1 tablespoon chopped fresh thyme leaves
3 pounds butternut squash, peeled, seeded, and cut into
    ¹/₂-inch chunks
4 cups chicken or vegetable broth (plus more, as needed)
1¹/₂ tablespoons chopped fresh sage
Salt
Black pepper
¹/₃ cup plain Greek yogurt

In a stockpot, heat the oil over medium-high heat. Add the onion and cook until softened, about 5 minutes. Add the garlic and thyme and cook for 3 minutes. Add the squash and cook, stirring frequently, until the squash begins to caramelize. Add the broth and bring to a boil. Reduce the heat to medium-low, cover, and simmer until the squash is tender, about 20 minutes. Add the sage.

Carefully transfer the soup to a blender or food processor, in batches if necessary. Remove the feed tube's cap from the center of the blender or food processor top, hold a clean towel over the hole, then puree the soup. If the soup is closer to the consistency of baby food than a smooth, creamy soup, add more broth, ¹/₄ cup at a time.

Return the soup to the pot and reheat. Season to taste with salt and pepper and serve with a dollop of yogurt.

Makes 6 (1-cup) servings
Per serving: 177 calories, 24 g carbohydrates,
4 g protein, 9 g fat, 6 g fi ber

Note: This soup allows for a lot of freedom in the kitchen. Here are some ideas for variations:

- Replace the thyme and sage with 2 tablespoons curry powder, 1/2 tablespoon minced fresh ginger, and 1/3 cup chopped cilantro, and top with yogurt and toasted cashews.
- Use coconut milk to replace half of the broth.
- Add other vegetables such as cauliflower, carrots, or sweet potatoes.
- Replace the thyme with 1 tablespoon minced fresh ginger, add 1 green apple along with the squash, and top with yogurt and cashews.

RightBites

Squash is bursting with beta-carotene, an antioxidant that helps protect you from cancer and heart disease. Your body takes beta-carotene from foods and turns it into vitamin A, but any beta-carotene that is left over serves as an antioxidant to keep cells healthy. It's important to get this key nutrient from food because beta-carotene in supplements doesn't offer the same protection and might even be harmful in high doses.

In addition to beta-carotene, winter squashes such as acorn, butternut, pumpkin, spaghetti, turban, hubbard, and delicata also provide vitamin C, iron, and fiber.

Hearty Chili

Contributed by Rallie McAllister, MD, MPH. "This chili has a lot of ingredients, but it's easy to make for dinner or a party."

2 cans (14.5 ounces each) stewed tomatoes
2 cans (6 ounces each) tomato paste
2 carrots, thinly sliced
1 white onion, chopped
2 stalks celery, chopped
¼ cup white wine
Pinch of crushed red–pepper flakes
1 green bell pepper, chopped
1 red bell pepper, chopped
⅓ cup steak sauce
5 slices bacon
1½ pounds extra-lean ground beef
1 package (1.25 ounces) chili seasoning
2 cans (15 ounces each) light red kidney beans, rinsed and drained

In a large pot, combine the tomatoes, tomato paste, carrots, onion, celery, wine, pepper flakes, green and red peppers, and steak sauce. Bring to a boil over medium-high heat, then reduce the heat to medium-low. Simmer for about 30 minutes.

Meanwhile, in a large skillet, cook the bacon until crisp. Drain and crumble. Set aside.

In the same skillet over medium heat, cook the beef in the bacon drippings, breaking it up with a wooden spoon, until the beef is cooked through, about 8 minutes. Stir in the chili seasoning. Stir the bacon and beef into the vegetables. Add the beans and cook until heated through.

Makes 6 servings
Per serving: **411 calories, 43 g carbohydrates, 37 g protein, 10 g fat, 10 g fiber**

Sa-Weet Potatoes

Contributed by Jennifer Hanes, DO. "In this yummy dish, sweet potatoes could move from merely a side dish to a healthy, delicious dessert. The flavors blend for a treat to satisfy any sweet tooth—even kiddos'! Food is medicine: The cinnamon is great to stabilize blood sugar, while the cayenne pepper helps speed metabolism. The sweet potatoes are full of vitamin A and fiber to keep you full longer."

½ cup water
2 sweet potatoes, scrubbed
¼ cup slivered almonds
½ teaspoon ground cinnamon
⅛ teaspoon cayenne pepper (optional)
1 large apple, cored and diced

Pour the water into a slow cooker and add the sweet potatoes. Cover and cook on high for 2 hours. (This technique is easy and does not require cooking the potatoes in the microwave for 20 minutes.)

When the sweet potatoes are soft, remove them from the slow cooker and allow them to cool slightly before peeling.

Meanwhile, in a small skillet over low heat, lightly toast the almonds, about 10 minutes, or until fragrant. Turn off the burner but leave them in the pan to stay warm while you prepare the rest of the dish.

Place the peeled sweet potatoes in a medium bowl and mash them with a fork or an electric mixer. As you mash them, sprinkle in the cinnamon and cayenne pepper, if using, adjusting the spices to taste.

Place the mashed potatoes on four plates and top with the diced apple and warm slivered almonds.

Makes 4 servings
Per serving: **120 calories, 21 g carbohydrates, 3 g protein, 4 g fat, 4 g fiber**

Roasted Vegetables

Contributed by Antoinette Cheney, DO. "These vegetables are especially delicious in wintertime. I like the way they make the house smell—although my husband is not a big fan of the odor of cooking broccoli."

1 small head cauliflower, cored
1 crown broccoli
2 carrots
1 onion
2 sweet potatoes, scrubbed
3 tablespoons olive oil, divided
1 teaspoon sea salt, divided
1 teaspoon Montreal Steak Seasoning (or other spice blend), divided
1 cup frozen corn kernels
1 bunch kale, inner stems removed

Preheat the oven to 350°F.

Cut all the vegetables into 1-inch chunks. Tear the kale into 1-inch pieces.

In a large bowl, toss the cauliflower, broccoli, carrots, onion, and sweet potatoes in 2 tablespoons of the oil, 3/4 teaspoon of the salt, and 3/4 teaspoon of the seasoning. Place the vegetables in a single layer on a baking sheet and roast for 25 to 30 minutes.

Meanwhile, toss the corn and kale in the remaining 1 tablespoon oil, 1/4 teaspoon salt, and 1/4 teaspoon seasoning. Midway through roasting, stir the vegetables and add the kale and corn. Continue to roast, until all the vegetables are tender and golden brown.

Makes 4 servings
Per serving: 251 calories, 36 g carbohydrates, 7 g protein, 12 g fat, 8 g fiber

Black Bean "Lasagna"

Contributed by Allison Bailey, MD. "When made with reduced-fat cheese, this is a healthy and yummy dish that the whole family enjoys. Best of all, it is super easy and quick to put together, and leftovers work well for lunches too. I like to serve this with some 'homemade' guacamole (avocado mixed with Trader Joe's fresh salsa) on the side!"

1 can (15 ounces) black beans, rinsed and drained
1 can (14 ounces) diced tomatoes
2 cups frozen corn, thawed
2 scallions, minced
½ teaspoon ground cumin
½ teaspoon dried oregano
8 corn tortillas (6" diameter)
6 ounces (1½ cups) grated reduced–fat Mexican cheese blend

Preheat the oven to 400°F.

In a medium bowl, combine the beans, tomatoes, corn, scallions, cumin, and oregano.

Line a 2-quart casserole dish or 13" x 9" baking dish with 4 of the tortillas. Spread with half of the bean mixture and half of the cheese. Repeat a layer with the remaining ingredients.

Bake for 15 to 20 minutes. Let stand for 1 to 2 minutes before serving.

Makes 4 servings
Per serving: **401 calories, 59 g carbohydrates, 19 g protein, 11 g fat, 7 g fiber**

Zesty-Zippy Barbecue Chicken

Contributed by Rallie McAllister, MD, MPH. "This is a quick and easy dish that's packed with protein and low in fat. My family loves it, and cleanup is a snap."

1 cup barbecue sauce, any flavor
4 boneless, skinless chicken breasts (6 ounces each)
1 small onion, thinly sliced
1 green pepper, thinly sliced

Preheat the oven to 350°F.

In a small mixing bowl, pour the barbecue sauce. Dip the chicken into the sauce, covering completely. Transfer the chicken into an oven browning bag. (Discard the remainder of the sauce.) Add the onion and pepper to the bag. Bake for 45 minutes, or until the chicken is cooked through.

 Makes 4 servings
Per serving: 312 calories, 28 g carbohydrates, 37 g protein, 5 g fat, 1 g fiber

Chicken Adobo

Contributed by Jennifer Bacani McKenney, MD. "This delicious recipe is from my parents' restaurant, the Bacani Plaza Grille in Fredonia, Kansas (www.bacaniplaza.com)."

8 skinless chicken thighs
$\frac{1}{2}$ cup light soy sauce
$\frac{1}{2}$ cup white vinegar
1 teaspoon minced garlic
1 teaspoon black pepper
$\frac{2}{3}$ cup uncooked white rice or brown rice (or 2 cups cooked)

Place the chicken thighs in a large pot or Dutch oven and pour the soy sauce and vinegar over them. Add the garlic and pepper. Cook over medium-low heat for about 1 hour, or until the chicken is cooked through, turning the chicken occasionally. (If the vinegar and soy sauce cook off too soon, add $\frac{1}{2}$ cup water. There should be some sauce left in the pot after the chicken is done.)

Meanwhile, prepare the rice according to the package directions.

Serve the chicken with a bit of the remaining sauce over the rice.

 Makes 4 servings
Per serving: **309 calories, 28 g carbohydrates, 31 g protein, 6 g fat, 1 g fiber**

Butternut Squash and Wild Mushroom Risotto

Contributed by Rallie McAllister, MD, MPH. "What's great about risotto is that it's rich and creamy without a hint of cream. I found this recipe on LittleJudeOnFood.com, a food blog 'written' by a toddler and his chef mother. Change up the vegetables to whatever you have on hand: Roast root vegetables or apples along with squash in the fall; in the spring, skip the roasted veggies and instead add fresh garden peas and asparagus toward the end of the risotto's cooking time."

½ medium butternut squash, peeled, seeded, and chopped into ½-inch cubes

3 tablespoons olive oil, divided

½ teaspoon salt

¼ teaspoon black pepper

8 to 12 ounces assorted wild mushrooms, cleaned and sliced

4 cups vegetable or chicken broth (preferably homemade), plus more, as needed

1 yellow onion, finely chopped

2 cloves garlic, minced

1 cup uncooked Arborio rice

½ cup dry white wine (optional)

2 cups (packed) baby spinach

2 or 3 leaves fresh sage, minced

2 tablespoons grated Parmesan cheese (wedge, not canned)

Preheat the oven to 400°F.

In a shallow roasting pan or baking sheet, toss the squash with 1 tablespoon of the oil to coat. Season with the salt and pepper and roast, stirring once, until tender and beginning to brown, for 15 to 20 minutes.

Meanwhile, in a medium skillet over medium heat, add 1 tablespoon of the oil. Sauté the mushrooms until browned. Season with additional salt and pepper to taste and remove from the heat.

In a small saucepan, bring the broth to a simmer. Reduce the heat to low to keep the broth warm.

In a large deep skillet (with sides) or Dutch oven, heat the remaining 1 tablespoon oil over medium heat. Add the onion and cook until translucent, stirring occasionally. Add the garlic and cook for 1 minute. Add the rice and stir to combine. Let the rice cook for 3 to 4 minutes, stirring occasionally to keep it from sticking and the onions from burning.

Add a ladleful of broth to the rice. (It will send up a cloud of steam!) Add the wine, if using. Cook, stirring occasionally, until the rice absorbs nearly all of the liquid but without letting the pan dry out. Add another ladleful of broth, stir, and allow the rice to absorb the liquid. Keep adding broth a ladleful at a time and allowing the rice to nearly absorb it, for about 20 minutes total.

Taste the rice. It should have an ever-so-slight bite to it when it's done. Add the reserved mushrooms and squash, the spinach, sage, and 1 more ladleful of broth. (You might not use all of the broth. If you run out, you can add water.) Stir to heat through and just wilt the spinach. Sprinkle the Parmesan over the risotto and turn off the heat. Give it all a stir and taste to adjust the seasonings.

Makes 4 servings
Per serving: 345 calories, 54 g carbohydrates, 10 g protein, 12 g fat, 5 g fiber

Chicken with Artichoke Hearts and Sun-Dried Tomatoes

Contributed by Pam D'Amato, MD. "This recipe is quick, easy, and healthy. I literally throw this together!"

2 boneless, skinless halved chicken breasts (4 half breasts)
Salt
Black pepper
1 jar (12 ounces) marinated artichoke hearts, undrained
1 jar (3 ounces) oil-packed sun-dried tomatoes, drained and chopped
8 ounces sliced white button mushrooms
1 small sweet onion, sliced
1 teaspoon garlic powder
2 teaspoons balsamic vinegar
1 teaspoon dried basil (or more, if desired)

Preheat the oven to 375°F.

In a 13" x 9" baking dish, place the chicken breasts and sprinkle with salt and pepper. Top with the artichoke hearts and a few teaspoons of the artichoke marinade. Add the tomatoes, mushrooms, onion, garlic powder, vinegar, and basil.

Cover the dish loosely with foil. Bake for 45 minutes, then uncover and bake for an additional 10 to 15 minutes.

Serve each chicken breast with the vegetables piled on top.

Makes 4 servings
Per serving: 310 calories, 13 g carbohydrates, 28 g protein, 15 g fat, 2 g fiber

Turkey Piccata

Contributed by Rallie McAllister, MD, MPH. "This turkey is delicious, but even better is the velvety, rich-tasting sauce. Serve the sauce on the side as a dipper for fewer calories. Pair it with vegetables or a salad."

4 turkey cutlets (1½ to 2 pounds)
Salt
Black pepper
½ cup whole wheat flour or gluten-free flour blend
1 tablespoon extra-virgin olive oil
2 tablespoons finely chopped shallots
½ cup white wine
⅓ cup fresh lemon juice
2 tablespoons butter
1 to 2 tablespoons chopped fresh parsley

Preheat the oven to 200°F.

In a zip-top plastic bag or between two sheets of waxed paper, pound the turkey cutlets to no less than ⅛ inch. Season with salt and pepper.

Put the flour in a shallow dish. Season with salt and pepper. Dredge the turkey in the flour, shaking off any excess. Set the turkey aside.

In a large skillet over medium-high heat, heat the oil. Brown the turkey quickly, 2 minutes on each side, or until golden brown. Remove the turkey from the skillet, set on a baking sheet, and put in the oven to keep warm.

Using the same skillet, reduce the heat to low, add the shallots and sauté for 1 to 2 minutes. Add the wine and lemon juice and simmer for 2 minutes. Add the butter. Whisk until smooth. Add the parsley, and season with salt and pepper to taste. Serve the sauce over the turkey or on the side.

Makes 4 servings
Per serving: 320 calories, 8 g carbohydrates,
43 g protein, 10 g fat, 1 g fiber

Stuffed Peppers

Contributed by Rallie McAllister, MD, MPH. "This versatile recipe comes from a toddler who 'writes' a blog with his chef mother at LittleJudeOnFood.com. They say virtually anything can be stuffed into a pepper, especially things you happen to have on hand or left over, but I like the Southwest flavors they employ here. Serve with brown rice or quinoa and a side of homemade guacamole."

1 teaspoon + 1 tablespoon olive oil
12 ounces extra-lean ground beef, ground pork, or soy crumbles
4 sturdy bell peppers (any color)
1 yellow onion, finely chopped
1 pint cherry or grape tomatoes, halved
1 teaspoon ground cumin
1 teaspoon ground coriander
Salt
Black pepper
1 ear corn, kernels removed (or ¾ cup frozen corn kernels, thawed)
1 chipotle pepper in adobo sauce, chopped

Preheat the oven to 375°F.

In a medium skillet over medium heat, heat 1 teaspoon of the oil. Add the beef, pork, or soy and cook, stirring occasionally, until just barely cooked through, about 6 minutes. (If using soy crumbles, cook until heated through.)

Meanwhile, carefully cut around the top of each pepper, right below the "shoulder," then pull out the seedy core. (Save the tops.) Pull out any remaining ribs and seeds. Set the cored peppers aside. Break off the pepper tops from the stems and roughly chop.

To the skillet, add the remaining 1 tablespoon oil, if necessary. (If you cooked beef, there might be enough fat left in the pan.) Add the chopped pepper tops, onion, tomatoes, cumin, coriander, and salt and pepper to taste. Sauté, stirring occasionally, until the pepper and onion are soft and the tomatoes have cooked down, about 8 minutes.

Add the corn and the chipotle pepper with as much adobo sauce as clings to it. Stir to heat through.

Divide the mixture among the peppers, setting them in a baking dish just big enough to hold them, such as a pie plate or 8" x 8" baking pan. Loosely tent the peppers with foil, then bake for 20 minutes. Remove the foil, then bake for another 10 minutes, or until the peppers are softened and the tops are browned.

 Makes 4 servings
Per serving: **237 calories, 18 g carbohydrates, 21 g protein, 10 g fat, 3 g fiber**

🍴◉ **Right**Bites

One of your best choices for vitamin C and carotenoids (which the body converts to vitamin A) is sweet bell peppers, especially if you choose organic peppers. A study done in Poland found that growing sweet bell peppers organically increased their antioxidant content.

Ginger-Soy Glazed Salmon

Contributed by Sonali Ruder, DO. "Salmon is the star in this recipe. Packed with heart-healthy omega-3 fatty acids, protein, and plenty of other nutrients, this dish is bound to boost your energy. I top the salmon with a ginger-soy glaze that forms a lovely sweet and savory coating. For a well-rounded meal, I serve this dish with sautéed baby bok choy and brown rice."

¼ cup low-sodium soy sauce
3 tablespoons honey
1 teaspoon Dijon mustard
½ teaspoon grated fresh ginger
¼ teaspoon Sriracha hot chili sauce or other hot sauce (optional)
2 teaspoons olive oil
4 fillets (6 ounces each) salmon
Kosher salt
Black pepper
Sliced scallions for garnish

Preheat the oven to 400°F.

In a small bowl, whisk together the soy sauce, honey, mustard, ginger, and hot sauce, if using.

In a large oven-safe skillet, heat the oil over medium-high heat. When the pan is hot, season the salmon fillets with salt and pepper and add them to the pan, presentation side down. Cook for 2 to 3 minutes without moving, or until a golden crust forms. Turn the fillets over and transfer the pan to the oven. Cook 5 to 6 minutes, until the salmon is just cooked through but still slightly pink in the middle. Carefully remove the pan from the oven and transfer the salmon to a platter.

Pour off the drippings from the pan and heat the pan on the stove over medium-high heat. Add the soy sauce mixture and cook for 2 to 3 minutes, or until thickened. Pour the glaze over the salmon. Garnish with scallions, if desired.

Makes 4 servings
Per serving: 340 calories, 14 g carbohydrates,
38 g protein, 15 g fat, 0 g fiber

🍴|**Right**Bites

Before antibiotics became the drug du jour in the 1940s, honey was the go-to remedy for treating everything from colds to constipation. Honey contains hydrogen peroxide, which can kill disease-causing bacteria. Honey might even help fight superbugs that are resistant to antibiotics.

As a topical agent, honey can be applied to wounds such as burns to help prevent infection, reduce inflammation, and heal the skin.

Of course, honey also helps fight disease when eaten. In one study conducted at the University of California, Davis, researchers discovered that people who consumed four tablespoons of honey a day for one month had higher levels of disease-fighting antioxidants in their bloodstreams. The researchers concluded that honey might protect against oxidative stress from free radicals, which contributes to Alzheimer's disease, cancer, and heart disease.

As you enjoy honey in your drinks and foods, remember that you shouldn't share honey with children younger than one year old because of the risk of botulism, which is a rare illness that can be fatal in infants.

Salmon Quesadillas

Contributed by Rallie McAllister, MD, MPH. "Salmon is a rich, tasty source of protein and beneficial omega-3 fatty acids."

4 ounces fat-free cream cheese, softened
2 tablespoons fat-free sour cream
1 teaspoon dried dillweed
6 flour tortillas (7" diameter)
4 ounces smoked salmon, flaked into very small bits
8 ounces (2 cups) grated reduced-fat Cheddar cheese

In a small bowl, combine the cream cheese, sour cream, and dill.

Spray 1 side of each tortilla with olive oil cooking spray. Place a tortilla, sprayed side down, in a large skillet. With the back of a spoon, spread with one-third of the cream cheese mixture. Add one-third of the salmon. Sprinkle with one-third of the Cheddar. Top with another tortilla, sprayed side up. Cook over medium-low heat for 2 to 3 minutes, or until the tortilla is golden brown. Turn and cook for another 2 to 3 minutes, or until the Cheddar has melted. Cut into wedges.

Repeat with the remaining ingredients.

Makes 6 servings
Per serving: 341 calories, 27 g carbohydrates,
28 g protein, 14 g fat, 1 g fiber

¡©| RightBites

Go fish! Salmon might be best known for being rich in omega-3 fatty acids, which are great for your overall health and your eyesight in particular. Research shows that getting enough omega-3 fatty acids in your diet reduces the risk of developing age-related macular degeneration, the leading cause of vision loss in older Americans.

Strawberry-Yogurt Pudding

Contributed by Ann Kulze, MD. "Dessert is a regular and revered Sunday night tradition in my home."

1 envelope (0.25 ounce) unflavored gelatin
½ cup boiling water
2 tablespoons honey
1 teaspoon orange extract
1 cup low-fat plain yogurt
½ cup pureed strawberries
2 tablespoons graham cracker crumbs

In a medium bowl, dissolve the gelatin completely in the water. Mix in the honey. Add the orange extract, yogurt, and strawberries.

Divide among 4 dessert dishes, sprinkle each with graham cracker crumbs, and chill.

Makes 4 servings
Per serving: **97 calories, 17 g carbohydrates, 5 g protein, 1 g fat, 1 g fiber**

⊙ **Right**Bites

Yogurt contains probiotics, beneficial bacteria that aid digestion and boost immunity. Probiotics might even help prevent and treat gum disease, stomach ulcers, hay fever, and colon cancer. Scientists have found that probiotics in the gut act as a metabolic "organ" that helps regulate metabolism and positively impacts diseases such as diabetes and obesity.

Oatmeal-Banana Bites

Contributed by Stacey Ann Weiland, MD. "This recipe is from my nutritionist friend, Elizabeth DiBiase, RD, at OffTheMatNutrition.com."

3 medium ripe bananas
2 cups old-fashioned rolled oats
¼ cup butter, coconut oil, or soy-free oil blend, melted
1 teaspoon vanilla extract
1 teaspoon baking powder
½ teaspoon ground cinnamon
¼ teaspoon salt
6 large dates, pitted and chopped
¼ cup finely chopped walnuts (optional)

Preheat the oven to 350°F. Line 2 baking sheets with parchment paper.

In a large bowl, mash the bananas until smooth. Add the oats; butter, oil, or oil blend; vanilla; baking powder; cinnamon; and salt and mix until well combined. Fold in the dates and nuts, if using.

Drop 2-teaspoon dollops of dough onto the prepared baking sheets. (These cookies don't spread, so press down a bit to make them the preferred shape.)

Bake for 15 minutes, or until the cookies are golden brown on the bottom. Cool on the baking sheet for 1 minute before transferring them to a wire rack to cool completely. Store in an airtight container.

Makes 40 bites
Per bite: 44 calories, 7 g carbohydrates,
1 g protein, 2 g fat, 1 g fiber

Blueberry Crumble

Contributed by Ann Kulze, MD. "This recipe leverages the natural sweetness and disease-busting power of berries so you can indulge without the guilt!"

6 cups fresh or frozen blueberries (or berries of choice)
1/4 cup granulated sugar
1 tablespoon lemon juice
2 teaspoons ground cinnamon, divided
2/3 cup whole wheat flour
1/2 cup old-fashioned rolled oats
1/2 cup packed light brown sugar
1/3 cup coarsely chopped pecans or walnuts
1/4 cup canola oil

Preheat the oven to 375°F. Coat an 8" x 8" (2-quart) baking dish with cooking spray.

In a large bowl, toss the berries with the granulated sugar, lemon juice, and 1 teaspoon of the cinnamon. Transfer to the prepared baking dish, cover with foil, and bake for 30 minutes.

Meanwhile, in a medium bowl, combine the flour, oats, brown sugar, and the remaining 1 teaspoon cinnamon. Mix to blend. Stir in the nuts and oil; toss until evenly moistened and clumpy. Remove the foil from the baking dish and scatter the topping evenly over the berries. Bake, uncovered, until the topping has browned and the fruit is soft and bubbling, about 30 minutes.

Makes 6 servings
Per serving: **361 calories, 59 g carbohydrates, 5 g protein, 15 g fat, 9 g fiber**

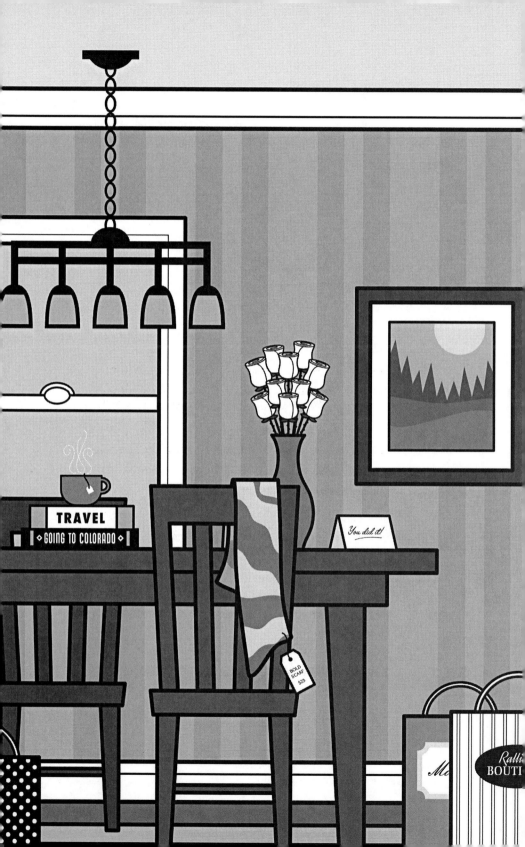

Chapter 3

Maintaining Weight

YOUR BODY

You did it! You set a goal, worked hard, and achieved it. Way to go!

You have joined a very special, elite group. The Centers for Disease Control and Prevention reports that more than 66 percent of Americans are either trying to lose weight or maintain their current weight. Despite our best efforts—and Americans spend an estimated *$42 billion* annually on weight loss foods, products, and services (yes, that's billion with a B!)—many dieters don't lose the weight. To make matters worse, just 5 percent of them manage to keep the weight off.

But *you* have gone against the grain, you've lost the weight, and now you can focus on a new goal—to maintain your new weight. We hope you can take some time to celebrate your success, and then begin the lifelong process of maintaining your weight. You deserve it!

JUSTIFICATION FOR A CELEBRATION

When you stand on that scale and the numbers reflect that goal you've been working toward, it's absolutely justification for a huge celebration!

> **If you can dream it, you can do it!**
> —*Walt Disney*

Celebrating Meeting Your Goals

How will you celebrate? One technique is to break a large goal into many smaller goals, and then celebrate meeting each one. Take some time to think about what motivates you—new clothes, pampering, cash? Then brainstorm ways to reward yourself in the most positive, motivating way that you can.

When I meet my goal, I'll celebrate by buying some new clothes because most of my pants and skirts are about to fall off.

> —*Lennox McNeary, MD, a mom of a four-year-old son, a specialist in physical medicine and rehabilitation at Carilion Clinic, and a cofounder of the Mommy Doctors Bakery (makers of Milkin' Cookies), in Roanoke, VA*

When I lost enough weight that I could fit into clothes that I had been wishing I could wear again, that was celebration enough for me!

> —*Kristin C. Lyle, MD, FAAP, a mom of 10-, 7-, and 5-year-old daughters, the disaster medical director at Arkansas Children's Hospital, and an assistant professor of pediatrics at the University of Arkansas for Medical Sciences, both in Little Rock*

When I finally lost my pregnancy weight, I went shopping to celebrate! It felt great to see a new outfit and think, *That is so cute.* And then to try it on and to think, *Oh my gosh, I feel really comfortable in this.* That's when I felt I finally had my body back!

> —*Christy Valentine, MD, a mom of a seven-year-old daughter, a specialist in pediatrics and internal medicine, and the founder of the Valentine Medical Center, in Gretna, LA*

FitBit

Watch out for "just a bite." A single French fry, a couple of potato chips, or a bite of cake all have at least 25 calories. Taking "just a bite" four or five times a day can add up.

> **The reward of a thing well done is to have done it.**
> —*Ralph Waldo Emerson*

Celebration now is being utterly present with family and friends, not food or wine. Of course, I love to celebrate with a rockin' pair of platforms, a new cashmere sweater, or hot sex with my husband. I'm blessed to have a great man whom I find wildly attractive and hysterically funny. Hurray for that.

> —*Sara Gottfried, MD, a mom of 13- and 8-year-old daughters, a board-certified gynecologist, and the author of* The Hormone Cure, *in Berkeley, CA*

I haven't celebrated my weight loss too much, but what I'm looking forward to celebrating is completing my first full marathon! That's when we'll celebrate—by going to a great restaurant here in Cincinnati. My running partner and her husband are good friends to me and my husband, and we resolved to go out on a couples' date to this great restaurant.

> —*Amy Thompson, MD, a mom of six-, four-, and two-year-old sons and an ob-gyn at the University of Cincinnati College of Medicine, in Ohio*

I've lost more than 70 pounds. Each time I hit a new size, and my clothes were too big, it was wonderful to have to go shopping again! Anytime I'd go down a size, I'd get rid of the too-big clothes. After all, I wasn't going to need them anymore!

That gets expensive, though. So I buy clothes that "shrink" with me, such as a shift dress, which is a dress that fits loosely and has elastic or an adjustable tie around the waist. Right now, I'm wearing a sweater dress that hugged my curves when I first bought it. It looked nice on me when I purchased it, but now that I've dropped a few more pounds, it's a bit looser and it looks even better. So while clothes with "give" can encourage one to overeat and indulge, if you're progressing

FitBit

Reward yourself for a job well done—without food! Give yourself a 10- to 15-minute treat of reading, listening to music, taking a relaxing bath, sitting in the sunshine, or just closing your eyes and dreaming.

downward in sizes, they can also be a great temporary "band-aid" until you reach your goal.

—*Jennifer Hanes, DO, a mom of a seven-year-old daughter and a four-year-old son, an emergency physician who's board certified in integrative medicine, and the author of* The Princess Plan: Shrink Your Waist, Expand Your Beauty, *in Austin, TX*

RALLIE'S TIP

I find it really helpful to reward myself regularly. The end result of change—weight loss in this case—is often reward enough, but sometimes, you need a little extra motivation along the way. Waiting for the numbers on the scale to change can seem to take forever, so it's nice to have some immediate gratification every once in a while.

Instead of waiting to celebrate a five-pound weight loss, I promise myself that if I walk three times a week for a month, I'll reward myself with a new pair of walking shoes. Or even a new pair of socks. If I say no to a dessert that I really, really wanted, but definitely didn't need, I might reward myself with an extra half hour of watching junk TV, when I should be answering e-mails. It's a great idea to reward yourself often, and for any positive behavior that you'd like to continue and that helps you achieve your ultimate goal.

Whenever I meet my overall weight loss goal, I reward myself by buying a pair of my favorite jeans. They're just expensive enough that I'm very motivated to maintain my weight loss so I can wear them for a long time. And every time I put them on, I remember that they have a special meaning for me. They symbolize my success. Wearing them helps remind me to keep doing the things I need to do to maintain a healthy weight.

Finally, when you're choosing your reward, make sure it's something that supports your new behavior. Don't reward yourself for eating more fruits and vegetables by buying yourself a giant cookie cake!

Maintaining Your Weight

Now that you've reached your goal and celebrated your achievement, you need to stick with the healthy habits that helped you to lose weight, so you don't gain it all back.

When researchers examined data from studies involving more than 14,000 people who lost weight and kept it off for at least a year, they found that only one in six maintained a weight loss of 10 percent or more. Is it just us, or is that not terribly encouraging?

More encouraging was a study that found that exercising for 80 minutes a week—that's just 11 minutes a day—after losing weight helped people avoid regaining the weight and kept belly fat off.

We love to focus on success, and who better to learn from than the people who joined the National Weight Control Registry. That organization was founded in 1994 to study more than 4,000 adults who have lost at least 30 pounds and kept the weight off for at least a year. The scientists recruit through newspaper and magazine articles, and weight loss winners enroll themselves. They're asked a battery of questions about how they lost the weight, and how they keep it off.

Not surprisingly, 89 percent of the folks said they lost weight using both dietary changes and exercise. They identified four "secrets" to maintaining their weight:

• They followed a low-calorie, low-fat diet.
• They exercised frequently.
• They weighed themselves regularly.
• They ate breakfast each day.

That's it: No magic lotion or potion. Just simple, healthy living. You can do it, too!

For me, it's important not to fall off the wagon, or at least not to wait too long before I get back *on* the wagon. For example, on Thanksgiving, I might eat whatever I want. But the next day, I get back to eating normally again. I try not to let holidays become holi*weeks*.

—*Michelle Spring, MD, a mom of a one-year-old son and two grown stepchildren and a board-certified plastic surgeon with Marina Plastic Surgery Associates, in Marina del Rey, CA*

Maintaining my weight is a work in progress. It can be as hard as losing weight. As I've gotten older, I'm more aware of which habits do me in: Picking at food and thoughtlessly getting seconds are the worst. Maintenance is all about not retreating to old habits.

—*Amy Baxter, MD, a mom of 15- and 12-year-old sons and a 10-year-old daughter; the CEO of Buzzy4Shots.com; and the director of emergency research, Scottish Rite, of Children's Healthcare of Atlanta, in Georgia*

Mommy MD Guides–Recommended Product
Yamax Digi SW200 Pedometer

"To maintain my weight, I aim to be active every day," says Jennifer A. Gardner, MD, a mom of a three-year-old son, a pediatrician, and the founder of an online child wellness and weight management company, HealthyKidsCompany.com, in Washington, DC. "I wear a simple, accurate, and inexpensive pedometer called the Yamax Digi SW200. My goal is to take 10,000 steps six days a week. My pedometer is really indispensable for my weight maintenance. I notice that when I stop wearing it, my activity goes down. It keeps me motivated by visually displaying how active I have been."

You can buy a Yamax Digi SW200 pedometer in stores and from online retailers such as **AMAZON.COM** for around $28.

Maintaining your goal weight can be every bit as hard as losing weight. I try to stick to a low-carb, high-protein diet as much as I can. When I stray from that and regain some weight, I kick my own butt.

Here you go again, I think. Back to square one.

Then I get back to eating my low-carb, high-protein diet again.

—*Judith Hellman, MD, a mom of a 15-year-old son, an associate clinical professor of dermatology at Mt. Sinai Hospital in New York City, and a dermatologist in private practice*

To maintain my goal weight, I try to eat whole grain, carbohydrate-rich foods, such as whole grain pasta and bread. I also limit myself to one serving of carbohydrate-rich foods per meal, such as one slice of bread or one cup of pasta.

—*Bola Oyeyipo-Ajumobi, MD, a mom of five- and two-year-old sons, a family physician at the Veterans Health Administration, and the owner of SlimyBookWorm.com, in San Antonio, TX*

To maintain my weight, I eat whole and organic foods as much as I can. I try to be conscious of what I am eating. Most importantly, I eat when I'm hungry, and I stop eating when I'm full. It's simple—and effective.

—*Kay Corpus, MD, a mom of a six-year-old daughter and a two-year-old son, a family physician, and the director of Owensboro Health Integrative Medicine, in Kentucky*

To maintain my weight, it helps a lot that I'm on my feet all day, seeing patients. I burn a lot of calories standing up and walking around the office all day!

I try not to undo all of that by eating healthy too. When I make food at home, I bake or grill foods, rather than frying them. I also bring healthy snacks to work, such as Greek yogurt and granola bars.

—*Jennifer Bacani McKenney, MD, a mom of a two-year-old daughter who's expecting another baby and a family physician, in Fredonia, KS*

I try to make fruit, vegetables, and protein-rich foods part of every meal. I'm also careful to eat enough at each meal so that I don't end up snacking on junk between meals or at night. I avoid anything with "lite" on the label. That just means the oil and fat have been replaced with carbohydrates. Oil is good! It keeps you full until the next meal. I use a huge amount of olive oil every day when I cook. I still wear clothes that I made myself in the 1970s. I owe it to olive oil and vegetables!

—*Elizabeth Berger, MD, a mom of a 30-year-old son and a 29-year-old daughter, a child psychiatrist, and the author of* Raising Kids with Character, *in New York City*

To maintain my weight, I eat a big breakfast, a meaningful lunch, and a small dinner each day. My family eats dinner together, and even though I cook foods with protein and starch, I don't eat much of them. I eat mainly vegetables. After dinner, I consider the kitchen to be closed. I usually don't eat anything in the four hours before bedtime.

—*Deborah Gilboa, MD, a mom of 11-, 9-, 7-, and 5-year-old sons, a family physician with Squirrel Hill Health Center in Pittsburgh, PA, and a parenting speaker whose advice is found at AskDoctorG.com*

Maintaining my weight is something I do consciously. It doesn't just happen, no matter whether I'm trying to keep 5 pounds off or 40 pounds off. So routine definitely plays a role here.

I don't put pressure on myself by weighing myself every day. When I used to do that, I got discouraged as my weight fluctuated day to day. So instead of using my scale as my weight police, I took out a pair of my favorite fitted jeans—the ones that I worked so hard to fit into! I wear these jeans once a week no matter what, especially on days I feel bloated from eating too much the night before.

Once I get these jeans on, they let me know, "yup, fitting me just right" or "no, things are getting snug." This way I catch myself before I put on too much weight without the stress of a number on the scale.

—*Arleen K. Lamba, MD, a mom of a three-month-old son, an anesthesiologist, the medical director of Blush Med Institute, and founder of the Blush Blends Skin Care line, in Washington, DC*

> **You may have to fight a battle more than once to win.**
> —*Margaret Thatcher*

One thing that is critical for weight control is to never skip breakfast! I'm not hungry at breakfast, but I eat it anyway. This morning, I stirred some thawed mixed berries into a dollop of 0% plain Greek yogurt and spread it on a healthy homemade bran muffin sprinkled with cinnamon and drizzled with a little molasses. It was delicious!

Also, I'm practically addicted to hot sauce. It triggers the release of endorphins and offers a subtle metabolic boost. It's not a lot, but every little bit helps. I check labels carefully because some hot sauces are high in sodium. I buy classic Tabasco.

—Ann Kulze, MD, a mom of 24- and 17-year-old daughters and 22- and 21-year-old sons; a nationally recognized nutrition expert, motivational speaker, and physician; and the author of the best-selling, award-winning Eat Right for Life *book series, in Charleston, SC*

I try to center my diet on fruits and vegetables. I don't like to buy imported fruits out of season, such as strawberries from South America, because I'm not sure about the pesticides they use and I feel like it has an enormous carbon footprint.

Instead, I buy a lot of frozen fruits and vegetables. They're always "in season." I buy frozen strawberries and blueberries, and I simply thaw them. I like to sprinkle a packet of powdered ranch dressing on frozen vegetables before cooking them as directed on the package. They're delicious!

—Lisa Campanella-Coppo, MD, a mom of a three-year-old daughter and an emergency physician with EMCARE and the Meridian Health System, in Monmouth, NJ

I find it very hard to maintain my weight loss. My husband and I enjoy eating delicious dinners with a glass of wine. Although I splurge on the

FitBit

weekends, it helps to have soup and a salad for dinner at least one night a week.

We like lentil soup or Mexican three-bean soup served with a grilled chicken salad and honey mustard dressing. Another lighter meal we enjoy is vegetarian chili. It's delicious, and it fills me up for hours.

—*Shilpa Amin-Shah, MD, a mom of a three-year-old son and a two-year-old daughter and an emergency physician and director of the recruiting team at Emergency Medical Associates, in Livingston, NJ*

As I got older, I realized that it's a myth that you can eat whatever's in sight and remain slim. Most of the people who are thin at 40, 50, and 60 watch what they eat. Svelte celebrities might create an aura of "I eat so much," but for most of us—and for most of them—it's just not true. As you age, it becomes harder and harder to maintain your weight.

I took the time to study what foods have more calories and what foods have fewer, what foods fill me up more, and what foods don't satisfy me. My go-to foods: veggies and fruit! They are great for improving your health and making your skin glow. They're also very filling and satisfying, but they have a very low caloric density. The best strategy to maintaining my weight is simply watching what I eat—all of the time. By now it's such a habit that I don't even notice that I'm doing it.

—*Ayala Laufer-Cahana, MD, a mom of 17- and 15-year-old sons and a 14-year-old daughter, a pediatrician, and the founder of Herbal Water Inc., in Wynnewood, PA*

I'm bad at following rules, so diets are very difficult for me. But the way that I've been able to maintain my weight and feel good is that I've always exercised. I haven't always taken formal exercise classes, but I'm a physical person and I don't sit still. When I'm talking on the phone, I walk around. I think our bodies and our brains need physicality. You can't be a happy person if you're sedentary.

I exercise because I want to be able to eat my favorite chocolate-covered doughnuts and to keep up with my kids and grandkids. It's the pits when your grandkids are able to outrun you!

—*Hana R. Solomon, MD, a mom who raised four children, a grandmom of three, a board-certified pediatrician, the president of BeWell Health, LLC, and the author of* Clearing the Air One Nose at a Time: Caring for Your Personal Filter, *in Columbia, MO*

Maintaining my weight has been part of my job description as a wellness educator for the past 17 years! For me, the key to maintaining weight is lifelong adherence to eating a healthy diet. What you eat has far more impact on what you weigh than how much you exercise.

A good guideline for me is limiting what I eat at any meal to what fits into my two hands cupped together—minus the fruits and non-starchy vegetables. I can eat as many of those as I want!

I'm also militant about avoiding the "great white hazards": white flour, white rice, white potatoes, white sugar, and sweets. Instead of dessert, I have a prudent portion of dark chocolate, which has loads of antioxidants but is very low in sugar.

—*Ann Kulze, MD*

I gained 70 pounds during my pregnancy. For me, breastfeeding was a terrific way to lose the weight, and it was a great bonding experience for me and my baby to boot. I was back to my normal weight within six months. But that's when the real challenge began.

For the first few years of my daughter's life, my eating and weight goals for her and my eating and weight goals for me were at opposite ends of the spectrum. My daughter needed to gain weight, me not so much.

I realized that it didn't make sense for me to eat the same meals as my daughter ate. Our meals instead overlap. For instance, I prepare a steak, a pork chop, or a chicken breast with a starchy food such as potatoes or rice for my daughter, and I make a big salad for me. I put a bit of salad on my daughter's plate, and I put a bit of meat and starch on mine. Yes, it might be easier to eat the same foods we prepare for our children, but I think it's essential not to.

In other cultures, a lot of traditional meals evolved in order to feed large families at different stages of their lives. Mexican meals are a great example. They include meat, beans, tortillas, and lettuce and other greens, and family members eat different combinations and amounts of foods, all at the same time. We've lost that in our culture.

—Dora Calott Wang, MD, a mom of a 10-year-old daughter, historian at the University of New Mexico School of Medicine, a unit director at Las Encinas Hospital in Pasadena, CA, and the author of The Kitchen Shrink: A Psychiatrist's Reflection on Healing in a Changing World

To maintain my weight, I try to eat out—and that includes "takeout"—fewer than three times a week, including breakfast, lunch, and dinner. I usually cook dinner at home five or six days each week.

I struggle with eating breakfast because I'm not often hungry in the morning. But I make eating breakfast a priority because I know that breakfast really is the most important meal of the day, and it stabilizes my blood sugar and leaves me less hungry later in the day.

I allow myself a small daily indulgence—usually dessert—because I believe that self-restriction inevitably leads to failure.

—Jennifer A. Gardner, MD, a mom of a three-year-old son, a pediatrician, and the founder of an online child wellness and weight management company, HealthyKidsCompany.com, in Washington, DC

A major challenge to maintaining my weight is what I call the "witching hour." It's that time after my sons are in bed, when I sit down to

Mommy MD Guides–Recommended Product
The Fresh 20

"After I changed my activity level, the other big part of my weight loss journey was changing my diet," says Lennox McNeary, MD, a mom of a four-year-old son, a specialist in physical medicine and rehabilitation at Carilion Clinic, and a cofounder of the Mommy Doctors Bakery (makers of Milkin' Cookies), in Roanoke, VA. "I know *how* to cook healthy, but figuring out what to cook each night was emotionally exhausting for me.

"A friend introduced me to the Fresh 20, which is a fabulous online meal-planning guide. I grocery shop on the weekend and then do most of my meal prep on Saturday or Sunday. I can have a good, healthy meal on the table in 10 to 20 minutes most nights, and I have healthy leftovers for lunch the next day. My husband lost a ridiculous amount of weight the first two weeks we did it, and it's definitely keeping our weights where they need to be. As a bonus, we're spending a lot less money on food, and we're wasting less too."

The Fresh 20 is online at **THEFRESH20.COM**. It's a subscription system, and you sign up for a membership. It costs $5 per month, billed at five-month increments. You receive weekly dinner menus, which are posted each Friday evening, so you can shop and organize and even do a lot of the cooking over the weekend and you don't have to worry about what's for dinner! The weekly menus feature complete meals with sides, a variety of cuisines to eliminate dinner boredom, seasonal ingredients, weekly prep guides to help you get organized, and balanced nutrition. They also have vegetarian and gluten-free menus.

Each week you also get shopping lists that are organized by category to make shopping easier. The lists include cost estimates to help with budgeting.

watch TV. No one sits on the couch watching *CSI* eating a bowl of broccoli!

To combat this, I plan out my meals and snacks each day. If I'm going to have a snack, I'm intentional about it. I consider what I've eaten so far, and then if I decide it's okay to have a treat, such as buttered popcorn, I do it. But it's not an every-night occurrence.

The trick to this is keeping my hands and my mind busy! I get the same buzz from scrapbooking, reading a good book, or checking out social media that I do from watching TV and eating a snack. And if my hands are busy scrapbooking or texting, I don't want to get them messy by eating a snack.

Losing myself in an activity, and losing all track of time, is the best way to distract myself from eating. When I'm doing those things, I don't feel hungry at all.

—*Deborah Gilboa, MD*

To maintain my weight, I have a list of superstar foods that I eat practically each and every day of my life. These foods include nuts and other high-quality protein foods, dark chocolate, dark leafy greens, berries, avocados, extra-virgin olive oil, and freshly brewed green tea.

FitBit

Snacking in front of the television leads to overeating. Researchers at the Smell and Taste Treatment and Research Foundation in Chicago found that when adults were given potato chips and asked to watch TV, they ate 42 percent more than when they were given potato chips and asked to sit in a quiet room.

Turning off your TV promotes weight loss. According to another study, this one published in the *American Journal of Public Health*, adults who watch television for three or more hours per day are significantly more likely to be overweight than those who watch for less than an hour per day.

I also eat a massive amount of whole plant foods—at least seven servings a day. I achieve that by eating a lot of salads and fruits or vegetables for snacks.

I'm also always striving to improve my diet. Right now, I'm working to incorporate more oily fish into my diet. It's a great source of the precious omega-3 fatty acids that are so important for heart health and to slow the aging process. I enjoy fresh salmon, but canned sockeye salmon is great too. I make a Quick Salmon Salad using canned salmon. (See the recipe on page 194.)

—*Ann Kulze, MD*

❧

I use a log to keep my weight on track. In the good old days, I wrote down what I ate in a notebook. Now I use a free app called FitDay. It lets me log my calories, daily activities, and even mood. The app has a search feature that I can use to look up foods, such as a blueberry muffin. It might not be 100 percent accurate, but it's close enough.

I think logging is beneficial for two reasons: It encourages me to think about what I'm eating and to set goals, and then it makes me write down what I actually ate.

I also monitor my weight pretty closely. I am a compulsive weigher; I weigh myself daily and adjust my calorie intake (a little) based on my daily weight. Like almost everyone, my weight goes up and down a few pounds from day to day. Right now, I'm not actively dieting. Everyone needs a break now and then. But I do have a calorie range I know I need to stay within to maintain my weight. If I see my weight creeping up, I'll get more serious about logging what I eat until my weight settles back down again.

—*Susan Besser, MD, a mom of six grown children, ages 28, 26, 24, 22, 21, and 19, a grandmom of two, a family physician, and the medical director of Doctors Express-Memphis, in Tennessee*

❧

A key to losing weight and keeping it off is having some easy, go-to snacks. Here are some of my favorite treats that have helped me maintain my 70-pound weight loss. They are easy to prepare, easy on the wallet, and even easier on the waistline. The best part is that they are so scrumptious, even my children like them.

Apple sandwich: Simply peel and slice the apple into thin sections and spread with peanut butter. This tastes so much better than simply putting peanut butter on apple slices because the peel is typically the bitter part of the fruit. Removing the skin results in a much sweeter crunch.

Kickin' sweet potato: Put your spuds in a slow cooker on high for a couple of hours (or if you poke holes with a fork, you can cook them in the microwave). When the potato is cooked, simply sprinkle with cinnamon and cayenne pepper. The taste is so rich, there is really no need for butter or sugar. Bonus: The cinnamon and cayenne pepper both are friendly to your metabolism and can help remove those unwanted pounds.

Avocado: So simple. Slice the avocado and add a squeeze of fresh lime juice and a pinch of salt. So creamy. The citrus and salt complement the healthy fats perfectly. These babies are bursting with vitamins and make a great snack after a hot yoga class to replace those lost electrolytes, sodium, and potassium.

Enjoy these tasty treats, knowing they will help you reach your size for success!

—*Jennifer Hanes, DO*

RALLIE'S TIP

Going to med school was one of the very worst things that ever happened to my weight. It wasn't just the long hours, the lack of sleep, the steady stream of sugary coffee and sodas, the bad food, or the stress. It was the scrub suits! Those big, roomy pants with the expanding drawstring waistbands allow you to grow, and grow, and grow, without ever even noticing!

After a couple of weeks of wearing nothing but scrub suits, I was shocked when I tried to squeeze back into a pair of my jeans. I couldn't even get the zipper halfway up!

After med school, I vowed that I would never again wear pants without a zipper and a snap on a regular basis. It's just too easy to gain weight without noticing unless you get feedback from snaps and zippers. Wearing jeans helps me maintain my weight. Like most women, I've got my skinny jeans, my acceptable-weight jeans, and my danger-zone fat jeans.

Whenever my fat jeans start getting a little tight, alarms start going off in my head. I know it's time to get serious about eating better and exercising more often. If I ever outgrow my fat jeans, I'll have no choice but to wear expanding scrub suits again!

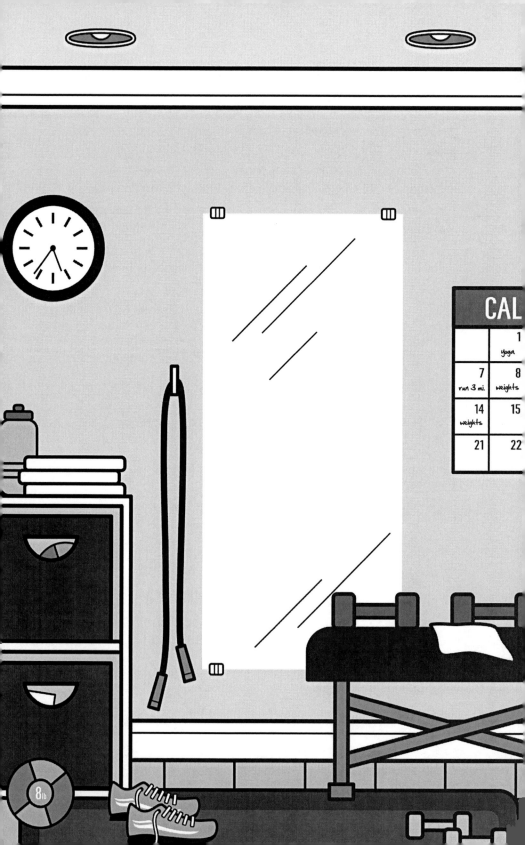

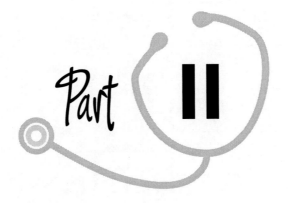

Part II

FEELING GREAT

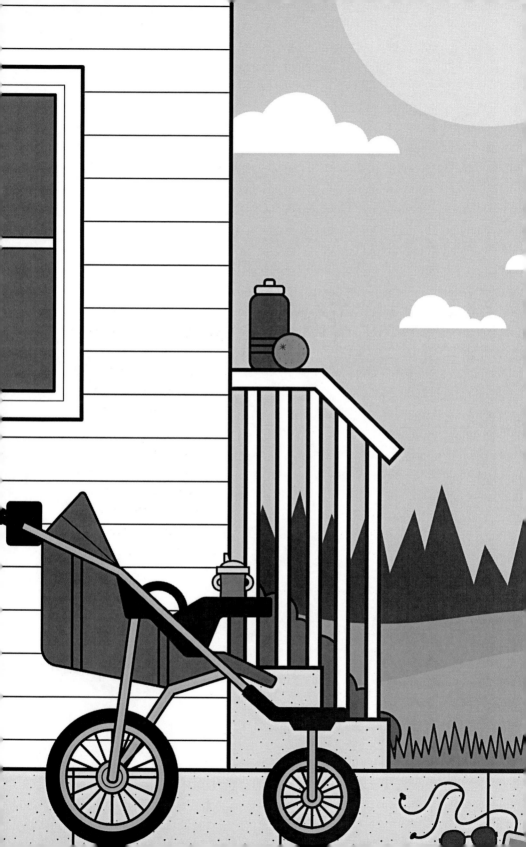

Chapter 4
Boosting Your Energy

YOUR BODY

Has your get up and go got up and left? You have lots of company. The Centers for Disease Control and Prevention in Atlanta asked people, "In the past 3 months, how often did you feel very tired or exhausted: never, some days, most days, or every day?"

More women than men said they felt very tired or exhausted most days or every day. Women ages 18 to 44 were almost twice as likely as men to feel wiped out: 16 percent versus 9 percent.

The reality is most of us feel tired a good deal of the time. In our overscheduled, 24/7, hurry-scurry lives, sleep is hard to come by. But not getting enough sleep can have serious consequences, including increased risk for accidents, impaired thinking and learning, increased risk of health problems, and decreased sex drive. All of these are good reasons to sleep better—tonight.

JUSTIFICATION FOR A CELEBRATION

Unlike the numbers on a scale and the size of your jeans, it's hard to measure how energetic you feel. When you feel the energy to scoop up your child, to run to greet a friend, to throw your arms up in celebration, and to laugh deep from your belly, those are all great reasons to celebrate—and to smile!

> **Energy and persistence conquer all things.**
> —*Benjamin Franklin*

Assessing Your Energy Levels

Before you set out to change something, such as increasing your energy, it helps to take stock of where you stand. Do you have energy to burn? Or are you too pooped to pop? Once you know where you are, it's a whole lot easier to get where you want to go.

Here's a simple quiz to gauge your energy levels. Weight loss expert and author of *The 7 Day Energy Surge* Jim Karas created this quiz. It's reprinted by permission of Rodale Inc.

I listen to music: ☐
   1 = Almost never
   2 = Sometimes when I am in my car
   3 = On the weekends when I am working around the house and remember to put something on
   4 = Most nights when I get home from work/my day with the kids and need to relax
   5 = All the time: in the morning, when I work out, at my office or computer, and at night, when it's time to wind down

My stress levels are: ☐
   1 = Out of control, because I live in a state of overwhelming stress
   2 = Pretty high during the week but somewhat better on the weekends
   3 = Up and down, depending on the day and the situation
   4 = Generally good, with an occasional dip due to family, work, relationships, kids, or illnesses, either my own or affecting someone I care a great deal about
   5 = Under complete control, because I know the warning signs when I am getting overly stressed up and have the coping skills to alleviate it

My overall mind-set is: ☐
   1 = Negative. I dwell far too much on the past.
   2 = Generally down, but I do try to minimize past failures
   3 = Okay. I have good and bad days, and they balance out in the long run.

4 = Upbeat, because I can usually talk myself out of a death spiral and try to live and look at the glass as half full rather than half empty

5 = Very up and people comment that my positive attitude makes me fun to be around

My sleeping habits are: ☐

1 = Terrible. I only sleep 4 or 5 hours a night and get up and go to bed at all different times.

2 = Pretty bad. I only sleep 5 or 6 hours a night and frequently awaken in the middle of the night.

3 = Okay. I sleep between 6 and 7 hours a night, but I almost always wish I had another hour in the morning to sleep. I have to use an alarm clock and hit the snooze button repeatedly. I also frequently try to catch up on sleep on the weekend.

4 = Better. I sleep between 7 and 8 hours five nights a week and around 6 or 7 the other two. I only use an alarm about 50 percent of the time.

5 = Great. I sleep between 7 and 8 hours every night, and I always go to bed and get up within the same 30-minute time period. I rarely, if ever, have to use an alarm.

My breathing habits are: ☐

1 = I'm barely breathing, because my chest and diaphragm hardly move and I never think about it.

2 = I breathe shallowly, but every now and then I sigh or yawn.

3 = My chest and shoulders slightly go up with each breath, and every now and then I try to take a few deeper breaths.

4 = With each breath, my chest expands and occasionally my belly fills. Every hour or so I check in with my breath.

5 = With each breath, my belly fills up with air that flows in my lungs and I am mindful and present.

My exercise habits are: ☐

    1 = Terrible. I haven't exercised consistently in years.

    2 = I try to walk most places, but don't usually do it except on the weekends.

    3 = I walk to and from my bus stop/train station/office every day and do a workout in my home or gym about once a week.

    4 = I get in two 45-minute workouts a week and meet a friend to walk an hour every Saturday.

    5 = I consistently get in three or four 30-minute workouts a week and do a combination of strength training and aerobics.

My drinking habits are: ☐

    1 = Terrible, because I am not drinking water and drink too much coffee, juice, soda, sports drinks, and alcohol.

    2 = Not so, so bad, but I don't drink more than two glasses of water, and I drink more than five cups of coffee a day.

    3 = Somewhat routine, because I do fill my 32-ounce water bottle once a day (and finish it) and have cut back on drinking wine, with the exception of weekends.

    4 = Much better, because I limit myself to two cups of coffee a day, more tea, less alcohol, and at least 50 ounces of water a day.

    5 = Really good, because I only have one cup of coffee first thing in the morning and drink more tea and at least 75 to 80 ounces of water a day. I've also cut my alcohol down to four total glasses of wine a week.

My eating habits are: ☐

    1 = Terrible. I just can't stop overeating all the time.

    2 = Good during the day but not so good on evenings and weekends.

    3 = About the same as they have been for a long time, up and down. I just can't get in a healthy and consistent routine for more than a day or two.

4 = Better than they have been in a long time, because I am making more careful choices and have eliminated a lot of junk.

5 = I'm making very good choices and can feel the difference in my weight and my energy levels.

My body weight is: ☐

1 = Terrible. I have gained a lot of weight and have kept it on

2 = Pretty bad. I struggle and can't stop losing and gaining the same weight.

3 = What it has been for a long time, higher than I want but not horrible

4 = I recently started a weight loss plan and have taken off several pounds.

5 = Pretty close to my ideal weight

I wake up every morning feeling: ☐

1 = Awful

2 = That I need another hour of sleep, at least

3 = Pretty much the same, not rested but not wiped out

4 = Ready to start the day with a cup of coffee

5 = Energized

I have sex with a partner: ☐

1 = Almost never

2 = Once every two weeks

3 = Once every week

4 = Two or three times a week

5 = More than four times a week

Tally up your scores, which will place you in one of the following three categories.

Low energy = 0 to 20
Moderate energy = 21 to 39
High energy = 40 to 60

I'm a very high-energy person. I have to juggle to balance everything that I need to do. In addition to work, I enjoy spending time with my family, traveling, and cooking. Without a great deal of energy, none of that is going to happen!

—*Pam D'Amato, MD, a mom of seven- and four-year-old daughters and an interventional pain management physician with University Spine Center, in Wayne, NJ*

I have a lot of energy. I think that's because I realize that any day could be my last day. I have survived cancer, and I understand how very blessed I am to be here this moment.

—*Hana R. Solomon, MD, a mom who raised four children, a grandmom of three, a board-certified pediatrician, the president of BeWell Health, LLC, and the author of* Clearing the Air One Nose at a Time: Caring for Your Personal Filter, *in Columbia, MO*

 When to Call Your Doctor

Low energy might seem par for the course when you have kids. However, persistent fatigue can be a sign of a medical condition, such as a thyroid problem that sometimes develops after giving birth and continues for months or even indefinitely without treatment. Depression, which is very common among new mothers, can also lower your energy levels. Or fatigue could point to a vitamin deficiency, sleep disorder, disease, or chronic infection. It could also be a side effect of a medication you're taking.

Eating more healthfully and exercising should lead to higher energy levels, not lower. If you're feeling run-down or you have a lack of motivation, make an appointment and talk about it with your doctor. In the meantime, pay attention to your energy levels—even keep a log. Identifying a pattern of fatigue—for example, maybe you feel energized in the morning but become tired easily once you're active—will help your doctor determine the cause.

> **Passion is energy. Feel the power that comes from focusing on what excites you.**
> **—*Oprah Winfrey***

I am an extremely high-energy person. I think I'm wired that way. I was a high-energy person from the get-go. My energy levels serve me well professionally and personally. It sustains me when I work long hours or run marathons.

> —*Nancy Rappaport, MD, a mom of 22- and 18-year-old daughters and a 20-year-old son, an associate professor of psychiatry at Harvard Medical School, an attending child and adolescent psychiatrist in the Cambridge, MA, public schools, and the author of* The Behavior Code

I'm both a high-energy and a low-key person! I'm generally calm and mellow, but at the same time, I like to do things and keep busy. I feel it's important to have downtime. I make a point to have an hour "off" each day when I get home from work to relax and de-stress.

> —*Debra Luftman, MD, a mom of a 22-year-old daughter and a 19-year-old son, a board-certified dermatologist in private practice, coauthor of* The Beauty Prescription, *developer of the skincare line of products Therapeutix, and a clinical instructor of skin surgery and general dermatology at UCLA*

I'm a "normal," go-with-the-flow type of person. I'm not the type of person who jumps out of bed and races out of the house to go to the gym. This understanding of my energy levels is helpful to me because I know that I have to schedule my gym time into my week, otherwise it will not happen.

> —*Jeannette Gonzalez Simon, MD, a mom of four- and one-year-old daughters and a pediatric gastroenterologist at Staten Island Pediatrics GI, in New York*

FitBit

Want to boost your energy instantly? Make a big lion-size yawn. It's nature's wake-up call!

I've come to realize that my mood, my energy levels, and my self-esteem are all intertwined. When I have more energy, I am more productive, and this boosts my mood and my self-esteem. I'm a real stickler about getting enough sleep because it's so critical to my energy, mood, and self-esteem. When I'm overtired, I feel very vulnerable.

—*Allison Bailey, MD, a mom of a nine-year-old son and a five-year-old daughter and founder and director of Integrated Health and Fitness Associates, in Cambridge, MA*

I think that energy, like happiness, has to do with your baseline levels of neurotransmitters in the brain. I've always had high energy levels. I think some of it has to do with my optimistic outlook on life, and some of it has to do with my propensity to bite off more than I can chew, which then forces me to deliver. I think people need to look at themselves and figure out how much activity they need to be happy. For example, I know that I don't do leisure well.

—*Amy Baxter, MD, a mom of 15- and 12-year-old sons and a 10-year-old daughter; the CEO of Buzzy4Shots.com; and the director of emergency research, Scottish Rite, of Children's Healthcare of Atlanta, in Georgia*

I'm blessed to be a high-energy person. I think that knowing your natural energy levels is very important. It's also helpful to know the time of day when you're most energetic. For instance, I know that I can't write at night because I have less energy in the evenings. If I try to write at night, it's total garbage! I do my best writing after breakfast.

—*Deborah Gilboa, MD, a mom of 11-, 9-, 7-, and 5-year-old sons, a family physician with Squirrel Hill Health Center in Pittsburgh, PA, and a parenting speaker whose advice is found at AskDoctorG.com*

RALLIE'S TIP

For most of my life, I've been bursting with energy. As a child, I'm sure it was a symptom of attention deficit/hyperactivity disorder, and it got me in a lot of trouble. As a young adult, I finally learned to channel my energy so that I could stop spinning in circles and start being more productive.

At a couple of points in my life, I found that I was drained and exhausted, and I couldn't accomplish as much as I was accustomed to, which in turn depressed me. That triggered a bit of a vicious cycle. On both occasions, there was a valid physical reason for my drastic drop in energy. Once was after I had two babies in two years while finishing my medical residency, and I became a bit anemic. The other was when I discovered I had developed hypothyroidism, or low levels of thyroid hormones.

Women who experience sudden—or even gradual—but significant changes in their normal energy levels shouldn't attribute it to aging, or think that it's all in their heads. It's really important to schedule an appointment with your physician to make sure there's not something serious causing the problem. It could be an infection, a metabolic disorder, or anemia.

Now I pay close attention to my energy levels, and I don't take it for granted. I try to nourish my body with all the nutrients, sleep, exercise, and water it needs for good health. If I notice that I'm feeling inexplicably tired or drained, I'll take a day or two to rest, relax, and take better care of myself. If I don't bounce back within a week or so, I make an appointment with my physician to make sure there's nothing serious going on.

Making Time for Yourself

You have 1,440 minutes in every day. Granted, you're probably sleeping about 480 of them. Still, that leaves you with almost 1,000 minutes of each and every day. No doubt you spend plenty of those minutes helping your children, your spouse, your boss, your friends, strangers in line at the grocery store, and others. But how many of those minutes do you use for yourself? Why not wrestle back some of those precious minutes for *you*?

I get up at 6:00 am so I can wake my kids up at 6:30. This gives me a little time for myself. I use that time to take a shower, get dressed, and do my hair.

> —*Heather Orman-Lubell, MD, a mom of 12- and 8-year-old sons and a pediatrician in private practice at Yardley Pediatrics of St. Christopher's Hospital for Children, in Pennsylvania*

My husband and my mother-in-law watch my son for me for a few hours every week. This way I can get a pedicure or massage or just

Mommy MD Guides–Recommended Product
DuraTowel

With kids, careers, and all of the chaos that ensues, who has time to deep clean, let alone spring clean? The key is to keep up with the little messes and prevent them from becoming big messes, which take even longer to clean up. Plus, catching a cold or flu can really throw a family's schedule into a tailspin. Who has time for *that*? It's important to clean surfaces completely to get rid of any germs.

"My life is super messy! My Great Dane can counter-surf without even trying, and my kids leave a stream of crumbs and spills behind them," says Sigrid Payne DaVeiga, MD, a mom of a seven-year-old son and a two-year-old daughter and a pediatric allergist with the Children's Hospital of Philadelphia, in Pennsylvania. "I am a complete nut about wiping my countertops. I also cannot stand the way my dish towels feel damp even when I hang them out to dry between uses. I bleach-wipe my counters at least once or twice daily, which is why I was shocked when I used a dampened DuraTowel on my soapstone countertop. There was a layer of dusty residue on the DuraTowel—as if my countertops hadn't been previously cleaned. It was awesome!

enjoy some time to myself so I don't feel exhausted all of the time.

—*Edna Ma, MD, a mom of a six-month-old son, an anesthesiologist at UCLA Olive View Medical Center, and the founder of BareEase pre-waxing numbing kit, in Los Angeles, CA*

Exercise is a great outlet for me, but my husband and my kids understand that about one night a week, I need to take a break for an hour or two. I usually go to the mall for some "retail therapy" or get a mani-pedi.

—*Martha Wittenberg, MD, MPH, a mom of an eight-year-old son and a six-year-old daughter and a family physician with Seal Beach Family Medicine, in California*

"DuraTowel is super-absorbent, has a really nice texture, and cleans up every spill in my kitchen," Dr. DaVeiga adds. "Plus, it actually left a super-nice look to the counter after it was wiped! Soapstone is strange in that it marks up so easily with cup rings and stains, and the DuraTowel smoothed all of that off!"

"I like using DuraTowel because it's really sturdy, and I can always count on it to work as hard as I do," adds Rallie McAllister, MD, MPH, a mom of three sons, a family physician, and the coauthor of *The Mommy MD Guide to the Toddler Years*, in Lexington, KY. "I get a lot of use out of each sheet, which appeals to my frugal nature. I can clean my kitchen counters with one DuraTowel—instead of five or six flimsy paper towels. I love knowing that I'm really cleaning my kitchen; I'm not just spreading germs from surface to surface with a dishcloth."

You can buy Bounty DuraTowel for $3.19 at food and grocery stores as well as mass retailers nationwide. For more information, visit **BountyTowels.com.**

⚫FitBit

> If you don't have time for a nutritious meal, consider using a meal replacement bar or shake. In terms of nutrition, they're usually far superior to many selections in vending machines or fast-food restaurants.

It's hard to have some battery-recharging time for me. One thing that I protect is my shower time. I take long showers! This gives me a few precious minutes to relax and recharge!

> —*Bola Oyeyipo-Ajumobi, MD, a mom of five- and two-year-old sons, a family physician at the Veterans Health Administration, and the owner of SlimyBookWorm.com, in San Antonio, TX*

My husband is also a pediatrician, and he works a 24-hour shift every Saturday, so I'm at home with our son. When my husband gets home Sunday morning, he takes over with our son, and I'm off. I usually leave the house to go do something to relax, such as get a massage. At the minimum, I go take a bath or shower with the door locked!

> —*Michelle Davis-Dash, MD, a mom of a 19-month-old son and a pediatrician in Baltimore, MD*

It's often hard for me to find the time to recharge my batteries. I like to take a long bath, sing loudly in the car, or watch a movie, but because these things rarely happen, I also look for ways to recharge that involve my family. This includes taking walks, playing hide-and-seek, singing and dancing with my son, or quietly reading him a story. But every once in a while I absolutely must make time to have lunch with my closest friends, and I always leave feeling positively giddy!

> —*Jennifer A. Gardner, MD, a mom of a three-year-old son, a pediatrician, and the founder of an online child wellness and weight management company, HealthyKidsCompany.com, in Washington, DC*

Making time for myself is something I really struggle with. I want to be everything to everyone—the best wife, mother, and doctor.

Sometimes, I have a difficult time transitioning from my busy office to my home life. I don't want to bring all of that work stress into my home! One thing that helps is sitting in my car outside my house for five minutes to calm down and get centered before going in. I don't check my phone messages, text, call, or read. Nothing. I just sit.

Another way I love to unwind is to take a bath or get in the hot tub for even 10 minutes and just let my mind quiet itself.

—*Michelle Spring, MD, a mom of a one-year-old son and two grown stepchildren and a board-certified plastic surgeon with Marina Plastic Surgery Associates, in Marina del Rey, CA*

If I feel tired, it's often because I haven't been doing enough self-care. I'm pretty religious about self-care because if I don't do it, I can get irritable. If my energy and time are stretched too thin, and I don't have enough downtime, I feel fried.

It's ironic that the more exhausted you are, the harder it is to

Clear Some Time for Friends

Have you ever gotten a call or an e-mail from a good friend and been so busy that it takes you weeks (or even months) to call or e-mail her back? And yet a good, long chat with a close friend is almost always uplifting. It can even energize you to stay on track and take care of yourself when your friend is working on weight loss as well.

Here's a plan: Say no to something less important so that you can say yes to a phone call with your BFF. Look at your calendar and identify ways to free up some time. And the next time you get a call to bake dozens of cookies for a bake sale or to volunteer your time when it means overfilling your calendar, say, "I'm sorry, but I don't have the time." Putting yourself first in this way means you'll open yourself up to the support you need as you're taking better care of yourself.

> **Love yourself first and everything else falls into line.**
> **You really have to love yourself**
> **to get anything done in this world.**
> **—*Lucille Ball***

figure out what you need. Sometimes when I'm overtired, I think that if I keep doing more and more, I'll catch up. That's probably okay in times of crisis. But over the long term, it's pretty corrosive. Instead, I make time—I actually *schedule* time—for self-care activities such as yoga.

—*Nancy Rappaport, MD*

After pregnancy and a few months of maternity leave, I felt compelled to rush back to work, almost like I had to make up for lost time and get busier than ever. Soon, I felt like my weekends were blurs of laundry, cleaning, and taking care of my daughter. In the evenings, I was catching up on administrative work from the office. By Sunday night, I was more exhausted than I was before the weekend!

About a year ago, I started taking Fridays off. I still am very busy at work, but I spend Fridays catching up on paperwork, doing errands, and spending time with my daughter while our nanny is here. We call them "Fabulous Fridays."

I've found that having this "cushion" at the end of the week makes the week *and* the weekend easier and more enjoyable. I've been much happier since I made this decision.

—*Rachel S. Rohde, MD, a mom of a two-year-old daughter, an assistant professor of orthopaedic surgery at the Oakland University William Beaumont School of Medicine, and an orthopaedic upper-extremity surgeon with Michigan Orthopaedic Institute, P.C., in Southfield, MI*

RALLIE'S TIP

Most moms I know will give and give of themselves until the well is dry! To prevent feeling physically and emotionally depleted, I think prioritiz-

ing is the key. One of the best ways to prioritize effectively is to list the areas of your life that are most important to you. I refer to this list as your "gardens" in life, because they have to be regularly tended to thrive and flourish. Most women list their children, their relationships with their partners, health, spirituality, fun, career, community service, friends, and parents.

Once you've created your list of "gardens," think of the activities you engage in on a regular basis to nurture these gardens. If you're not doing something very regularly to nurture your gardens, they'll never bear fruit: They'll just shrivel up and die.

If your health is important to you, but you never make time to exercise or relax or get enough sleep, you won't succeed in being healthy. If your relationship with your partner is important to you, but you never make time for fun and intimacy, you won't succeed in having a good relationship.

Understanding and listing your priorities makes it easier for you to avoid giving too much of yourself and helps you make the right decision when you're forced to choose between activities.

If, for example, your son's teacher invites you to her sister's baby shower, you might find it easier to say no when you realize that this activity doesn't support any of your priorities in life. You can say, "No, thank you" and go ride bikes with your son instead, an activity that supports three of your life priorities—your children, fun, and health.

I believe there is enough time for us to do it all in one lifetime, just not all at once! I think it's very challenging—and very stressful—to try to do it all and have it all at the same time. Of course many people are able to successfully juggle being a good parent and partner, having a demanding career, working out four days a week at the gym, and brushing and flossing vigorously twice a day. As long as everything's going smoothly, and as long as we're really careful, we can carry it off. But when we're juggling all these roles and responsibilities, it makes our life balance very precarious and very difficult to maintain. If we experience a shift in any one of these areas, such as when a child gets sick or we take on a big project with a looming deadline at work, it has a big impact on the other areas of our lives and quickly disrupts the tenuous balance.

As a physician, I see and treat women in the aftermath of "having and doing it all" on a daily basis. This has given me a great deal of insight about the high costs of having it all—emotionally, physically, and in terms of precious relationships. Life is a wonderful journey. Pace yourself!

Eating and Drinking for Energy

Imagine for a minute that you owned the vehicle of your dreams. Maybe it's a BMW. Or a yacht. Or a Cessna Skyhawk SP. Would you pinch some pennies and put el-cheapo fuel into your precious car, boat, or plane? No! You'd fill 'er up with the best fuel your money could buy.

Why do anything less for your body? What you eat and drink is *your* fuel to power your body to do the 2,431 things you need to do each and every day. Treat your body like the powerful machine it is, and fuel it right. After all, it's *your* ultimate driving machine.

❧

I have a morning espresso addiction. We have an espresso machine at home, and I love it. I try to limit myself to one coffee a day with just a half-teaspoon of sugar and soy or almond milk.
    —*Michelle Spring, MD*

❧

Sometimes in the afternoon if I have an energy slump, I'll drink a cup of green tea. I like it plain, no sweetener. It's very energizing.
    —*Pam D'Amato, MD*

❧

I don't drink caffeine. I ironically only crave caffeine when I'm pregnant. To keep my energy high, I sleep at least six hours a night and exercise.
    —*Bola Oyeyipo-Ajumobi, MD*

❧

I drink a cup of coffee every day, but every few months I'll do what I call a "detox." I stop drinking caffeine for a week. Then after that, it's surprising how much energy a cup of coffee gives me. I feel so much more energized by coffee after I take a short break from it.

—*Tiemdow Phumiruk, MD, a mom of 13-, 10-, and 7-year-old daughters, a pediatrician in the emergency department of Children's Hospital Colorado at Parker Adventist Hospital, and adjunct faculty at Rocky Vista University College of Osteopathic Medicine, in Parker, CO*

To fight fatigue, I know it's important to stay hydrated. Even being slightly dehydrated saps energy and compromises blood flow to the brain, so I'm not thinking as clearly as I should be. The best way to tell if you're dehydrated is to look at the color of your urine. It should be very pale yellow.

—*Ann Kulze, MD, a mom of 24- and 17-year-old daughters and 22- and 21-year-old sons; a nationally recognized nutrition expert, motivational speaker, and physician; and the author of the best-selling, award-winning* Eat Right for Life *book series, in Charleston, SC*

I find that keeping myself hydrated really helps keep my energy up. I set a goal for myself to make sure to drink at least 64 ounces of water a day, and I avoid caffeine because it can dehydrate you more.

—*Jennifer Bacani McKenney, MD, a mom of a two-year-old daughter who's expecting another baby and a family physician, in Fredonia, KS*

Last spring, I begged my husband for a Vitamix blender. "That's silly," he said. But he got it for me anyway!

I had been using a tiny blender that I feared might explode any

minute. But the Vitamix is much more powerful. Most mornings I drink a fruit smoothie for breakfast. I feel so good on those days.
—*Heather Orman-Lubell, MD*

Working long shifts at the hospital, it's hard not to notice that eating certain foods makes me feel tired. When we order out for hamburgers

Mommy MD Guides-Recommended Product
Dunkin' Donuts Coffee

"Time to make the donuts." Does that line conjure up images of old-fashioned orange stools at a Dunkin' Donuts counter?

Back in the 1980s and early '90s, Dunkin' Donuts touted that they made 52 varieties of donuts fresh every day. Today, Dunkin' Donuts has renewed its image with cheerful, clean restaurants full of bright colors and a friendly staff. There are no orange vinyl stools to be seen. While donuts are still their mainstay, they also serve bagels, sandwiches, oatmeal, and hot and iced coffee, latte, cappuccino, espresso, hot chocolate, and vanilla chai.

Dunkin' Donuts range in calories from 200 (for the French Crueller) to 550 (the chocolate coconut cake donut). There are plenty of other options on their DDSmart menu of items that provide guests with better-for-you options. It includes a multigrain bagel with 350 calories; a ham, egg, and cheese English muffin sandwich with 280 calories; two kinds of egg white flatbreads with 280 calories each; and oatmeal with dried fruit with 270 calories. You'll even find their lite line of lattes, such as a small iced caramel latte lite with 80 calories.

When the kids are begging for a sweet treat or if you're making plans to meet a friend for breakfast, Dunkin' Donuts can provide a nice break even when you've made a goal of eating healthfully. Sit down, realx, and sip a coffee or latte.

and French fries, I feel tired. Those foods wear me down. They're "comfort foods," and they're so comforting that they make me want to lie down and take a nap!

On the flip side, eating other foods gives me energy. Eggs are my most energizing foods. I love omelets. I also love to eat fruit, especially pears. Even the smell of a fresh pear gives me energy.

—Stephanie A. Wellington, MD, a mom of a 13-year-old son and an 11-year-old daughter, a hospitalist in the Level III NICU at Bellevue Hospital Center in New York City, and the medical coach and founder of PostpartumNeonatalCoaching.com

I'm a high-energy person, but 12-hour shifts can still be a challenge. By about 3 pm, I start to get tired.

One thing that really helps boost my energy levels is eating a good breakfast. It gives me long-lasting energy throughout the day. I used to skip breakfast because I was always in a hurry to get out the door for work. But I'd find myself getting very tired within a couple of hours. Now I eat a breakfast of oatmeal with fruit and nuts or eggs with whole grain toast.

I also bring snacks to work, and I eat a snack every few hours. Some of my favorite energizing snacks are a mixture of almonds and dried fruit and apple slices with peanut butter.

—Sonali Ruder, DO, a mom of a two-month-old daughter, an emergency physician at Coral Springs Medical Center near Fort Lauderdale, FL, and a recipe developer and blogger at TheFoodiePhysician.com

I have boundless energy. One thing that helps tremendously is eating protein at every meal. My top picks for protein foods include fish, shellfish, skinless poultry, beans, nuts, seeds, whole soy foods, omega-3-fortified eggs, and low-fat or fat-free dairy products.

If I'm hungry between meals, I know that I need to step up my protein intake a bit. Hunger is an indication of low blood sugar, which also zaps your energy!

—Ann Kulze, MD

FitBit

I snack on fruit all day long, especially fruits that are high in antioxidants, such as berries and oranges. I find that these foods are very energizing. Eating them makes me feel light on my feet.

I pack fruit from home in zipper-lock bags or plastic containers. This also motivates me to eat it, rather than snacking on vending machine foods, because I don't want to carry it back home with me, and I don't want it to go to waste.

—*Aline T. Tanios, MD, a mom of 10- and 4-year-old daughters and an 8-year-old son and a pediatric hospitalist and assistant professor at the Washington University School of Medicine, in St. Louis, MO*

One of the biggest challenges to my energy is being on call overnight and being wakened. Even receiving a phone call in the middle of the night affects my energy the next day. I don't feel completely normal. I feel sluggish and tired.

To combat the energy drain, I try to eat well 80 percent of the time. I eat a lot of fresh fruit, Greek yogurt, and nuts. One of my favorite breakfasts is a whole grain waffle spread with crunchy peanut butter. I try to focus on eating well for energy.

On Friday and Saturday nights, my family slacks off, and we'll eat out and maybe even get dessert.

—*Amy Barton, MD, a mom of an 11-year-old daughter and 8- and 5-year-old sons and a pediatrician at St. Luke's Children's Hospital, in Boise, ID*

A few years ago, I switched to a gluten-free diet. I was having skin sensitivity issues and digestion problems, and I noticed that both got worse when I ate wheat, in particular.

I avoid pastas, breads, and other foods containing gluten.

Occasionally, I still eat a gluten-free pasta dish. (Trader Joe's Brown Rice Pastas are my favorite.) But for most meals, now I eat a lot of lean protein, fruits, and vegetables. I snack on trail mix made of dried fruit, seeds, and nuts. Since changing my diet, my allergy and digestive problems have gone away, and as side benefits, I feel healthier, and I have a lot more energy.

—*Allison Bailey, MD*

I'm very conscious of how foods affect me—whether they deplete me or energize me. I try to pay attention. I eat a lot of green vegetables. I also make sure I get beneficial fats such as coconut oil and olive oil and those from foods such as avocados and olives. I also eat "clean" protein from organic meats and poultry, grass-fed beef, and wild-caught Alaskan salmon.

Mommy MD Guides–Recommended Product
Celestial Seasonings Tea

"After my morning coffee, my favorite get-up-and-get-going drink is Celestial Seasonings Green Tea," says Allison Bailey, MD, a mom of a nine-year-old son and a five-year-old daughter and founder and director of Integrated Health and Fitness Associates, in Cambridge, MA. "It has some caffeine, but less than coffee so I don't get as jittery. And as an added benefit, it contains antioxidant vitamin C and naturally occurring flavonoid antioxidants to help maintain my everyday well being. It's a great, healthy pick-me-up in the middle of the day."

You can buy Celestial Seasonings Green Tea directly from the company at **CELESTIALSEASONINGS.COM**, as well as at stores such as Walmart and Target and online retailers such as **AMAZON.COM**. The price is around $2.99 for 20 teabags. It can also be found in K-cups at select retailers. It's available in many different flavors, both regular and decaf.

I notice that eating foods high in simple carbs, such as bread, crackers, and refined grains, makes me feel bloated and tired, so I avoid them most of the time.

—*Kay Corpus, MD, a mom of a six-year-old daughter and a two-year-old son, a family physician, and the director of Owensboro Health Integrative Medicine, in Kentucky*

A few years ago, I gave up coffee for 10 days. I confess I'm attached to the aroma of coffee, and it's the jolt I need to jump-start my day. I like being caught in a cycle of sugar and caffeine euphoria. When I gave up coffee, I also took a hiatus from processed sugars, red meat, and refined foods such as pasta and bread.

With the help of a yoga teacher who is also a nutritionist, I went with seven of my colleagues on a 10-day quest to find out what foods "best serve us." During this journey, I became aware of all the people who stroll down the streets cradling their Starbucks cups. When I mentioned to my friends that I was caffeine free for 10 days as part of a spring fast, I might as well have said that I was volunteering to go on a forced march through Siberia. I wondered if caffeine is our security blanket that provides the energy for us to scramble from one momentous task to another. I worried that I might not be able to write without my caffeine jolt.

Even though this started out as a 10-day hiatus from coffee, I've kept it up for two years. I found out that I don't crave it or need it to keep my energy up. From this experience I discovered that you can change a habit, even if it involves something that you think you can't live without. And I got to experience what it must be like for my patients when I ask them to try to change a habit.

—*Nancy Rappaport, MD*

To keep my energy levels up, I eat plenty of fresh fruit. I seek out fresh berries, and I also supplement fresh with frozen fruit when necessary.

I make yogurt smoothies with plain or fruit-flavored yogurt and add the frozen fruit and swirl it in a blender. You can freeze this mixture to make yogurt pops. Sometimes I defrost the fruit overnight and just add the fruit to my yogurt without mixing it in the blender. For my son, I add frozen strawberries to orange juice and whirl the combo in the blender.

I love making fruit sauces with frozen berries by cooking the berries with a little sugar and lemon juice. I put this on oatmeal in the morning.

A lot of people don't think about incorporating frozen fruit into their diets, but it can be less expensive than fresh fruit. Frozen fruit is actually pretty flavorful when it's flash frozen at the peak of ripeness. Consider that a lot of "fresh fruit" sits around in the grocery store for a long time and has traveled thousands of miles from another country!

—*Jennifer A. Gardner, MD*

⌒⌒

I try to make wise eating choices and think of food as fuel. I find that if I focus on eating to nourish and energize myself, rather than eating whatever I want, it makes a huge difference in how I feel. I have so much more energy. If I eat a lot of junk food that I'm craving on the weekends, I don't feel as good. It might taste great, but I know I'll pay for it later.

I eat a lot of nutritious, high-protein foods, such as nuts and seeds. In the fall, I roast pumpkin seeds. I buy turkey jerky in bulk at Costco or Sam's Club, and I also shop at Whole Foods or Sprouts, where you can buy foods in bulk. I like to buy reasonably priced protein foods such as lean cuts of turkey, Greek yogurt, and cottage cheese. I also love roasting vegetables and making kale chips from fresh kale. (See the recipes on pages 202 and 302.)

FitBit

I make homemade granola sweetened with maple syrup or applesauce instead of sugar, and it's so much tastier and more nutritious than the store-bought kind. I also make a wonderful dish with chia seeds. I mix them with a bit of vanilla soy milk and let them soak overnight. The end result tastes a bit like tapioca pudding. I have to admit, it's an acquired taste!

I think that eating a variety of healthful foods is the key. When people try to eat the same selection of foods over and over, they get bored and give up.

—*Antoinette Cheney, DO, a mom of a seven-year-old son and a six-year-old daughter and a family physician with Rocky Vista University College of Osteopathic Medicine, in Parker, CO*

RALLIE'S TIP

Sometimes when I'm really tired, I crave the very foods that will make me feel worse in the long run. It's body betrayal! When we're tired, we seem to be drawn to foods that are loaded with sugar, salt, unhealthy fats (trans and saturated), and empty calories. Cravings for carbohydrates are common, and for a good reason. Carbohydrate-laden foods are known to help increase levels of serotonin, a mood-enhancing neurotransmitter in the brain, so carbohydrate cravings might be a sign that you're innately trying to self-medicate. (Many antidepressants work by increasing serotonin levels in the brain and body.)

Although chips, chocolate bars, giant bowls of pasta, and deluxe, double-crust pizzas might be my first and favorite choices of carbohydrates, eating too many of these types of foods inevitably leads to weight gain, which can be even more depressing. Eating carbohydrate-rich foods is fine, but it's important to choose those that support your good health and a healthy weight. Good carbohydrate choices include whole fruits and vegetables and low-fat, whole grain breads, cereals, and grains.

Exercising for Energy

One-third of Americans consider themselves to be inactive. We suspect if more were being honest, the number would be even higher! Yet, exercise can help increase your energy.

It seems ironic that exercise increases energy. Shouldn't working out make you tired? Actually, energy begets energy, and exercise will boost—not sap—your energy. Exercise leads to higher energy levels by improving the delivery of blood and nutrients to your tissues, helping your heart and lungs work more efficiently, and strengthening your muscles. That primes your body to be better able to handle your daily tasks—picking up a toddler a hundred times a day, lugging groceries in from the car, and meeting the 2,131 daily demands of being a mom.

Also, exercise can help increase your energy because it can improve chronic conditions that drain your energy, such as arthritis, high blood pressure, diabetes, and heart disease.

❦

Exercise is the single most powerful means you have to fight fatigue. The more energy you expend, the more energy your body is capable of producing. I am honestly never, ever tired. I know that my daily exercise is the key to my boundless energy.

—*Ann Kulze, MD*

❦

To work in my high-stress job, I need plenty of energy. I set my alarm to wake me up early each morning so I can go for a two-mile run. That really boosts my energy.

—*Shilpa Amin-Shah, MD, a mom of a three-year-old son and a two-year-old daughter and an emergency physician and director of the recruiting team at Emergency Medical Associates, in Livingston, NJ*

I find that I'm most energetic when I take a walk each day. In the winter when this is harder, I bundle up my son and take him to the playground and make a point to play with him, rather than watching him play. Usually there are few other kids around, so he's happy to oblige. I always feel better on sunny days in the winter!

—*Jennifer A. Gardner, MD*

No matter how tired I am, I feel so much better if I get even 10 minutes of activity. I think it's due to a combination of the endorphin rush from exercise plus the knowledge that I'm doing something good for myself. If I'm tired, I'll take a break and do 10 minutes of stretching or go for a walk.

—*Michelle Spring, MD*

Mommy MD Guides-Recommended Product
iPod Shuffle

The power of music when you exercise is big. One study found that people who listened to motivating, upbeat music while working out on a treadmill had 15 percent more endurance and enjoyed the exercise more.

When it only takes a few good tracks to make you feel energized and great during your workout, why not get out your earbuds? The iPod shuffle is a great choice because it's small, and you can clip it to your clothes during a walk or jog. The quality of the sound can't be beat, and it might be the only time you can listen to music you want to hear—assuming your kids have hijacked your car's CD player. An iPod shuffle is also very affordable, only around $45, but you'll need a computer with the latest version of iTunes to get it up and running. The iPod shuffle comes in seven colors.

You can buy an iPod shuffle in the electronics departments of stores such as Walmart and Target, in Apple stores, or online here: **APPLE.COM/IPOD-SHUFFLE**.

> **The more you lose yourself in something bigger than yourself, the more energy you will have.**
> **—*Norman Vincent Peale*,**
> ***author of* The Power of Positive Thinking**

Exercise is a huge energy booster for me. Even after trying so many different types of exercise, I still can't say that I truly enjoy exercise. But it never fails to make me feel energized and vital. I try to exercise every day. This way every day is already a good one.

> —*Ayala Laufer-Cahana, MD, a mom of 17- and 15-year-old sons and a 14-year-old daughter, a pediatrician, and the founder of Herbal Water Inc., in Wynnewood, PA*

I'm lucky in that I'm on my feet all day at work, moving around. That helps me stay active and keeps my energy levels high. If I had a desk job, I would get up and move around every few hours. Activity begets energy!

> —*Sonali Ruder, DO*

Exercise boosts my energy because it helps me to sleep. I work alternating shifts, and so I work an overnight shift, then two days later I work a day shift.

After I get home from an overnight shift, no matter how exhausted I am, I do cardio training for 30 minutes. The exercise tires me out and "unkinks my chi" enough so I can get to bed on time and reset my sleep schedule.

> —*Lisa Campanella-Coppo, MD, a mom of a three-year-old daughter and an emergency physician with EMCARE and the Meridian Health System, in Monmouth, NJ*

Sometimes when I'm tired, doing a few yoga poses boosts my energy. For example, the sun salutation series that involves forward and back bends is a great energizing routine. The series can be done just once or twice, when I don't have much time, or several times with different variations if I have more time.

—*Allison Bailey, MD*

⤳⤺

I have an hour-long commute each way to work. It's horrible. Sitting for that long in the car is hard on your body—not to mention on your spirits.

By the time I get home each night, I feel like a carcass. Fortunately, I have a very supportive husband. He knows if I don't do something for myself to recharge my batteries, I'll go crazy. I like to do yoga or go for a run. We often have scattered and demanding lives at home and work, and it can be hard to find a set time to exercise. My husband and I always work together to find a couple of times each week when he can watch the kids so that I can exercise. I try to run on the treadmill at our local YMCA once or twice a week and go to a power yoga or hot yoga class once a week. I also enjoy walking our dog, but it's so challenging to walk a dog with a toddler now that I don't do that as much as I used to.

—*Sigrid Payne DaVeiga, MD, a mom of a seven-year-old son and a two-year-old daughter and a pediatric allergist with the Children's Hospital of Philadelphia, in Pennsylvania*

⤳⤺

Even when I'm really, really tired, or when I have a cold, I still exercise. That wasn't always the case. Usually, when I got sick, exercising was the first thing to go. I remember one time, I was very sick with a cold.

"I can't go work out," I told my husband. "I can hardly finish a sentence without coughing. How am I going to exercise?"

My husband urged me to give it a try.

"If you don't go, you'll never know," he said. "But if you go, and you don't cough, you'll be pleasantly surprised."

I was amazed to find out that he was right. The workout made me feel better. Exercise expands your lungs and opens up your airways. I didn't cough at all!

—Amy Thompson, MD, a mom of six-, four-, and two-year-old sons and an ob-gyn at the University of Cincinnati College of Medicine, in Ohio

⌒⌒

I believe it's a myth that exercising gives you energy. When I exercise, it makes me tired! Of course, this is different for different people. After I exercise, I feel good that I've done it, but for me the best part of exercise is the enjoyment I feel after being done with it.

—Judith Hellman, MD, a mom of a 15-year-old son, an associate clinical professor of dermatology at Mt. Sinai Hospital in New York City, and a dermatologist in private practice

Supplementing for Energy

Can you get an energy boost in a bottle? Manufacturers seem to think so. According to the Council for Responsible Nutrition, energy drinks have become one of the fastest-growing categories of supplement. It's not surprising when you consider we're a nation of sleep-deprived caffeine fiends.

Speaking of caffeine, it's the most widely used drug not just here in the land that runs on Dunkin', but in the entire world. Caffeine is found in the leaves, seeds, or fruit of a number of plant species, such as coffee and tea plants. It acts by speeding up the messages to and from the brain. Literally, it makes you think faster. Isn't that amazing?

⌒⌒

I believe that all women of child-bearing age should take prenatal vitamins, just in case a little "accident" happens. I take mine as my daily multivitamin, and it's helpful with my energy levels and immune system.

—Jeannette Gonzalez Simon, MD

I take an iron supplement, which can help boost energy in someone who's anemic. It can be difficult to get enough iron in your diet unless you eat a lot of red meat. (Be sure to talk with your doctor before taking iron supplements because taking too much can cause medical problems.)

—*Nancy Rappaport, MD*

RALLIE'S TIP

One thing that really energizes me is green tea. I love the taste of it, and it always seems to give me a little energy boost whenever I drink it, without giving me insomnia later on. Green tea has been shown to promote weight loss by increasing the metabolism of both fat and calories.

Identifying Energy Busters

Have you ever felt like you're merrily moving along through your day—when all of a sudden something happens that causes you to feel as if you've smacked into a brick wall? Your energy goes from higher than high to lower than low. *Is it possible to die from being this tired?* you might wonder. You feel like a paler shade of yourself. A ghost of you.

No doubt there are many different energy busters, and different people are probably susceptible to different ones. Interestingly, according to a survey by the American Psychological Association, people who are obese have higher levels of energy-depleting stress. Turns out that weight and energy go hand in hand—just like marshmallows and chocolate.

◦◦◦

I avoid energy-zapping protein foods: fatty cuts of red meat, such as beef, pork, and lamb, and full-fat dairy products.
—*Ann Kulze, MD*

◦◦◦

I try not to eat too many carbohydrates, such as white grains and simple sugars. I love them, but I feel sluggish when I eat too many.
—*Heather Orman-Lubell, MD*

◦◦◦

I avoid eating heavy, calorie-dense foods. If you gave me a hamburger to eat right now, I would love it. But then I'd want to lie down on the couch and take a nap.
—*Aline T. Tanios, MD*

◦◦◦

I try to be happy. I think that being unhappy is a huge energy drain. Also, I find that clerical tasks really drain my energy. I delegate them as much as possible.
—*Eva Ritvo, MD, a mom of 22- and 17-year-old daughters, a psychiatrist, and a coauthor of* The Beauty Prescription, *in Miami Beach, FL*

◦◦◦

One thing I find that drains my energy is multitasking—trying to do too many things at once. Instead, I try to focus on one thing at a time, especially when I'm tired. I find that it better concentrates my energy.
—*Edna Ma, MD*

I've become aware of things that decrease my energy. One is seeing gray skies for more than three days at a time. My residential choices are the west and southwestern parts of the United States for that reason.

—*Bola Oyeyipo-Ajumobi, MD*

I've always observed that the biggest energy drains are actually problematic psychological situations rather than simple physical overwork. Unresolved issues of this kind can eat up peace of mind and lead to exhaustion before you lift a finger! Being perfectionistic or needing to be in control in unrealistic ways—I see these ambitions tiring out a lot of moms!

—*Elizabeth Berger, MD, a mom of a 30-year-old son and a 29-year-old daughter, a child psychiatrist, and the author of* Raising Kids with Character, *in New York City*

When my kids were little, I was exhausted. On the weekends, I'd come home from an activity and take a two-hour nap. I thought I was just tired from motherhood and work.

But something told me that I should have some blood work done. I did, and it turned out my thyroid hormone levels were lower than they should be. My doctor prescribed medication, and I felt so much better. Women who are unusually tired can also have imbalances with their estrogen, progesterone, or cortisol.

—*Martha Wittenberg, MD, MPH*

My biggest energy drains are stress and worry. My children are in college, and they stress me out sometimes. I worry about them, and that worrying saps my energy.

To combat that, I try to talk through my feelings. I let my kids know that I'm available to them anytime they need me. I also exercise to deal with stress. That helps me through and keeps me moving forward.

—*Debra Luftman, MD*

⚫FitBit

Just because a food is low in fat and sugar doesn't mean it's good for you. A single serving of baked chips isn't all that bad for you—it's just not that good for you. It has nothing valuable to offer in terms of nutrition. Make sure that every food you eat contributes to your good health. Choose foods that serve as high-quality fuel rather than just filler.

If I put on extra weight, I feel tired and sluggish. I think that's partly because it's hard work carrying around more weight. But also I think it's a mind-set, a feeling that I'm not being healthy. When some extra pounds creep on, I don't feel the same way about myself as I do when I'm at my goal weight.

When I'm at—or at least near—my goal weight, which is what I weighed between my two pregnancies, I feel most energized. I feel phenomenal—like I can do anything!

—*Stephanie A. Wellington, MD*

I find that before my menstrual cycle, PMS makes me really tired. It's challenging now that my cycle is irregular. It's hard to anticipate when my period is coming and when I might be more tired.

If I'm tired, I sometimes make myself lie down and take an after-noon nap. I also try to be patient with myself. Even though I'm very OCD and want to get things done, I try to let some things go when I'm tired and accept the fact that I'm not going to get everything done that I want to accomplish.

—*Tiemdow Phumiruk, MD*

I've learned that about once a month, there will be two to three days that I just don't want to do anything on my to-do list. I also feel more "snacky" and hungrier than usual. I imagine this is related to my menstrual cycle.

I really don't do anything to fight this; I've found it's best to ride

> **In times of great stress or adversity,
> it's always best to keep busy, to plow your anger
> and your energy into something positive.**
> —*Lee Iacocca*

it out. The less I beat myself up about these phases, the faster they go away. I give myself permission not to worry about crossing items off my to-do list, and I simply add new items to the list when I think of them.

I try to enjoy these respites! I like to read romance novels. They're brain candy!

—*Deborah Gilboa, MD*

I find that unpleasant coverage of news events, such as what occurred during the nastiness of the latest election, drains me of energy. I was upset by the way the candidates handled themselves and how the campaigns were conducted. The news coverage was deplorable.

Watching the news made me feel awful and fatigued. So I turned it off! Instead, I started to watch classic movies. I enjoy watching them, and they increase, rather than decrease, my energy. I love movies, and I have discovered a whole new interest.

—*Linda Brodsky, MD, a mom of a 30-year-old son and 28-and 25-year-old daughters, the president of WomenMDResources.com, a physician in private practice with Pediatric ENT Associates, and a retired professor of otolaryngology and pediatrics, in Buffalo, NY*

I'm a type A, high-energy person. But the older I get, the harder it is for me to be on call for work. When I'm on call, I receive phone calls throughout the night. After that, I'm tired for two days.

I've learned to cut myself some slack. I usually set my alarm for 5 am to work out before my kids wake up, but for a night or two after being on call, I don't set my alarm. I let myself sleep in to try to catch up on my rest.

I also don't put as much pressure on myself to exercise on those days. If exercise feels good to me, I do it. If not, I skip it. We moms put so much pressure on ourselves to do everything, 100 percent, all of the time. That's just not realistic!

—*Eva Mayer, MD, a mom of a nine-year-old daughter and an eight-year-old son, an associate professor of pediatrics at Temple University, and a pediatrician with St. Luke's Pediatrics Associates, in Bethlehem, PA*

❧

Working late puts a drain on my energy. This happens a lot. My shifts are supposed to end at 10 pm, but sometimes I don't leave until 1 am.

I have to get up at 6 am the next morning to get my kids ready for school. Those days are hard. It might sound silly, but some mornings, I take a moment and pray, "Please, Lord, help me get through this day. I need your help today!"

I find this really helps. It's calming, and it helps me to acknowledge that it's going to be a rough day. Then I'm able to muster the energy.

—*Kristin C. Lyle, MD, FAAP, a mom of 10-, 7-, and 5-year-old daughters, the disaster medical director at Arkansas Children's Hospital, and an assistant professor of pediatrics at the University of Arkansas for Medical Sciences, both in Little Rock*

❧

When I really thought about my energy and what was sapping it, I realized that I have a few friends who are really a drag. They complain all of the time about how things aren't going right. I made a decision to limit my interactions with people like that. I didn't cut them out of my life entirely, but I do limit my time with them.

You have to realize that you're not obligated to everyone, all of the time. Find people to spend time with who are positive and happy. I make sure to save my energy for supporting friends when they are really in need.

—*Linda Brodsky, MD*

❧

When I was younger, I felt like I had so much energy, and I tried to do everything to the max. I went to college, then medical school, then residency. I was chief resident and then I went on to a fellowship program. I achieved everything I set out to do.

But having kids is a humbling experience. Suddenly, I wasn't able to do everything I wanted to do, all of the time. Sometimes I wish I could videotape our lives to capture all of the requests I receive from my kids and my dog and how quickly the requests come flying at me; I feel like a whirling dervish.

"Mom, can I have some milk?"

"Mom, can I have a pencil?"

I have so many requests to meet that sometimes it feels hard to get anything else done. For my children, and also for my patients, I put a lot of effort into letting them know that I'm very invested in helping them. It's a major energy drain. To combat this, I do the best I can to stay upbeat and be positive. I try to keep things light.

"I think you're mistaking me for the maid we don't have," I say to my son, one of his favorite lines from Calvin and Hobbes.

—*Sigrid Payne DaVeiga, MD*

At one point, I was so exhausted and nonfunctional that I basically could not do much more than sit on the couch. This went on for about seven years. I met a naturopath, and she said that my adrenal glands were "burned out." Your adrenal glands are considered your stress glands because they secrete cortisol, known as the stress hormone. Anything that stresses your body, including pain, insomnia, allergies, illness or injury, emotional stress, and excessive exercise, signals your adrenal glands to secrete cortisol so that you'll be ready to fight or flee. After prolonged stress, your adrenal glands can't continue to produce enough cortisol, and the levels fall low, which leads to a burnout situation. Cortisol is essentially your life force, so when your levels are really low, you might feel like you're dying. You might find that you have no motivation, no energy, and no joy, but you can't figure out why. This is a condition that is completely correctable with natural therapies and easily diagnosed with the proper testing. Once I knew what was wrong, I didn't feel such despair. After I was treated, it wasn't long before I began to feel like myself again.

I began taking adrenal extracts, and I started eating differently. I went an entire year without eating grains, and I felt so much better. I believe that eating wheat had damaged my intestines and had stressed my adrenal glands. I also began to take natural thyroid extract, which also made a huge difference in my energy levels.

Now I eat what I call "clean" foods—meats, vegetables, nuts, and good fats. I choose organically grown food as much as possible. I avoid aspartame and other artificial sweeteners. I use only natural sweeteners, such as maple syrup, honey, or even raw, unprocessed sugar. At least your body knows what to do with that!

—*Marie Dam, MD, a mom of 24- and 20-year-old daughters and an anti-aging medicine specialist in private practice in Naples, FL, and Danbury, CT*

RALLIE'S TIP

Time pressure puts a huge drain on my energy. It seems that there's always too much to do, and never enough time to do it all. Every day when I wake up, I realize that I've got about 16 beautiful, precious hours to do all of the things that are important to me and the people who count on me. I don't want to squander a single minute of my day doing things that don't matter to anyone!

To help me stay on track, and to make good use of my time, I start each day with a to-do list. I write down all of the things that I would love to accomplish during the day, and then I prioritize them. If something is really important, and I feel that I must get it done, I don't leave it to chance. Even if it's something as simple as calling a friend to check on her, I write it down and make time for it. I start with the most important things on my list, and work as far down the list as I comfortably can. If I don't make it all the way down the list to number 15, which might be cleaning the trash out of the backseat of my truck, it's no big deal. I can always do that another day.

Identifying Energy Boosters

Need to add a little pep to your step? There are dozens of things that you could try—some you might never have thought of. Consider these, which target each of your five senses.

Taste: Something high in magnesium. Studies show that women with magnesium deficiencies had higher heart rates and required more oxygen to do physical tasks than they did after their magnesium levels were restored to normal. If your magnesium level is low, your body needs to work harder to do the most basic tasks, which can make you feel tired.

The recommended daily intake of magnesium is around 300 milligrams for women and 350 milligrams for men. One way to get more magnesium is to eat a handful of almonds, hazelnuts, or cashews. Or try Natural Calm. (See page 341.)

Smell: Some peppermint. In a study at Wheeling Jesuit University in West Virginia, peppermint vapors gave college basketball players more motivation, energy, speed, and confidence. Some athletes use peppermint inhalers, and at one time Reebok even built a peppermint smell into some sports bras.

Hear: Some upbeat music. It will boost your energy.

Feel: The wind in your hair and sunshine on your face. In studies at California State University, a brisk 10-minute walk increased energy, and the effects lasted for an incredible two hours. When the study participants walked just 10 minutes a day for three weeks, their overall energy and mood were both boosted.

See: Photos of your family, or your "happy place," or better yet, your family in your happy place. If you have a favorite photo of your family in your favorite place, such as your kids at Walt Disney World, put it on your desk. Just looking at a photo can "transport" you to that happy time and place and boost your energy—and spirits.

∞

As part of my prayers each night before bed, I pray to have enough energy the next day to get through the day and to feel good.

—*Kristin C. Lyle, MD, FAAP*

When I find myself falling into a midday lull, I take a nice warm bath and soak and relax. I find myself really energized afterward.

—*Shilpa Amin-Shah, MD*

Spending time with my friends boosts my energy. I try to schedule social events into my week to get an energy boost. Of course, that's what extroverts do! For introverts, that might have the opposite effect. You have to know yourself and what works for you!

—*Katherine Dee, MD, a mom of eight-year-old twin daughters and a six-year-old son and a radiologist at the Seattle Breast Center, in Washington*

I'm a very optimistic person, and I think that keeps my energy high. Also when I take good care of myself—by eating better, exercising, and sleeping enough—I feel better. Otherwise I'm sluggish, cranky, and miserable.

—*Heather Orman-Lubell, MD*

To keep my energy levels up, I try to keep up with my hobbies—gardening, sewing, and reading. My husband and I also do a lot with

Play Online Games

Your kids shouldn't be the only ones who play games! If you need an energy boost, morale improver, or quick pick-me-up, distract yourself by playing Mahjongg, Angry Birds, Words with Friends, Bubble Shoot, Solitaire, or the dozens of other free games available online or on your phone. You'll forget about those candy bars, junky chips, and leftover cake tucked away in the cupboard in no time.

Go to Yahoo! Games at **GAMES.YAHOO.COM** to find a game that appeals to you, or you could search your phone's app store.

> **The higher your energy level,
> the more efficient your body. The more efficient
> your body, the better you feel and the more you will
> use your talent to produce outstanding results.**
> —*Tony Robbins, an author and motivational speaker*

our kids, and we try to stay involved with their lives. Being around kids, who are so full of energy, is energizing!

— *Stacey Ann Weiland, MD, a mom of a 14-year-old daughter and 9- and 7-year-old sons and an internist/gastroenterologist, in Denver, CO*

⌒⌒

I find that when I'm out and about with other people, I have much more energy. If I'm alone at home and feeling sluggish, I grab my little dog, put her on a leash, and we go for a walk. That makes us both feel good. I feel good because I've done a good thing for myself and for my dog, and my dog feels good because she loves being outdoors. It's so nice to sit on a bench, put my dog on my lap, and people—and dog—watch.

— *Judith Hellman, MD*

⌒⌒

Exercise helps wake me up in the morning. If I don't work out, I feel sluggish the rest of the day.

But I'm not going to lie. I use caffeine when I have to! Ironically, I didn't drink coffee in medical school, not until I became a mom. I'm a better mom some days with caffeine.

— *Antoinette Cheney, DO*

⌒⌒

I find that being in nature boosts my energy. In fact, I think exposure to nature is essential for good health. I love to walk in a park or on a beach. I also love watching birds. They are simply magical, and I can find them just about anywhere, just about any time!

— *Ann Kulze, MD*

If at all possible, find something you love to do—and do it! I went to medical school and became a pediatrician. Later in my career, I specialized in medical disaster. When I did that, it was like a part of my brain that had been turned off was suddenly switched on! It was so exciting and energizing! I couldn't get enough of it. It was a tremendous boost to my energy.

—*Kristin C. Lyle, MD, FAAP*

When I'm tired, I try to change my environment, even if it's only for 10 or 15 minutes. I find that if I've been doing something for a long time, such as sitting at the computer, I feel like I'm in a rut, but if I go do something else, it's very energizing.

It's best if I do something physical, such as go outside for a walk. That way I get some sunlight on my face and in my eyes, and it helps to wake me up. After that, if I go back to my desk, I don't feel tired anymore.

—*Edna Ma, MD*

One thing that helps to keep my energy levels high is moving constantly. I work in an urgent care center, and I move around all day, 12 hours a day. If I had a job where I sat a lot, I'd have to get up and move frequently to keep from getting sluggish. On slower days, I keep a step bench in my office and march while reading journals to keep alert.

—*Susan Besser, MD, a mom of six grown children, ages 28, 26, 24, 22, 21, and 19, a grandmom of two, a family physician, and the medical director of Doctors Express-Memphis, in Tennessee*

Being a new mom, wife, anesthesiologist, business owner, and medical director keeps my plate very full. A good cup of coffee really gets my day going, but coffee alone can't give me the energy to get through my busy life—emotionally or physically.

I boost my energy and fight fatigue by having maintenance facials every two weeks. These targeted facials help me fight fatigue by hydrating my skin, increasing blood flow to my face, and keeping me energized. If I'm fatigued, I choose an energy booster facial with eucalyptus aromatherapy. This lifts my spirits and boosts my energy.

—*Arleen K. Lamba, MD, a mom of a three-month-old son, an anesthesiologist, the medical director of Blush Med Institute, and founder of the Blush Blends Skin Care line, in Washington, DC*

I have an extremely high energy level. I find that making time to do the things that I love energizes me. I love to read, and I'm always in the middle of three or four books. I also love to talk to people, and so I really enjoy my work where I have to spend a lot of time talking. I love to share my love of books with others, so I started a book club, which meets 9 or 10 times a year. We spend time catching up on other things as well. Going to the movies and out to eat with friends also helps to re-energize me. I also love to create things. I love to write, and blogging keeps my energy levels up. Having new ideas, writing them down, and sharing them helps to keep me involved. I especially love it when someone responds to something I've written and tells me it was helpful. I get a real kick out of that.

—*Linda Brodsky, MD*

No matter how tired or busy I am, I always put on at least the bare minimum of makeup: lip gloss and eyeliner. That makes me look like I had two or three more hours of sleep than I actually did. Plus, perceptions are reality: If I look tired, and people tell me how tired I look, it's going to make me feel even more tired! If I look refreshed, I'll *feel* refreshed too.

—*Edna Ma, MD*

To keep up my energy, I try to drink as much water as I can, but I don't think I ever will be able to stay as hydrated as I think I should be. The other drinks that I like have caffeine in them, so I try to limit those to two or three a day. You won't drink it if it isn't there, so I keep the water in front of me at my office station as I see patients.

I find that when I'm completely exhausted, if I force myself to dress nicely and do my hair and makeup, I feel more energized.

●FitBit

Dietary protein is a source of long-lasting energy. Try to include a little protein in each meal and snack. Just adding a few almonds or a slice of low-fat cheese will help satisfy your hunger and keep your blood sugar levels stable for much longer than if you ate a high-carbohydrate meal or snack.

My next goal is to get back to working out. I know it makes me feel better, but it's fallen by the wayside in the past few years.

—*Rachel S. Rohde, MD*

⁓

I really enjoy doing yoga and running. When I have the time, I also like to go to the Koresh Dance Studio in Philadelphia and take classes with the more advanced dancers. For me, all of these activities are very singular. I go alone. I am friendly and pleasant, but I do not go out of my way to make friends because these are spaces that I need to keep personal and for myself.

In these spaces, I don't compare myself to others around me. I just push myself to concentrate on the task at hand. I love listening to music and getting a bit of a rush from some good music and the physical activity at the same time. My head feels so much clearer after I do this, like I can start fresh on the next 15 tasks that face me at home or work.

—*Sigrid Payne DaVeiga, MD*

⁓

I drink an enormous amount of coffee. I find it extremely validating and gratifying that studies on coffee find that it has mostly neutral or positive health benefits.

People like me, who have some ADHD, often self-medicate with coffee. That might have been the genesis of my love affair with the bean.

I used to make a pot of coffee each morning and take it with me to work—even on overnight shifts. As long as I stop drinking coffee by 4 am, I can still sleep when I get home. I think I burned out all of my caffeine receptors in medical school. On night shifts, at 3 am or so,

I would go down to the snack bar and buy the coffee dregs at the bottom of the pot that had been cooking away all night. I'd put the full cup of nastiness by my bed so when I woke up 2 hours later, I could chug it. I don't recommend this, just full disclosure.

—*Amy Baxter, MD*

☙❧

On a recent trip to New York City, I realized how fortunate my family is to be so connected to nature. Despite living in the suburbs, we listen to the birds every morning, chase lizards several times a week, grow some of our own food, spend time outdoors every day, and have a blanket of stars at night. However, until recently, there was an element missing. Incorporating this missing element has greatly enhanced our lives.

The missing ingredient: barefoot time outside. As an emergency physician, I always encouraged footwear outdoors to avoid cuts and twigs impaled between toes that I have treated while at work. And, living in the South, one can be surprised by a hill of fire ants. I previously thought it best to wear shoes and avoid these potential risks. But it turns out we really were missing a wonderful opportunity to bond with nature, ourselves, and each other.

Piles of data support the health benefits of connecting with nature. Houseplants help purify and oxygenate the air while serving as a calming presence. Fresh foods have greater health benefits, especially when eaten after literally plucking them from the plant. Finally, time outdoors is connected to better sleep and reduced anxiety. In a spiritual or metaphysical realm, all forms of life are connected, and increasing our respect and gratitude for all life, in turn, improves our own. Some naturalists even claim spending time outside helps promote weight loss, which might, in fact, be true.

The new solution for improving your life: barefoot time in the grass. I realized our lawn is generally free of twigs, dog excrement, and fire ants. Yes, there could be a risk to playing barefoot outdoors, but I have found the benefits to be unbelievable. Our family began spending 10 to 15 minutes barefoot outdoors each evening after dinner playing Frisbee. It's a fun, easy game that provides the opportunity to discuss other topics of the day. My children are four and seven years old, and Frisbee has become so popular they now ask for it in the morning as well.

Starting our day by feeling the cold, wet grass beneath our feet somehow puts it all in perspective. I find it calming and relaxing. My children find it energizing, and I believe the outdoor activity helps them to concentrate better during other morning activities. I realize time before school can be hectic, but you might just find this activity offers the reward of getting your kids ready faster. It's as simple as preparing for school and playing in the yard for a few minutes before the bus arrives or before you begin the morning commute. Yes, feet can get dirty, but they are easily cleaned by wiping with a small towel.

As a mom and doctor, I believe the focused bonding and connection to nature helps me and my family feel more supported and ready to face the challenges of the day. As an adult, I find tranquility in noticing the different soil textures and feel of the grass while appreciating the morning breeze or watching a beautiful sunset. This easy, free daily commune with nature might truly improve your life. Try it.

—*Jennifer Hanes, DO, a mom of a seven-year-old daughter and a four-year-old son, an emergency physician who's board certified in integrative medicine, and the author of* The Princess Plan: Shrink Your Waist, Expand Your Beauty, *in Austin, TX*

RALLIE'S TIP

As often as possible, I listen to music that I know will energize me and lift my spirits. Depending on my mood, I'll listen to rock, country music, and sometimes even opera or polka!

I also make good use of scented candles, body lotions, air fresheners, and fragrances with invigorating aromas, such as ginger, orange, lemon, peppermint, and cinnamon, to give my energy levels and moods a little boost throughout the day.

Sleeping Better

"To sleep, perchance to dream" sounded a whole heck of a lot easier before kids. We can only imagine Shakespeare wrote this *before* his three children—including a set of twins!—were born.

Creating an inviting environment in your bedroom is a key to getting good sleep, according to a poll by the National Sleep Foundation. A good mattress, comfortable pillows, and soft bedding are important, and also a dark, cool, clean room helps people go to sleep.

In general, we spend about one-third of our lives asleep. But the exact amount of shut-eye you need is actually unique to you. Some people need six hours of sleep a night, while others need nine. Sleep experts say you'll know you're getting the right amount when you wake up on your own feeling refreshed. No kidding!

I take a calcium supplement at night before bedtime. I think it helps me to sleep better. Think about it: For generations people have been drinking warm milk to fall asleep!

—*Nancy Rappaport, MD*

When to Call Your Doctor

First it was the baby (or babies) that kept you awake. But if by now everyone else in your family is sleeping through the night and you're still not getting enough shut-eye, what should you do?

Insomnia could be the sign of a sleep disorder such as sleep apnea or of a condition such as depression or anxiety. It could even be caused by a medication, such as birth control pills or drugs used to treat pain, cold symptoms, high blood pressure, allergies, heart disease, thyroid disease, or asthma. Insomnia makes you miserable, and it can make it harder to keep up with healthy eating and exercise. It can even lead to overall poor health.

If your sleep problems last longer than a few weeks or if poor sleep is causing distress in your life, call your doctor or a sleep expert. If you're still not sure, take a look at the following common signs of sleep disorders. Schedule an appointment with your doctor if you have any of the following symptoms.

• It takes more than 30 minutes to fall asleep.

I turn off my laptop and tablets by sundown. They disrupt your melatonin production. You've got to master your sleep routine by your thirties, or you'll start to fall down a hormonal flight of stairs. I take an herb called ashwagandha and a supplement called phosphatidyl serine to wrangle cortisol at night.

—*Sara Gottfried, MD, a mom of 13- and 8-year-old daughters, a board-certified gynecologist, and the author of* The Hormone Cure, *in Berkeley, CA*

If I don't get a good night's sleep, the next day won't be what it should be! I occasionally take a melatonin supplement to help me fall asleep. I don't take a lot: I break a three-milligram tablet in half. I find that helps me to sleep better.

—*Pam D'Amato, MD*

- As you fall asleep, you have vivid dreams.
- You're a chronic snorer.
- Your partner tells you that you seem to quit breathing during sleep.
- You wake up during the night and can't go back to sleep.
- You experience tingling or crawling sensations in your legs at night that won't go away unless you move or rub them.
- Your partner tells you that you jerk your legs or arms during sleep.
- You feel like you can't move when you first wake up.
- You don't feel refreshed in the mornings.
- You're sleepy during the day even when you went to bed early the night before.
- You need caffeine to stay awake during the day.
- You fall asleep in the daytime or within five minutes of lying down to nap.
- Your muscles suddenly become weak when you're emotional, such as when you're angry, afraid, or when you laugh.

⚫**Fit**Bit

Make time for sleep. Sleep deprivation triggers hormonal changes that can lead to overeating and weight gain. In a 15-year study, University of Wisconsin researchers found that loss of sleep results in lower levels of leptin, which is a hormone that plays a key role in regulating appetite.

I'm a big believer in the medical school philosophy "Sleep while you can." If I'm very tired, I'll take a nap. I make sure that someone else is watching my son, and I use sensory deprivation techniques, such as wearing ear plugs and eye shades.

—*Edna Ma, MD*

I work in a very high-stress job, and I need to get enough sleep. If I don't get six to seven hours of sleep, I'm exhausted the next day. If I'm very tired, I ask my husband to take our kids out of the house for a few hours in the afternoon so I can take a nap.

—*Shilpa Amin-Shah, MD*

I limit the amount of water I drink before bedtime. Otherwise I have to wake up to go to the bathroom, and it disrupts my sleep.

—*Eva Ritvo, MD*

If I'm ever having trouble falling asleep, or if I've had a stressful day and fear I might have trouble falling asleep, I'll take a shower or bath before bed. That relaxes my body—and my mind—a bit and helps me fall asleep.

—*Sonali Ruder, DO*

The best way to have enough energy is to get enough sleep. I have to make sleep a priority. Each night, I have a routine, and I have certain benchmarks I need to meet to get to bed on time. For example, we eat dinner each night by 5:30. Then I need to clean up the house, get my kids to bed, and get into the shower myself by 9 pm. Some nights

I have to tell myself, *I'm not going to get to that tonight; it can wait until tomorrow* because getting enough sleep is more important.

—*Kristin C. Lyle, MD, FAAP*

⌀⌀

It is well recognized that insufficient sleep and an irregular sleep schedule lead to fatigue. I personally try to set a regular bedtime and regular time to get up in the morning, although the exact times may require adjustment for work situations, travel, houseguests, and other scheduling irregularities. And I love coffee!

—*Elizabeth Berger, MD*

⌀⌀

I recently joined the "mommy club" when I gave birth to my baby boy. I'm just getting out of my "fourth trimester." I love mommyhood, but I do miss my sleep.

To get better sleep, I use aromatherapy with a lavender-based body lotion from Blush Blends called Underneath It All. Lavender has great soothing and relaxing properties, and it has been shown to help people who suffer from insomnia. In this way, I'm always relaxed, and my skin is soft and smooth!

Another great option is to use lavender candles. Taking a nice warm bath surrounded by some lavender candles helps me relax and unwind just in time for a good rest!

—*Arleen K. Lamba, MD*

⌀⌀

I'm expecting my second child, and so getting enough sleep is especially important—and challenging. I try to get eight hours of sleep, but often I'll have work to do after my daughter goes to bed or before she wakes up. Those tend to be my most productive times, but I also have to balance that with spending some alone time with my husband. Balancing health, work, and family time is always a challenge!

—*Jennifer Bacani McKenney, MD*

⌀⌀

I have learned that I can't fall asleep if I'm trying to remember things that I need to do. I keep a to-do list on my phone. It's an app that allows you to group items into categories. I set up categories for the days of the week. When I add an item to my to-do list, I also "slot" it into which day I plan to accomplish it. This helps me better manage my to-dos. And getting those items out of my head and onto my list helps me to sleep.

—*Deborah Gilboa, MD*

❧

I never lie, I work hard, and I always try my best. I think that helps me sleep well at night! If I'm thinking of a patient I saw earlier, or I'm replaying a conversation I had, I know that I must "attend to it." I need to do something about the patient or the conversation. My brain tells me that this issue still requires some attention. Once I've settled this, I fall asleep because I now have a plan.

—*Hana R. Solomon, MD*

❧

To me, a good night's sleep is a must. When good sleep is compromised, the quality of the next workday is suboptimal, and mental health, alertness, and efficiency suffer.

Mommy MD Guides-Recommended Product
Cloud B Plush Aroma Pillow

"When my daughter was five, she started having trouble sleeping. We had no clue why," says Debra Jaliman, MD, a mom of a 21-year-old daughter, a dermatologist in private practice, an assistant professor of dermatology at Mt. Sinai School of Medicine in New York City, and the author of *Skin Rules: Trade Secrets from a Top New York Dermatologist.* "I bought her a lavender-scented pillow, and her sleep improved immediately."

The herb lavender reduces the stress hormone cortisol and improves sleep quality.

You can buy a Cloud B Plush Aroma Pillow in stores such as Target and Babies R Us and at online retailers such as **AMAZON.COM** for around $17.

> **A well-spent day brings happy sleep.**
> —*Leonardo da Vinci*

I've found it helpful to limit screen time at night. The TV, computer, and iPad are all stimulating. Just as I help my kids to wind down at night before bed, I realized I need to let myself wind down too. I try to turn off all screens two hours before bedtime.

—*Aline T. Tanios, MD*

༄

I have sleep apnea. It's a common medical condition that often goes undiagnosed. If you've been told you have a characteristic snoring pattern, you might have sleep apnea. Many people with the disorder snore louder and louder and then suddenly stop and gasp for breath. If you have sleep apnea, you might be waking up dozens or hundreds of times each night without even knowing it, and this leaves you feeling exhausted the next day. Definitely go to see a doctor.

A lot of children with untreated sleep apnea can't focus during the day, and they might be misdiagnosed with ADHD.

When I realized that I might have sleep apnea, I went to see my physician. To manage my apnea, I try to sleep on my stomach. When you sleep on your back, you're more likely to have problems with apnea. I also wear a mouth guard at night to facilitate easy breathing.

—*Eva Ritvo, MD*

༄

I'm a very high-energy person, and it sometimes can be hard to wind down enough to go to sleep. I find that meditating and doing yoga at night help to "switch" my brain off. I think these activities are especially helpful for people who have too much frenetic energy, who feel "jagged." Yoga and meditation help me to make the transition to sleep.

I do 20 to 30 minutes of meditation about three times a week and yoga once or twice a week.

Even though meditation has been around for more than

FitBit

Sometimes we use food to provide a quick pick-me-up, when what we really need is more sleep. Try to make time for seven to eight hours of sleep each night. If you're tired and you have a choice between a bite to eat and a 20-minute nap, take the nap!

2,000 years, it's amazing how few people know how to do it. I simply sit quietly in a comfortable place. I let my eyes and body relax. Sometimes I choose a word—a mantra—to focus on, and other times I merely focus on my breathing.

For me, meditating is like taking a wash towel and wringing it out. It helps me to bring focus into my day.

—*Nancy Rappaport, MD*

How do I boost my energy? I sleep! I think it's a myth when people say they don't have time to sleep. I say you don't have time *not* to sleep.

I aim for seven hours of sleep each night. Being well rested makes me more productive. It boosts my energy and my mental clarity. Also, it helps me with my weight. If you're tired, it saps your willpower to eat well and exercise. Getting good sleep is a huge piece of the weight loss puzzle.

To help get to sleep, I turn off all TVs and social media sites a few hours before bedtime. Some people take an Epsom salt bath before bed, and studies support that magnesium, which in this case is absorbed through your skin, can help you sleep. I find going to bed with a good book or magazine unwinds me and helps me to sleep.

—*Jennifer Hanes, DO*

I've never been able to function well without sleep. I have no idea how I made it through surgical residency, especially when there were no work hour restrictions.

I make sure that I go to bed early enough so that I can get at least seven to eight hours of sleep each night. I can't turn my phone off because I need to be available through the answering service in case patients call, but most people know not to call or text me after around 9 pm. I don't do the laundry until the weekend, and I've found that it's still there waiting for me just as I left it!

I've had to let go of my self-imposed perfectionistic rules about straightening up everything in the house before going to bed. My "to-do list" never gets cleared, and it took me a while to come to terms with that. But if you don't care for yourself, you have a very hard time taking care of anyone else.

—*Rachel S. Rohde, MD*

RALLIE'S TIP

Everyone in our family has busy schedules, and this often causes me to miss out on much-needed sleep. Of course, missing sleep drains me, and when I'm tired, I tend to eat more to try to boost my energy levels. The more sleep I miss, the more difficult it becomes to maintain my weight, and it seems nearly impossible to lose weight.

Mounting scientific evidence supports the notion that sleep deprivation significantly increases the risk for becoming overweight or obese. While the reasons for this phenomenon aren't entirely clear, experts have several theories. One theory is that sleep loss produces changes in the body that ultimately lead to an increase in food consumption. Over the past decade, several studies have shown that sleep restriction suppresses blood levels of the appetite-suppressing hormone, leptin, while increasing levels of ghrelin, a hormone that stimulates hunger.

I try to get at least seven hours of sleep each night, and I stick to a regular sleep schedule as much as possible.

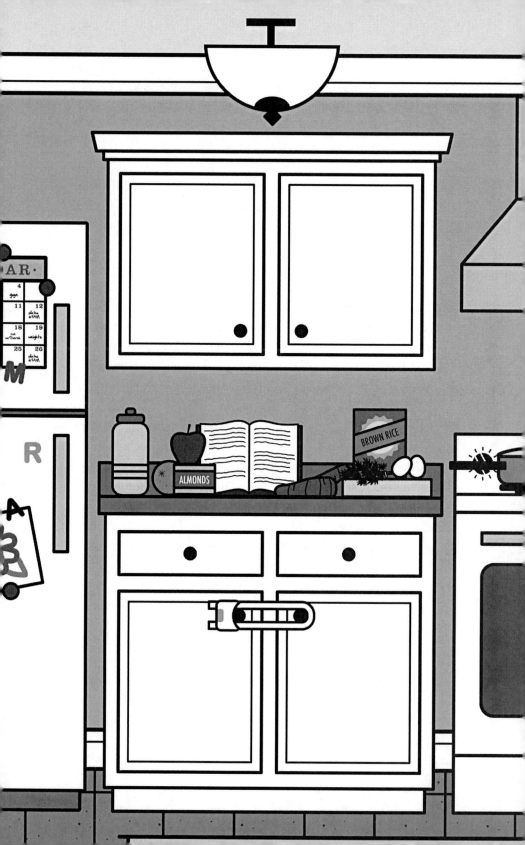

Chapter 5
Recipes for Feeling Great

What makes a recipe a favorite? Is it because the recipe's easy, inexpensive, and proven? We think so!

We asked our Mommy MD Guides for their family favorites, and here are our top picks that will boost energy and make you feel great! These recipes are all filled with energizing, health-boosting nutrients.

Because we've included the carbohydrates, protein, fat, and fiber counts for each, you can use any of these recipes with our Take Five! program with ease.

We prepare each of these recipes in our kitchens. Our families loved them, and we hope yours will too!

Bon appetit!

> **The only time to eat diet food is
> while you're waiting for the steak to cook.**
> —*Julia Child*

Bulletproof Coffee

Contributed by Sara Gottfried, MD. "This recipe was inspired by Dave Asprey, an author, biohacker, and entrepreneur. Try to find the highest-quality, most toxin-free [coffee] beans you can."

1½ to 2 cups brewed black coffee
2 tablespoons coconut oil

In a countertop blender or with a hand blender, blend the coffee with the coconut oil.

Makes 1 serving
Per serving: **238 calories, 0 g carbohydrates, 0 g protein, 27 g fat, 0 g fiber**

RightBites

Coffee is made by brewing beans, which means it's plant-based and has disease-fighting antioxidants just as other plant foods do. Although the antioxidant power of coffee isn't as great as many fruits and vegetables, it does pack a punch. Research suggessts that coffee helps improve concentration, memory, and learning immediately after drinking it. There is evidence to suggest that people who drink coffee regularly might have a lower risk for Alzheimer's and Parkinson's disease.

Being a coffee drinker also might help reduce your risk of cancer, including cancer of the breast and colon. In addition, it might help protect against diabetes. An 18-year Harvard study of more than 120,000 people found that drinking coffee regularly significantly lowered risk of type 2 diabetes.

Energy-Boosting Smoothie

Contributed by Rallie McAllister, MD, MPH. "For moms on the go, a smoothie is a quick and easy, nutrition-packed meal that will boost your health and keep you energized and satisfied for hours. When it comes to creating your favorite smoothie, use the most wholesome and nutritious ingredients available—and your imagination!"

½ cup blueberry or pomegranate juice
½ cup fat-free yogurt with probiotics (any flavor)
½ cup fresh fruit such as blueberries, chopped apples,
    or chopped pineapple
3 rounded tablespoons flavored protein powder made from soy,
    peas, or whey
2 tablespoons ground flaxseeds
½ teaspoon ground cinnamon
1 cup ice

In a blender, place the juice, yogurt, fruit, protein powder, ground flaxseeds, cinnamon, and ice, and blend until smooth.

Makes 1 serving (approximately 2¾ cups)
Per serving: 374 calories, 55 g carbohydrates, 25 g protein, 7 g fat, 7 grams fiber

🍽 RightBites

Flaxseed is high in fiber, with three grams per tablespoon, and it contains protein and plenty of vitamins and minerals. Flax also contains lignans, which are plant estrogens with a chemical structure similar to the hormone estrogen. Plant estrogens act as weak estrogens in the body, and they have been found to have anti-tumor properties and might help lower the risk of breast and colon cancers.

Choose ground flaxseed or flaxseed oil, which your body can digest better than whole seeds.

Green Machine Chocolate Smoothie

Contributed by Stacey Ann Weiland, MD. "This recipe is from my nutritionist friend, Elizabeth DiBiase, RD, at OffTheMatNutrition.com. It's a wonderful way to get children to eat greens and fruit. The chocolate and blueberries hide the color and taste of spinach. You can try other greens, such as kale, for a stronger green flavor and more nutrition."

1 cup milk, almond milk, or soy milk

1 cup spinach

1 banana

½ cup unsweetened frozen blueberries

1 to 2 teaspoons unsweetened cocoa powder (or to taste, depending on how much chocolate is wanted)

2 drops liquid stevia or 1 dollop maple syrup or honey

In a high-powered blender, place the milk, spinach, banana, blueberries, cocoa powder, and sweetener and blend for up to 1 minute, or until the smoothie is frothy and well blended.

Makes 1 serving

Per serving: 302 calories, 50 g carbohydrates, 10 g protein, 9 g fat, 6 g fiber

RightBites

Drinking milk is an easy way to get calcium, a mineral that strengthens your bones and helps keep your muscles, blood vessels, and nerves healthy. Women should get about three cups of dairy a day.

Oatmeal-Banana-Berry Pancake

Contributed by Rallie McAllister, MD, MPH. "This isn't your Grandma's pancake recipe. These pancakes are hearty, moist, and very satisfying."

2 eggs
1 banana, mashed
¼ cup coconut milk
½ cup quick-cooking rolled oats
2 tablespoons flour
¼ teaspoon almond extract
¼ teaspoon ground cardamom
¼ cup fresh blueberries

In a small bowl, lightly beat the eggs with a fork. Add the banana and stir with the fork to combine. Add the coconut milk and blend.

In a medium bowl, combine the oats, flour, almond extract, and cardamom. Pour the egg mixture into the oat mixture and stir just until combined.

Heat a 10-inch nonstick skillet over medium-high heat. Pour in the batter and drop the berries on top. Cover, reduce the heat to medium-low, and cook for 5 minutes. Flip the pancake, cover, and cook until firm, 1 to 2 minutes.

Makes 1 (10-inch) pancake
Per serving: **599 calories, 73 g carbohydrates, 23 g protein, 26 g fat, 9 g fiber**

RightBites

Potassium, a mineral found in bananas, has been shown to help reduce blood pressure. A report by the World Health Organization suggests that people with high potassium consumption have a 24 percent lower risk of stroke compared to people with low potassium consumption.

Jump-Start-Your-Day Breakfast Burritos

Contributed by Sonali Ruder, DO. "These burritos are a hearty and nutritious meal to start your day and set you on the right path for healthy eating all day long. The best part is that if you're not a morning person, you can prepare a whole batch of them ahead of time and freeze them. Then when you want to eat one, you just unwrap, pop it in the microwave, and take it to go! Serve the burritos alone or with reduced-fat sour cream, if desired."

2 teaspoons olive oil
1 small yellow onion, chopped
1 red bell pepper, chopped
Kosher salt
Black pepper
1 cup canned black beans, rinsed and drained
1 teaspoon chili powder
6 eggs
6 egg whites
2 ounces (½ cup) grated reduced-fat Cheddar cheese
6 whole grain wraps (9" diameter) (I use La Tortilla Factory
    Smart Delicious Whole Grain Soft Wraps)
¾ cup prepared salsa
¼ cup sliced scallions
Hot sauce (optional)

In a large nonstick skillet, heat the oil over medium heat. Add the onion and bell pepper and season with salt and black pepper. Cook, stirring occasionally, 7 to 8 minutes or until softened. Stir in the beans and chili powder and cook another for 2 to 3 minutes, or until heated through. Pour the contents of the skillet into a bowl and set aside. Wipe the skillet clean.

In a large bowl, whisk the eggs and egg whites together with ½ teaspoon salt and ¼ teaspoon black pepper.

Spray the skillet with cooking spray and heat over medium heat. Add the eggs and cook them, stirring occasionally, until soft curds form. Stir in the cheese and cook another minute, or until melted. Remove from the heat.

Spread each tortilla with equal amounts of the veggie-bean mixture and top with the scrambled eggs. Spread 2 tablespoons salsa, some sliced scallions, and hot sauce, if using, on top. Roll the tortillas up burrito style: Fold the side closest to you over the filling, then fold both sides in toward the center and roll up.

If not eating right away, wrap each burrito in plastic wrap or foil and freeze. To reheat, unwrap and microwave until warm, about 2 minutes, turning over halfway through. For a crispier wrapping, heat in the microwave, then bake in a 450°F oven for 5 to 10 minutes.

Makes 6 burritos
Per serving: **209 calories, 19 g carbohydrates, 19 g protein, 9 g fat, 9 g fiber**

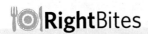 **Right**Bites

As a monounsaturated fat, olive oil can help reduce cholesterol levels, improve blood sugar regulation, and lower the risk of heart disease. A French study of more than 7,500 people age 65 and older showed that those who regularly consumed olive oil had a 41 percent lower risk of stroke compared with people who never consumed it.

Dr. Ann's Homemade Granola

Contributed by Ann Kulze, MD. "Homemade granola is so easy to make. When it comes to taste, value, and healthfulness, this recipe puts the store-bought varieties to shame. Feel free to omit or add any nuts, seeds, or dried fruit to your liking."

5 cups old-fashioned rolled oats

1 cup shredded coconut (optional)

½ cup walnuts, coarsely chopped

½ cup pine nuts

½ cup pecans, coarsely chopped

1½ cups dried fruit of choice (such as raisins, apricots, or cranberries)

½ cup molasses

¼ cup extra virgin olive oil or canola oil

3 teaspoons ground cinnamon

1 teaspoon vanilla extract

Preheat the oven to 325°F.

In a large mixing bowl, place the oats, coconut (if using), nuts, and dried fruit. Stir until thoroughly combined. Add the molasses, oil, cinnamon, and vanilla and stir until the dry ingredients are evenly coated. Spread the mixture evenly on a baking sheet with sides and bake for 25 to 30 minutes, or until light brown and toasted. (For even cooking, carefully stir the granola mixture every 10 minutes.)

Remove the granola from the oven and allow it to cool. (It will become crunchier as it cools.)

Store the granola in an airtight container at room temperature or in the freezer in a zipper-lock plastic bag.

Makes about 8 cups, or 12 (²/₃-cup) servings
***Per serving:* 358 calories, 48 g carbohydrates, 8 g protein, 16 g fat, 5 g fiber**

Doctor Dip

Contributed by Jennifer Hanes, DO. "If you eat this dip every day, it could keep us [doctors] away. This dip is a delight of high-protein goodness. If you use local honey, and eat this daily, it might help reduce your seasonal allergy symptoms. Apples are a great fruit to use as a dipper. Other healthy choices include bananas, grapes, and even pears."

1 cup plain Greek yogurt
1 cup creamy peanut butter
1 teaspoon honey

In a small bowl, combine the yogurt, peanut butter, and honey. Serve with cut fruit. Store any remaining dip in an airtight container in the refrigerator for up to 1 week.

Makes 8 (¼-cup) servings
Per serving: **228 calories, 8 g carbohydrates, 10 g protein, 19 g fat, 2 g fiber**

RightBites

Antibiotics are notorious for causing diarrhea, but eating a daily serving of yogurt can help you avoid this unwelcome side effect. Antibiotics are designed to kill bacteria that are making you sick, but they also attack friendly microbes in your gut. As a result, your body has a harder time digesting food. Nearly a quarter of people taking antibiotics experience diarrhea, and as many as one in five doesn't finish antibiotic therapy for that reason.

Probiotics, which are found in yogurt and kefir, replenish the good bacteria in your gut, helping your digestive system work properly while you're taking antibiotics.

Kale Chips

Contributed by Antoinette Cheney, DO. "I like to make these chips when I'm craving something crunchy and salty but want to eat something healthier than from a box or bag."

1 bunch kale (about 10 cups), washed and spun or patted dry
2 tablespoons olive oil
1 teaspoon kosher salt (or other seasoning)

Preheat the oven to 350°F.

Remove the center stem from the kale leaves, then tear the leaves into equal-size pieces. (The smaller the pieces, the crisper the final chips will be.) Place the kale in a single layer on a baking sheet. (Use 2 sheets, if necessary, but bake them separately.) Drizzle the kale with the oil, and mix it with your hands to distribute the oil. Sprinkle the kale with the salt. Bake for 12 minutes, or until crispy and starting to brown. Allow to cool before snacking. Store in an airtight container at room temperature for up to 2 days.

Makes 4 servings
Per serving: 76 calories, 3 g carbohydrates,
1 g protein, 7 g fat, 1 g fiber

RightBites

Cruciferous vegetables such as kale, broccoli, cabbage, and collard greens contain cancer-fighting compounds called isothiocyanates (ITCs), which help destroy cancer cells, and sulforaphanes, which appear to strengthen the body's defense against cancer.

Findings from another study suggest that kale, garlic, and strawberries appear to protect the body from injury caused by nitrites. Found in hot dogs and other processed foods, nitrites are food preservatives that have been linked to the development of certain cancers.

Kale is high in fiber, which is filling and helps to lower cholesterol levels, regulate blood sugar, and prevent constipation.

Tabbouleh

Contributed by Hana R. Solomon, MD. "My husband often prepares this, and we enjoy it, as well as other dishes, all week."

1 cup fine-grind (#1) bulgur
2 large tomatoes, chopped
1 teaspoon salt
3 to 5 large bunches flat-leaf parsley, finely chopped (about 2 to
   3 cups)
2 tablespoons dried mint
$\frac{1}{4}$ to $\frac{1}{2}$ cup olive oil
$\frac{1}{2}$ cup fresh lemon juice

Rinse the bulgur and drain off the excess water. Place the bulgur in a medium bowl. Let it stand for 30 to 60 minutes to soften, stirring every now and then.

Add the tomatoes, salt, parlsey, and mint and mix thoroughly. Add the oil and lemon juice and taste for seasoning. Add more salt, if desired. Store, covered, in the refrigerator.

Makes 10 ($\frac{1}{2}$-cup) servings
Per serving: **110 calories, 14 g carbohydrates,
3 g protein, 6 g fat, 4 g fiber**

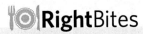 **Right**Bites

Research at the University of Missouri found that a compound in parsley called apigenin delayed the formation of tumors in rats with breast cancer, leading the scientists to theorize that the compound might also help prevent breast cancer in human.

Herbed Chickpea Salad

Contributed by Rallie McAllister, MD, MPH. "This recipe comes from LittleJudeOnFood.com, which is 'written' by a toddler and his chef mother. It's quick and easy to prepare and makes great use of summer's freshest herbs. Add more (or less) of them to suit your taste."

2 cans (15 ounces each) chickpeas, rinsed and drained
1 cup fresh parsley, finely chopped
1 cup fresh basil, finely chopped
2 cloves garlic, minced
Juice of 1 lemon (or more, to taste)
2½ tablespoons olive oil
2 ounces (½ cup) freshly grated Parmesan cheese
Kosher salt
Black pepper

In a medium bowl, gently combine the chickpeas, parsley, basil, garlic, lemon juice, oil, and cheese. Season with salt and pepper to taste. Serve at once or chill, covered, before serving. Store tightly covered in the refrigerator for up to 3 days.

Makes 4 servings
Per serving: 294 calories, 34 g carbohydrates, 11 g protein, 13 g fat, 7 g fiber

⦿ RightBites

Chickpeas offer a healthy dose of almost all of the essential amino acids (the building blocks of protein), beneficial unsaturated fats, and vitamins, including beta-carotene, folate, thiamin, riboflavin, and niacin. Research suggests that chickpeas might help lower the risk for heart disease, type 2 diabetes, certain cancers, and digestive disorders.

Aunt Joy's Curried Chicken Salad

Contributed by Martha Wittenberg, MD, MPH. "This salad is really pretty and colorful. You can leave out the chicken, sprinkle with cilantro, and serve with fish. I brought this to a party recently, and even my friends who are caterers loved it! You can make this one day ahead."

1/2 cup light mayonnaise
1 teaspoon curry powder
1/2 teaspoon salt
1/8 teaspoon black pepper
2 cups cubed cooked chicken, cooled
1 1/2 cups cooked rice pilaf, brown rice, or quinoa, cooled
1/2 cup chopped red or green bell pepper
1 can (11 ounces) mandarin oranges, drained
1/4 cup sliced scallions
1/2 cup golden raisins

In a large bowl, mix together the mayonnaise, curry powder, salt, black pepper, chicken, rice or quinoa, bell pepper, oranges, scallions, and raisins. Chill for at least 2 hours before serving.

Makes 4 servings
Per serving: 401 calories, 41 g carbohydrates, 25 g protein, 15 g fat, 3 g fiber

Carola's Thai Bouillabaisse

Contributed by Nancy Rappaport, MD. "This dish is great for entertaining a group of friends. It's relatively easy to prepare. It's important to note that eating with friends can help with self-care and replenishing energy."

1 tablespoon canola or coconut oil
1 stalk lemongrass, lightly smashed and cut into 3" pieces (to be removed later)
1 piece (1") fresh ginger, peeled and minced
4 shallots, minced
8 cloves garlic, minced
2 leeks, washed and sliced (white part and very light green parts only)
4 cups fish stock or vegetable broth
2 cans (13.5 ounces each) coconut milk
1 cup white wine
1 tablespoon fish sauce
1 chile pepper (such as red Chinese chile pepper), seeds removed and minced (or ½ teaspoon chili powder, or to taste)
½ to 1 teaspoon Thai red curry paste
Pinch saffron
1 cup uncooked basmati or jasmine rice
2 tomatoes, chopped
12 ounces skinless salmon, cut into 1" chunks
1 pound mussels, rinsed and debearded (discard any cracked shells)
1 pound peeled and deveined medium or large shrimp
1 cup fresh cilantro, roughly chopped
1 cup fresh basil, cut into ribbons
2 limes, cut into wedges

In a large soup pot, heat the oil over medium heat. Add the lemongrass, ginger, shallots, garlic, and leeks and cook, stirring occasionally, for about 5 minutes, or until the vegetables begin to soften.

Add the stock or broth, coconut milk, wine, fish sauce, chile pepper, curry paste, and saffron. Bring to a boil, reduce the heat to medium-low, and simmer for 30 minutes.

Meanwhile, prepare the rice according to the package directions.

Remove the lemongrass from the broth. Add the tomatoes and salmon and cook for 2 minutes. Add the mussels and cook for 2 more minutes. Add the shrimp, and cook for 2 to 3 more minutes, or until the salmon is just cooked through, the mussels have opened, and the shrimp are pink and their tails are curled. Discard any mussels that have not opened.

Divide the rice among 8 bowls. Ladle the bouillabaisse over. Sprinkle the cilantro and basil on top. Serve with the lime wedges.

Makes 8 (1½-cups) servings
Per serving: **571 calories, 40 g carbohydrates, 37 g protein, 29 g fat, 2 g fiber**

🍽 **Right**Bites

About 10.5 ounces of shrimp deliver 1.5 grams of heart-healthy omega-3 fatty acids. In fact, the American Heart Association recommends that people with heart disease consume at least one gram of omega-3s a day. The results of several clinical trials showed that heart patients who boosted their consumption of omega-3s lowered their risk of heart attack and death.

Omega-3 fatty acids improve heart health by helping to reduce triglyceride levels, normalize blood pressure, and prevent abnormal heart rhythms.

Chicken Soup

Contributed by Hana R. Solomon, MD. "This is my mom's chicken soup recipe. It's the best in the world! Parsley root, or petrushka in my family, looks like a large white/light gray carrot or parsnip. Its peak season is between November and February. If you can't find it, substitute the same amount of fresh parsnips or turnips."

1 chicken (3 to 4 pounds)
2 carrots, peeled and cut into small pieces
2 stalks celery, cut into small pieces
1 small onion (whole)
1 parsley root, cut into small pieces
¼ cup fresh dill (uncut)
Salt

Cut the chicken into quarters and wash well. Place in a large pot and cover with cold water. Bring to a boil.

Add the carrots, celery, onion, and parsley root. Simmer over medium heat for 15 minutes, occasionally skimming the foam from the top of the water. Remove the chicken, allow it to cool, remove the skin and bones, and return the chicken to the pot. Remove the onion. Simmer for another 15 minutes, then add the dill. Season to taste with salt.

Makes 4 servings
Per serving: **511 calories, 6 g carbohydrates, 43 g protein, 34 g fat, 2 g fiber**

🍴◉ RightBites

Adults get on average two to four colds a year, each time spending 8 to 10 miserable days suffering. When it happens to you, enjoy a bowl of chicken soup. Researchers at the Nebraska Medical Center in Omaha found that eating chicken soup can help reduce the severity and duration of the common cold.

Southwest Soup

Contributed by Jennifer Hanes, DO. "This satisfying Southwest-inspired soup will shock you with flavor and stick-to-your-ribs yumminess, without adding inches to your thighs. The smoky flavor of the peppers and onions in the southwestern corn adds interest and depth to the flavor. For those bold enough, you can kick it up to eye-watering superspicy to encourage drinking extra water with dinner."

1 pound boneless, skinless chicken breasts
1 or 2 chicken bouillon cubes (optional)
1 can (10 ounces) regular or hot Ro–Tel
    (tomatoes and diced green chiles)
1 can (16 ounces) fat-free refried beans
2 cans (16 ounces each) red kidney beans, rinsed and drained
16 ounces frozen southwestern corn, or 16 ounces frozen corn
    and 1 teaspoon southwestern seasoning

Put the chicken in a saucepan and add enough water to cover by 1 to 2 inches. Bring to a boil, and add the bouillon, if using, for additional flavor. Boil for around 10 to 15 minutes.

Meanwhile, in a blender, combine the tomatoes and refried beans. Blend until smooth. (This will serve as the base of your soup.)

Transfer the tomato mixture to a large soup pot and add the kidney beans and corn. Add water from the saucepan, if desired, to thin the soup. Bring to a simmer.

Once the chicken is cooked through (white in the center), remove and rinse under cold water to freshen. When cool enough to handle, chop into bite-size pieces and add to the soup.

 Makes 8 (1-cup) servings
Per serving: **216 calories, 26 g carbohydrates, 20 g protein, 3 g fat, 7 grams fiber**

Thai-Style Congee (Rice Stew)

Contributed by Tiemdow Phumiruk, MD. "This is Asian comfort food. It's very much like chicken noodle soup, with a lot of rice. If it sits for a while, the rice will soak up all the soup. Just add more broth and seasonings (for example, for leftovers the next day)."

2 tablespoons vegetable oil

3 or 4 cloves garlic, minced

1/2 to 3/4 cup ground chicken or shrimp,
    or any leftover cooked meat

4 cups chicken broth (homemade is best, but canned is fine)

2 cups cooked white rice, or 3/4 cup uncooked

6 shakes (2 tablespoons) fish sauce

1 to 2 tablespoons white vinegar

1 teaspoon salt

Black pepper

1/4 cup chopped cilantro, divided

1/4 cup chopped scallions for garnish

In a large skillet over high heat, heat the oil. Add the garlic and stir-fry for 30 seconds. Add the chicken or shrimp and cook until just cooked through. (If it is already cooked, add it last.)

Pour in the broth and bring to a boil. Add the rice. (If using uncooked rice, you'll have to monitor the pot and keep stirring until it's cooked.) Add the fish sauce and vinegar and salt and pepper to taste and bring to a boil. Add half the cilantro while cooking, then add the remainder for garnish. Garnish with scallions, if desired.

Ideally, the texture should be soupy. The rice shouldn't soak up all the liquid.

Makes 4 servings
Per serving: 246 calories, 29 g carbohydrates, 11 g protein, 10 g fat, 1 g fiber

Coconut Rice

Contributed by Jeannette Gonzalez Simon, MD. "This is the best coconut rice recipe! It's excellent as a side for Thai and Indian dishes, such as curries or seafood recipes. This is also a super kid-friendly dish!"

2 cups coconut milk
1 cup cream of coconut
½ teaspoon salt
2 cups uncooked Thai jasmine white rice
2 heaping tablespoons unsweetened shredded coconut
(the type used for baking)

In a medium saucepan over medium-high heat, bring the coconut milk, cream of coconut, and salt to boil. Stir in the rice and coconut and stir occasionally to keep the rice from sticking to the bottom of the saucepan and burning.

Once the liquid has begun to gently bubble, stop stirring and reduce the heat to low (just above minimum). Cover tightly and let simmer for 20 minutes, or until the rice is soft and most of the liquid has been absorbed by the rice. (If the liquid is absorbed before the rice is of desired tenderness, remove the saucepan from the heat and let sit, covered, for 5 minutes before serving.)

When ready to serve, remove the lid and fluff the rice with a fork. If desired, add a bit more shredded coconut or toasted coconut, to taste.

Makes 8 servings
Per serving: **407 calories, 58 g carbohydrates, 5 g protein, 18 g fat, 2 g fiber**

To toast coconut: Place 1 tablespoon shredded coconut in a skillet over medium-high heat and stir ("dry fry") until light golden brown.

Roasted French String Beans with Toasted Sesame Seeds

Contributed by Ayala Laufer-Cahana, MD. "You can serve this delicious side dish hot or at room temperature."

1 pound haricots verts (thin French green beans), ends trimmed
2 tablespoons toasted sesame oil or olive oil
2 tablespoons sesame seeds
Pinch or two of red pepper flakes (optional)
Salt
Black pepper

Preheat the oven to 400°F with a baking sheet in the oven.

In a medium bowl, toss the string beans with the oil, sesame seeds, and red pepper, if using.

Spread the beans in a single layer on the preheated baking sheet.

Bake for 3 to 5 minutes, or until the beans become slightly brown and are sizzling, but are still very crunchy and vibrant.

Season to taste with salt and pepper.

Makes 8 servings
Per serving: **65 calories, 4 g carbohydrates, 1 g protein, 4 g fat, 2 g fiber**

Vegetable Lasagna

Contributed by Ann Kulze, MD. "Even lasagna can be great for you."

3 tablespoons extra-virgin olive oil
8 ounces sliced mushrooms
1 cup prepackaged shredded carrots
1 yellow onion, chopped
1 can (15 ounces) tomato sauce
2 cans (6 ounces each) tomato paste
1 can (2.25 ounces) sliced black olives, drained
10 ounces frozen chopped spinach, thawed and squeezed
3 tablespoons chopped fresh basil
1½ teaspoons dried oregano
1 cup low-fat cottage cheese
1 cup part-skim ricotta cheese
16 ounces (4 cups) shredded mozzarella cheese
3 ounces (¾ cup) grated Parmesan cheese
9 oven-ready (no-boil) lasagna noodles

Preheat the oven to 375°F. In a large skillet over medium heat, heat the oil, add the mushrooms, carrots, and onion and sauté for 8 minutes, or until tender. Stir in the tomato sauce, paste, olives, spinach, basil, and oregano. Cook for 10 minutes, to allow the flavors to blend. In a small bowl, mix together the cottage cheese and ricotta cheese. In a separate bowl, combine the mozzarella and Parmesan.

Coat a 13" x 9" baking dish with cooking spray. Place 3 lasagna noodles in a single layer in the dish. Spread with one-third of the cottage cheese mixture, one-third of the tomato mixture, and one-third of the mozzarella mixture to cover the noodles. Repeat the layers two more times.

Bake for about 30 minutes, or until the cheese is melted and the sauce is bubbling. Let stand for a few minutes before serving.

Makes 8 servings
Per serving: 486 calories, 36 g carbohydrates,
31 g protein, 25 g fat, 6 g fiber

Mediterranean Chicken

Contributed by Ann Kulze, MD. "This dish is loaded with superstar foods, and all of my kids love it. Serve the chicken over brown rice, multigrain pasta, or quinoa, along with a tossed salad."

2 tablespoons extra-virgin olive oil, divided
1 yellow onion, chopped
4 cloves garlic, chopped
2 cans (14.5 ounces each) diced tomatoes with juice
3 tablespoons drained capers
1/4 cup chopped fresh parsley (or 1 1/2 tablespoons dried)
3 tablespoons chopped fresh basil (or 1 teaspoon dried)
3 tablespoons chopped fresh oregano (or 1 teaspoon dried)
1 1/2 pounds boneless, skinless chicken thighs, cut into pieces

In a heavy skillet, heat 1 tablespoon of the oil over medium heat. Add the onion and garlic and sauté until a bit soft, about 5 minutes. Add the tomatoes, capers, and herbs. Bring to a boil. Reduce the heat to low and continue cooking, stirring occasionally, for about 25 minutes, until the mixture thickens a bit.

In a separate large skillet, heat the remaining 1 tablespoon oil. Sear the chicken on both sides until golden brown. Add the chicken to the tomato mixture and continue cooking, uncovered, for 7 to 10 minutes, or until cooked through.

Makes 4 servings
Per serving: **374 calories, 14 g carbohydrates, 33 g protein, 20 g fat, 2 g fiber**

Slow-Cooker Ham Tetrazzini

Contributed by Rallie McAllister, MD, MPH. "This dish is yummy and filling, with lots of protein and just a little fat."

1 can (10.5 ounces) reduced-fat condensed
   cream of mushroom soup
2½ ounces (1 cup) sliced mushrooms
1 cup cubed cooked lean ham
½ cup fat-free evaporated milk
2 tablespoons water
8 ounces spaghetti
2 ounces (½ cup) grated Parmesan cheese

In a slow cooker, combine the soup, mushrooms, ham, milk, and water. Cover and cook on low for 4 hours.

Toward the end of the cooking time, prepare the spaghetti according to the package directions; drain. Add the spaghetti and cheese to the slow cooker. Toss to coat.

Makes 4 servings
Per serving: **379 calories, 53 g carbohydrates, 23 g protein, 8 g fat, 3 g fiber**

Mediterranean Potato, Onion, Tomato, and Fresh Herb Bake

Contributed by Ayala Laufer-Cahana, MD. "This easy, vegan, hearty dish combines the comfort of potatoes, with the light freshness of fresh basil and parsley and the lovely redness of tomatoes and red spices. Serve it with warm rustic bread to soak up the juices at the bottom of the baking dish."

7 medium potatoes, (preferably Yukon Gold) peeled and sliced
5 large tomatoes, sliced
4 yellow onions, sliced
2 scallions, sliced
3/4 cup chopped fresh basil
2 tablespoons chopped fresh parsley
2 teaspoons dry basil
1 teaspoon paprika
Dash of cayenne pepper (to taste)
Salt
Black pepper
1/2 cup extra virgin olive oil
1/4 cup chopped fresh basil (optional)

Preheat the oven to 400°F.

In a large bowl, combine all of the ingredients. Taste a tomato slice and correct seasoning as needed.

In a large, deep baking dish, arrange the ingredients, cover with foil, and bake for 1 1/2 to 2 hours, until golden and the potatoes are soft. (Do not overfill the dish; place it on a baking sheet if it might overflow.) Remove the dish from the oven and stir the mixture a few times during baking. Remove the foil 10 minutes before the dish is ready. Garnish with the fresh basil (if using).

Makes 6 servings
Per serving: 389 calories, 53 g carbohydrates, 6 g protein, 19 g fat, 7 g fiber

Lemon-Herb Salmon

Contributed by Jeannette Gonzalez Simon, MD. "Fish is one of the fastest, easiest things to cook."

2 fillets (4 ounces each) salmon
2 sprigs fresh rosemary or dill, divided
Salt
Black pepper
2 teaspoons butter, divided
2 lemons

Preheat the oven to 400°F.

Tear off a piece of foil a little larger than twice the size of 1 salmon fillet. Coat the foil with cooking spray or rub with olive oil. Place half of the rosemary or dill in the middle of the foil.

Sprinkle 1 fillet with salt and pepper to taste and place it on top of the herbs. Add 1 teaspoon of the butter.

Thinly slice half of 1 lemon and place the slices on top of the salmon. Squeeze the juice of the remaining half lemon over the fillet.

Fold the foil by bringing the ends together over the salmon, folding tightly several times. Repeat with the two ends of the foil, sealing them tightly also.

Repeat with the remaining salmon fillet, herbs, butter, and lemon.

Place the foil-wrapped salmon packets on a baking sheet and bake for 10 to 12 minutes, or until the fish is just cooked in the center.

Makes 2 servings
Per serving: 225 calories, 5 g carbohydrates,
25 g protein, 12 g fat, 1 g fiber

Sweet and Salty Trail Mix

Contributed by Rallie McAllister, MD, MPH. "I like to make my own trail mix. I keep it handy in my cooler, my car, or my desk so I can grab a handful whenever I need a quick burst of long-lasting energy."

½ cup blanched almonds
½ cup raisins
1 cup low-fat granola cereal
½ cup dried cranberries
½ cup dried blueberries
½ cup shelled sunflower seeds

In a container with a tight-fitting lid, mix the almonds, raisins, granola, cranberries, blueberries, and sunflower seeds. Store, tightly covered, at room temperature.

Makes 14 (¼-cup) servings
***Per serving:* 132 calories, 19 g carbohydrates, 3 g protein, 5 g fat, 3 g fiber**

RightBites

Nuts might be high in fat, but they're the healthy fats: mono-unsaturated and polyunsaturated. These fats don't elevate cholesterol levels, and they might lower your risk for heart disease. In a study that followed 86,000 women over 14 years, Harvard researchers found that women who ate five ounces of nuts each week lowered their risk of a heart attack by 35 percent compared to women who ate less than one ounce a month.

Nuts can also help with weight loss. In one study of 65 people who were overweight or obese, those who ate a diet that included three ounces of raw almonds every day lost 62 percent more weight than those who ate a diet without nuts.

Mocha Espresso Granita

Contributed by Sonali Ruder, DO. "If you're looking for a refreshing caffeine hit on a hot day, this dish is for you. Try it plain or, for a slightly more decadent treat, top it with some lightly sweetened whipped cream or fat-free whipped topping and chocolate shavings."

4 cups brewed espresso or strong coffee
1/3 cup natural Demerara sugar or turbinado sugar
2 tablespoons unsweetened cocoa powder
3/4 teaspoon ground cinnamon
Fat-free whipped topping or freshly whipped cream (optional)
Dark chocolate shavings (optional)

In a large bowl, stir together the espresso, sugar, cocoa powder, and cinnamon until the sugar is dissolved. Taste and adjust the level of sweetness, as desired. Pour the mixture into a 13" x 9" glass baking dish. Place the dish in the freezer.

Freeze for 30 minutes. Remove the dish and use a fork to scrape the mixture, breaking up any icy clumps. Return the dish to the freezer. Repeat the process every 30 minutes or so, scraping the mixture with a fork to break up the ice crystals and create a light and fluffy texture. (It should take 2 to 2½ hours total.)

Scoop the granita into dessert bowls. Serve plain or garnish with whipped topping or whipped cream, chocolate shavings, and a sprinkling of cinnamon, if desired. Serve immediately.

 Makes 8 servings
Per serving: 45 calories, 11 g carbohydrates,
0 g protein, 0 g fat, 1 g fiber

Super Chocolatey Cookies

Contributed by Ayala Laufer-Cahana, MD. "*These cookies are perfect for the serious chocolate lover and great for cookie fans too. I've received a recipe request from every recipient of this cookie gift who dares to bake. These cookies are as close as it comes to eating pure chocolate while still serving a dessert. They're rich, chunky, delicious, and decadent, and they hit the chocolate-craving spot right on.*"

17.6 ounces (500 grams) dark chocolate (72% cacao),
    broken into pieces
17.6 ounces (500 grams) milk chocolate, broken into pieces
²/₃ cup all-purpose flour
1 teaspoon baking powder
Pinch salt
1 cup sugar
4 tablespoons unsalted butter, at room temperature
4 eggs
2 teaspoons vanilla extract
1 cup chopped walnuts (optional)

Preheat the oven to 350°F.

Set up a double boiler by placing a glass or metal bowl over a saucepan with 1 to 2 inches of barely simmering water (do not let the bowl touch the water). Place the bittersweet and milk chocolate in the bowl, and melt it, stirring occasionally until smooth. (Be careful of the steam that will come out of the saucepan when you remove the bowl.)

In a small bowl, sift together the flour, baking powder, and salt.

In a large bowl, use an electric mixer to cream the sugar and butter. Add the eggs, one at a time, until thoroughly incorporated. Then add the vanilla and continue beating until well combined.

Beat in the flour mixture, and then mix in the melted chocolate and nuts, if using. (The final batter is thick and dark.)

Line 2 baking sheets with parchment paper or Silpat baking mats. Using 2 tablespoons, drop 12 cookies onto each baking sheet, 2 inches apart.

Bake for 9 to 11 minutes, or until the cookie tops get glossy and crack a bit. Cool the cookies for a few minutes before removing from the baking sheets. Repeat with the remaining batter.

Store the cookies in an airtight container.

Makes 48 cookies
Per cookie: **150 calories, 17 g carbohydrates, 2 g protein, 8 g fat, 2 g fiber**

RightBites

Chocolate is made from cocoa beans, which are a great source of natural antioxidant, called flavonoids. Flavonoids combat cell damage caused by free radicals, reducing the risk of cancer, heart disease, and Alzheimer's disease.

Because raw cocoa beans are much too bitter to eat, chocolate manufacturers add sugar and fat to create a treat that tastes good. In the process, the beans lose some of their health benefits.

When you're in the mood for a nutritious sweet treat, dark chocolate is your best bet because it contains 23 percent fat-free cocoa solids. Look for dark chocolate made with unsweetened, 100 percent cocoa powder. And be sure to keep the calories in check by limiting your portion.

Blueberry-Zucchini Muffins

Contributed by Rallie McAllister, MD, MPH. "These delicious, dairy-free muffins are a great way to savor summer's bumper crop of zucchini and blueberries, but they can be enjoyed year-round. I found them on LittleJudeOnFood.com, where the toddler who 'blogs' with his chef mother notes that these also freeze very well."

2 cups unbleached all-purpose flour
1 cup whole wheat flour
1 teaspoon ground cinnamon
½ teaspoon ground nutmeg
2 eggs
⅓ cup packed brown sugar
2 teaspoons vanilla extract
3 cups freshly grated zucchini, drained
⅔ cup canola oil
2 teaspoons baking soda
½ teaspoon salt
1 cup fresh blueberries, frozen (so they don't crush and stain the
    batter)

Preheat the oven to 350°F. Line 18 muffin tins with paper liners, or coat the tins with cooking spray or melted butter.

In a large bowl, whisk together the flours, cinnamon, and nutmeg.

In a separate bowl, whisk together the eggs, brown sugar, and vanilla. Stir in the zucchini. Add the oil, baking soda, and salt, and stir to combine.

Add the wet ingredients to the dry, and stir until just combined and all the flour is moistened. Gently stir in the blueberries.

Fill the prepared muffin tins two-thirds full and bake for 15 to 20 minutes. (If you're making mini muffins, check them at 15 minutes.) The muffins should be firm to the touch, and a toothpick inserted in the center of one should come out clean. Cool the muffins in the tins for 5 minutes, then remove to a wire rack to cool completely.

**Makes 18 regular muffins
or 12 regular muffins + 12 mini muffins**
Per regular muffin: **180 calories, 21 g carbohydrates, 3 g protein, 9 g fat, 2 g fiber**

🍽 **Right**Bites

When it comes to zucchini or any type of summer squash, go ahead and indulge. Squash has a high water content, just 20 calories per cup, and nourishes your body with vitamins C and B_6, the mineral potassium, and fiber.

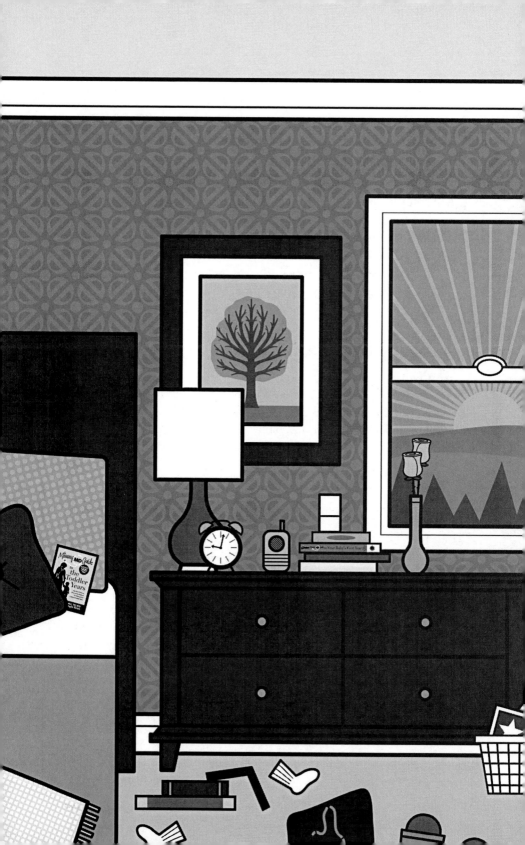

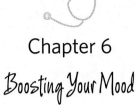

Chapter 6
Boosting Your Mood

YOUR BODY

Anyone can feel sad or depressed at times. Sometimes stresses and problems in life can trigger depression. But it's fascinating to think that women are 50 percent more likely than men to experience an actual mood disorder over their lifetime, according to the National Institute of Mental Health (NIMH). Mood disorders include all types of depression and bipolar disorder.

As many as two-thirds of women try to soldier on with a mood disorder, trying to suffer in silence. It's important to realize though that once a person has been diagnosed with depression or bipolar disorder, the chance for her children to have the same diagnosis is increased. Extensive research has shown that a mother's depression, especially when untreated, can interfere with her child's social, emotional, and cognitive development. Getting treatment is essential for your health—and for that of your family.

JUSTIFICATION FOR A CELEBRATION

Feeling great is reason to celebrate and the celebration all in one! If you feel great, you'll want to celebrate, and if you're celebrating, you're probably feeling great. Celebrate good times—c'mon!

> **While we may not be able to control all that happens to us, we can control what happens inside us.**
> —*Benjamin Franklin*

Assessing Your Mood

Bet you have a mug of coffee, glass of water, or (gasp) bottle of soda sitting nearby. Take a look: Is it half full or half empty? In general, are you an optimist or a pessimist? It's helpful to know if your mood tends toward the sunny or the saturnine.

The Goldberg Depression Questionnaire below was developed by Ivan Goldberg, MD, a psychiatrist and clinical psychopharmacologist in private practice in New York City who was formerly on the staff of the National Institute of Mental Health and the departments of psychiatry of the Columbia-Presbyterian Medical Center and Columbia University's College of Physicians and Surgeons. This assessment is reprinted here with permission by Dr. Goldberg.

For each question, ask yourself how you have felt and behaved during the past week.

0 = Not at all

1 = Just a little

2 = Somewhat

3 = Moderately

4 = Quite a lot

5 = Very much

I do things slowly. ☐

My future seems hopeless. ☐

It is hard for me to concentrate on reading. ☐

The pleasure and joy have gone out of my life. ☐

I have difficulty making decisions. ☐

I have lost interest in aspects of life that used to be important to me. ☐

I feel sad, blue, and unhappy. □

I am agitated and keep moving around. □

I feel fatigued. □

It takes great effort for me to do simple things. □

I feel that I am a guilty person who deserves to be punished. □

I feel like a failure. □

I feel lifeless—more dead than alive. □

My sleep has been disturbed (too little, too much, or broken sleep). □

I spend time thinking about HOW I might kill myself. □

I feel trapped or caught. □

I feel depressed even when good things happen to me. □

Without trying to diet, I have lost, or gained, weight. □

Add up your answers: □
The highest possible score is 90. Record your score, then take the test in another week and watch for changes.

I'm an upbeat and positive person. Mellow has never been an adjective for me!
—*Pam D'Amato, MD, a mom of seven- and four-year-old daughters and an interventional pain management physician with University Spine Center, in Wayne, NJ*

> **Our lives improve only when we take chances,
> and the first and most difficult risk we can take
> is to be honest with ourselves.**
> —*Walter Anderson, a German writer*

When I think about my mood, I find that if I'm tired, I am a lower-mood person. If I've had a good night's sleep, I'm a higher-mood person. My mood level and energy levels are closely related.

> —*Nancy Rappaport, MD, a mom of 22- and 18-year-old daughters and a 20-year-old son, an associate professor of psychiatry at Harvard Medical School, an attending child and adolescent psychiatrist in the Cambridge, MA, public schools, and the author of* The Behavior Code

I know that my moods are related to my hormonal cycle. I find that I'm most creative around the time of ovulation, and my mood is lower when it's time for my period. I've learned to accept this and work with my body, not against it. I acknowledge it, and I let it be.

For example, I have noticed creative activities such as planning a birthday party or scrapbooking or writing blogs come much easier around the time of ovulation. Of course I engage in these activities during other times, but when possible, I allow myself to be swept away. I am also really good at organizing closets and drawers during ovulation, although I abhor doing it the rest of the month.

> —*Jennifer Hanes, DO, a mom of a seven-year-old daughter and a four-year-old son, an emergency physician who's board certified in integrative medicine, and the author of* The Princess Plan: Shrink Your Waist, Expand Your Beauty, *in Austin, TX*

Sadly, I'm a "glass-half-empty" person. The good news is that my approach to life makes me a better surgeon because I notice the details that are out of place. That combined with my Virgo sign makes me a perfectionist. That is beneficial to the outcomes of my surgeries.

The bad side of this is that I'm very critical of myself. I don't always think positive thoughts! I've really struggled with that and have come to realize the value of positive internal dialogue.

—Michelle Yagoda, MD, a mom of an 11-year-old son, a facial plastic surgeon, the CEO of Opus Skincare, LLC, and cofounder of BeautyScoop, a patented and clinically proven supplement for skin, hair, and nails, in New York City

When to Call Your Doctor

According to the Centers for Disease Control and Prevention in Atlanta, an estimated 1 in 10 U.S. adults report depression.

In particular, feeling sad, anxious, or empty happens to about 13 percent of women after pregnancy, thanks to a steep drop in estrogen and progesterone after childbirth.

To feel great—and you most certainly can even if you have depression—you need to get treatment. Call your doctor or seek immediate help if you have thoughts of hurting yourself or your child.

Call your doctor if you have the following signs of depression for longer than two weeks.

- You don't have interest in your child.
- You feel restless.
- You're moody.
- You're sad and cry often.
- You feel hopeless or overwhelmed.
- You feel worthless.
- You're fatigued and lack motivation.
- You're not eating enough or you're eating too much.
- You can't focus or you have trouble making decisions.
- You can't count on your memory.
- You don't enjoy activities that used to bring you pleasure.
- You find yourself withdrawing from family and friends.
- You're experiencing persistent stomach issues, headaches, or body aches and pains.

FitBit

Most women are master multitaskers. So why not find a way to boost your mood and fitness at the same time? One way is to get some exercise. It might be the last thing you feel like doing when you're depressed, but going for a run or hitting the gym can actually make you feel better.

Studies support the fact that exercise is a mood booster. In one study, people who worked out regularly on a treadmill or stationary bike for 12 weeks saw the severity of their depressive symptoms reduced by nearly 50 percent.

Need a quick fix? Exercise is good for that too. Another study found that workouts can boost your mood for up to 12 hours.

RALLIE'S TIP

I've always tried to maintain a happy, grateful attitude. I struggled to stay happy and positive when I was younger, but with years of practice, it's now second nature. It's who I am.

If I do need to feel grumpy, peeved, resentful, or sorry for myself for some reason, I put a time limit on it—maybe 5 to 10 minutes. If it's something minor going on, that's usually enough time to get it out of my system! And more importantly, I don't end up wasting an entire day accomplishing nothing because I'm in a bad mood.

It's not always the easiest thing to do to maintain a positive, happy outlook. It actually takes a little effort and a lot of practice. Sometimes it's not even the most beneficial thing to do. It seems that occasionally, other people suspect that you might be a little dim-witted if you appear to be joyful most of the time. Or they don't take you seriously. Or they might think, Sure, it's easy for you to be happy. You don't have any problems! Of course that's not the case. Everyone has problems, and at any given time, we could all find at least a dozen things to be unhappy about.

Fortunately, it's just as easy to find two dozen things to be happy about. A couple of times each week, I make a mental list of all the things that are going right in my life, and of everything that I'm grateful for. When things pop into my mind that aren't going right, or that I'm not grateful for, I focus on what I can do to change them for the better, rather than how unhappy they make me. I can't always change everything or everyone in my life, but I always have the power to change the way I feel about anything.

Making Time for Yourself

It's simple math: If you give and give and give and never get anything back, you will run out. Your well of patience and strength isn't endless at all. Take some time to do what you need for you, to refill your well. It's like they say on airplanes: Put on your own oxygen mask first. Who can you help if you're passed out?

∽

The key to finding time for yourself is to integrate it into your life. I drive to pick up kids for many hours every day, and I always have something to read. That way when I have some time waiting for them in the car, I can read and relax.

—*Stacey Ann Weiland, MD, a mom of a 14-year-old daughter and 9- and 7-year-old sons and an internist/gastroenterologist, in Denver, CO*

∽

I've started to call Saturdays my "slump days." I like to spend time hanging out with my son, such as going to see a movie. Or I'll just read in bed and try to have some downtime. By Sunday, I start to relax and feel like it's really a weekend. And then, too quickly, it's over.

—*Judith Hellman, MD, a mom of a 15-year-old son, an associate clinical professor of dermatology at Mt. Sinai Hospital in New York City, and a dermatologist in private practice*

∽

It's essential for parents to have a little bit of time to themselves each day. This needs to be time not working, not doing chores, and not caring for others. This helps parents not lose sight of who they are, and what their needs are.

> **Now is the time.**
> —*Martin Luther King Jr.*

Based on my years of counseling patients, I have come up with concrete recommendations. I advise parents that they need to have 30 minutes each day and a four-hour block each week—to themselves. For people who aren't parents, this seems pretty minimal. Even people with full-time jobs, who aren't parents, get four-hour blocks "off" each day. But it's amazing how challenging it can be for parents to find even this small amount of time to ourselves.

—Dora Calott Wang, MD, a mom of a 10-year-old daughter, historian at the University of New Mexico School of Medicine, a unit director at Las Encinas Hospital in Pasadena, CA, and the author of The Kitchen Shrink: A Psychiatrist's Reflection on Healing in a Changing World

After my kids gave up their naps, I instituted "quiet time." My girls didn't have to actually nap, but they had to do something quietly in their rooms for about 45 minutes.

This gave me some much-needed quiet time. You can't be a mommy 24/7. Everyone needs a break.

—Tiemdow Phumiruk, MD, a mom of 13-, 10-, and 7-year-old daughters, a pediatrician in the emergency department of Children's Hospital Colorado at Parker Adventist Hospital, and adjunct faculty at Rocky Vista University College of Osteopathic Medicine, in Parker, CO

I've learned that I need to assign time for myself. I assign time for everything else, why not myself? At first it felt selfish to take time for myself, but I realized that if you don't take care of yourself, you can't take care of others.

I started to schedule time for myself, such as a pedicure or manicure. I always bring my calendar along, and when I finish one appointment, I schedule the next one.

—*Aline T. Tanios, MD, a mom of 10- and 4-year-old daughters and an 8-year-old son and a pediatric hospitalist and assistant professor at the Washington University School of Medicine, in St. Louis, MO*

∞∕∞

I think sometimes rather than making time, it's helpful to reframe time that you already have as "me" time. I have about an hour commute to work. I could resent that time "wasted" in the car. But instead, I consider that time for myself. Driving is relaxing for me. I listen to music or audiobooks while I drive. I can take several different routes to work, and I choose whichever suits my mood. My driving time is my time to decompress and the only time I really have alone.

—*Christy Valentine, MD, a mom of a seven-year-old daughter, a specialist in pediatrics and internal medicine, and the founder of the Valentine Medical Center, in Gretna, LA*

∞∕∞

Who doesn't need to save time? Here's a simple tip: I do a lot of shopping online, and Amazon has "Amazon Mom" and "subscribe and save" options. I have "subscriptions" for diapers, wipes, Diaper Genie refills, and even face cream. You can set up your shipment preferences, such as the frequency or dates to order, and you can

✎FitBit

Scientists at the University of Missouri came up with a model for happiness based on their research. If you want to maintain happiness, look for positive and life-changing experiences whenever possible *and* make a conscious effort to appreciate what you already have. They also noted that life changes that bring happiness are more often experiences rather than buying new things.

cancel or expedite shipments easily. This service is a huge help for busy moms.

Another time-saver is my DVR. I love a few shows, and I record them so that I can zip through commercials and watch an hour show in about 40 minutes! I'm sure advertisers would not like that, but it sure saves time and keeps me from staying up late to catch my shows.

—*Rachel S. Rohde, MD, a mom of a two-year-old daughter, an assistant professor of orthopaedic surgery at the Oakland University William Beaumont School of Medicine, and an orthopaedic upper-extremity surgeon with Michigan Orthopaedic Institute, P.C., in Southfield, MI*

Changing Your Mind-Set

People often joke that it's a woman's prerogative to change her mind—though they don't consider that to be a good thing. So why not consider it permission instead to change your mind-*set*?

Interestingly, when it comes to boosting your mood and being happy, having high expectations can backfire. Psychologists say that when people worry too much about being happy, they end up disappointed. The key is likely *high* expectations. Try to set reasonable ones instead.

⌒⌒

Exercise is my sanity. I find I can bust out of a bad mood if I get some sort of workout in.

—*Katherine Dee, MD, a mom of eight-year-old twin daughters and a six-year-old son and a radiologist at the Seattle Breast Center, in Washington*

⌒⌒

Sometimes when my mood gets low, I try to remember that I have to take responsibility for my mood. It's my responsibility to create a world that works for me, where I can be productive and constructive.

—*Eva Ritvo, MD, a mom of 22- and 17-year-old daughters, a psychiatrist, and a coauthor of* The Beauty Prescription, *in Miami Beach, FL*

> ## Life is a series of problems.
> ## Do we want to moan about them or solve them?
> —*M. Scott Peck,*
> *an American psychiatrist and author of*
> ### The Road Less Traveled

Recently I discovered a technique that has really changed my life. Before I go anywhere, such as into a meeting, I take a few seconds to set my intentions for what I want the coming interaction to be. For example, if I'm going to pick up my son from school, I might think, *I want my child to feel welcome and loved.* Or if I'm going to a meeting, I might think, *I want my colleague to feel comfortable and relaxed.*

I find that setting my intentions like this results in much less stress and much more positive interactions.

—*Jennifer Hanes, DO*

I had a revelation a few weeks ago. I realized that I needed to improve my mood. Especially at work, there were times I'd rather have been home with my daughter. It was time to make a change.

I realized that everyone—my family, my friends, my patients—deserves the best of me. They deserve for me to be a happy, positive person. That realization helped me to turn my mood around.

—*Jennifer Bacani McKenney, MD, a mom of a two-year-old*
daughter who's expecting another baby and a family physician,
in Fredonia, KS

I try to be a glass-half-full person. But, I'm not like that all of the time. I do a lot of "internal" talking to myself. If something bad happens, I tell myself, *This is just a temporary situation.* I'll reframe it in my mind, thinking, *How bad will this seem looking back on it in five years when my daughter is in high school? Will it even be an issue then? Probably not!*

—*Amy Barton, MD, a mom of an 11-year-old daughter and*
8- and 5-year-old sons and a pediatrician at St. Luke's Children's
Hospital, in Boise, ID

FitBit

If you're not in the mood to exercise, maybe you'll feel like dancing. Crank up the music and put your body in motion. Dancing is a great way to burn calories and increase cardio-vascular fitness. Plus, it'll likely pick up your mood right along with your heart rate!

My parents were Holocaust survivors, and we were very poor. We ate meat only once a week, and I put cardboard in my shoes to cover the holes in the soles. I always would pray that no one would walk up the stairs behind me in school and see the holes in my shoes!

Despite all of our struggles, my mother taught my sister and me to remember how lucky we are. She taught us to think, *We have a warm place to live, and we have the opportunity to work.* My mother really pounded into our heads how lucky we are. Nothing is owed to us; we have to earn it. And we have to make our own happiness.

—*Hana R. Solomon, MD, a mom who raised four children, a grandmom of three, a board-certified pediatrician, the president of BeWell Health, LLC, and the author of* Clearing the Air One Nose at a Time: Caring for Your Personal Filter, *in Columbia, MO*

I've learned that in any situation, what's important is attitude. When you're very busy, as I was at the end of my pregnancy—still operating on patients at 38 weeks, hunting for a new home, and running around trying to get everything ready for my baby to be born—it's easy to feel overwhelmed and exhausted. But if you commit to keeping a positive mind-set and thinking of everything as fun, you can find a way to enjoy all the numerous tasks that must be done.

Luckily, my husband is also a great partner in that he brings joy to everything we do and go through together instead of getting stressed out. Focusing on and getting overwhelmed by the negative only slows you down and makes every second drag out even longer.

During the challenging, busiest times in life, I focus on what's good, fun, and positive, rather than dwelling on what's bad, unpleasant, and negative.

—*Catherine Begovic, MD, a mom of a six-month-old daughter and a plastic surgeon at Make You Perfect, Inc., in Beverly Hills, CA*

I'm a generally happy person, but life is so busy that I've found I had to change my mind-set. I had to learn to let some things go. I've come to terms with the fact that my house isn't going to be perfectly clean all of the time. I don't think it's realistic to have a family

Paint Some Pottery

In the '80s, ceramics classes were very popular. Women met each week to paint some pottery, catch up on their families and careers, and share their hopes and dreams. Who has time for that these days?

Even if you can't carve out an hour each week, maybe you can find one hour to visit a paint-your-own-pottery place. These unique stores are popping up all over the country with names like Color Me Mine. You don't even need to register—just pop in, plop down, and paint.

At these friendly stores, you can choose a piece of unfired pottery from more than 400 choices, such as a pot, figurine, or mug. Even if you are art-challenged, you can use the stencils and rubber stamps provided. Staff is on hand to help and offer suggestions. They even have a design computer with thousands of designs you can trace or transfer.

All of their paints are nontoxic, free of lead, and food-safe. They are dishwasher-safe too, in case you want to make something such as a mug or an "it's your special day" plate. (Is that a cheer we hear?)

It's very inexpensive art therapy! Generally you'll pay a visit fee of $9 to $10 and have to buy the piece you'd like to paint. They start at about $12. Visit **ColorMeMine.com** for more information.

and a job and believe that everything is going to be finished all of the time.

For example, I used to do the laundry and have it all folded and put away all of the time. Now I might have time to wash and dry a load, but it might sit for a while in the dryer. I might let dirty dishes sit in the sink for a bit. I'm a very neat person, but I have to accept that my life is going to have some clutter in it now.

I also allocate my time carefully. For example, I like to volunteer at my kids' school. I know that I can't take on the role of room mother or team parent, but I can at least sponsor the team or help in the classroom for an hour once or twice a month. Along the same lines, my husband volunteered to be the assistant coach, not the head coach, of my son's baseball team.

—*Martha Wittenberg, MD, MPH, a mom of an eight-year-old son and a six-year-old daughter and a family physician with Seal Beach Family Medicine, in California*

Reducing Stress

A few decades ago, did we even talk about stress? Life seemed so much slower, calmer, happier. Today, we seem to be obsessed with stress.

But here's good (and surprising!) news: The American Psychological Association (APA) says that Americans reported lower stress levels in 2011 compared to four years earlier.

Interestingly, what causes and relieves stress is very individual. What might be stressful for one person (organizing a messy closet!) might be invigorating for someone else (hurrah, order!). Sometime when you're not stressed, or at least *less* stressed, try brainstorming some ways to help yourself to de-stress.

According to the APA, the most common ways people manage stress and feel better include listening to music, walking, exercising, reading, visiting with friends or family, and napping.

Along the same lines, the best ways to deal with stress, according to those surveyed, were being better time managers, saying no to some opportunities, being willing to compromise, adjusting expectations, avoiding stressful people or situations, and expressing emotions.

When to Call Your Doctor

Stressed? Join the club, right? You need only survive your kids' vomiting virus at home at the same time a work deadline is looming to know stress levels unique to parents. Then, of course, there are stresses specific to you and your life circumstances, whether it's a family illness or a job loss.

At some times, the pressure of stress can help push you to rise up and do some of your best work. At other times, when stress and demands don't let up, the constant pressure and anxiety can have serious effects on your health and life. Even worse, after a while it can be easy to miss the signs of chronic stress—such as lack of energy, extreme emotions, tension headaches, or back pain—because you've gotten so used to them.

How do you know when it's time to seek medical help because of stress? Seek immediate medical help if you've been thinking about hurting yourself or others.

Call your family doctor or a mental health professional if you're experiencing any of the following stress symptoms.

- You're abusing drugs or alcohol.
- You have physical symptoms that won't go away.
- You're perpetually withdrawn.
- You're underperforming at work.
- You feel as if you can't cope with life's demands.
- You're feeling extremely anxious or you have irrational fears.
- Your sleeping habits have changed.
- Your eating habits have changed, or you're becoming obsessed with food.
- You're self-destructive, or you're engaging in dangerous behaviors.

My dog is a wonderful stress reducer. When I get home from work, he's happy to see me. He's a golden retriever, so he's all about pleasing me, and he likes to cuddle up with me. That definitely reduces my stress, and I'm always happy to be with him.

> —Debra Luftman, MD, a mom of a 22-year-old daughter and a 19-year-old son, a board-certified dermatologist in private practice, coauthor of The Beauty Prescription, developer of the skincare line of products Therapeutix, and a clinical instructor of skin surgery and general dermatology at UCLA

It's so important to take some time out for yourself—for your overall health and beauty. Having an occasional glass of red wine is a great way for me to relieve stress. Plus, the antioxidant benefits of red wine are undisputed. I have a glass of red wine with dinner a few nights a week, when the meal lends itself to it.

> —Michelle Yagoda, MD

For me, the best way to handle stress is by working to change the things that are stressing me out. For instance, it's stressful to have a waiting room full of patients. So I work steadily to see them as efficiently as possible. I might never get to an empty waiting room, but knowing that I'm working toward the goal is helpful. I know that I'm doing the best that I can.

> —Kristin C. Lyle, MD, FAAP, a mom of 10-, 7-, and 5-year-old daughters, the disaster medical director at Arkansas Children's Hospital, and an assistant professor of pediatrics at the University of Arkansas for Medical Sciences, both in Little Rock

I find that trying to remember things takes up a lot of brainpower and causes a lot of stress. If I'm trying to keep track of which days my kids need to bring their library books to school, who needs to bring what sports gear to which practice when, and topics I need to talk to my sons' teachers and coaches about, I'll lose my mind.

I write all of these things down. That really reduces my stress level. In addition to my to-do list, I like to make my phone calendar a note-taker as well, especially since there I can set an alarm.

—*Deborah Gilboa, MD, a mom of 11-, 9-, 7-, and 5-year-old sons, a family physician with Squirrel Hill Health Center in Pittsburgh, PA, and a parenting speaker whose advice is found at AskDoctorG.com*

My greatest stress reliever is cooking! I started cooking when I was in my residency in New York City. I was working really long hours and a

FitBit

Skipping meals is stressful to the brain and body, and it can make losing weight difficult. In response to stress, the adrenal glands release cortisol, a stress hormone that triggers the desire for sweet foods. Cortisol also promotes weight gain, especially in the abdominal region.

lot of night shifts. I'd often come home from the hospital and watch cooking shows on the Food Network. At one point I realized, *I could do that!*

So when I'm stressed, I put on upbeat music and cook something. I forget about everything else when I cook. I find it very relaxing.

—*Sonali Ruder, DO, a mom of a two-month-old daughter, an emergency physician at Coral Springs Medical Center near Fort Lauderdale, FL, and a recipe developer and blogger at TheFoodiePhysician.com*

It wasn't until I trained as a Certified Professional Coach and Energy Leadership Index Master Practitioner that I really understood the need for me to recharge my batteries daily, rather than waiting until I scheduled a vacation. I wake up 30 minutes before the rest of my family. That's the time I set aside to focus on me. I enjoy a cup of tea, and I read inspirational and spiritual literature.

Before I go to bed at night, I do a similar process with prayer, journaling, and daily gratitude. I do my best to maintain this practice even when I'm working in the hospital.

—*Stephanie A. Wellington, MD, a mom of a 13-year-old son and an 11-year-old daughter, a hospitalist in the Level III NICU at Bellevue Hospital Center in New York City, and the medical coach and founder of PostpartumNeonatalCoaching.com*

I've learned that I need to address the stress in my life so that I can control it, rather than letting it control *me.*

Reading self-help books helps. Some books that have helped me include *Time Management from the Inside Out, Don't Sweat the Small Stuff,* and *The 7 Habits of Highly Effective Families.*
    —*Aline T. Tanios, MD*

When I finished my residency training, I was the typical overworked, overprogrammed, type A person. I was teaching at New York University part-time, working a full-time clinical emergency department job, and also working part-time as a lobbyist with our New Jersey American College of Emergency Physicians chapter. Despite this frenzy of activity, I remember being terribly lonely. I was always working when everyone else was off and was "bored" when everyone else was working and I was off.

When I met my husband, I finally had a buddy who liked to do all of

Pray and Meditate

If you are a religious person, taking some time to pray at church, synagogue, or even at home can help you feel more connected to your environment and less stressed. A Philadelphia-based researcher, Andrew Newberg, MD, conducted studies in which he analyzed scans of people's brains while they prayed. No matter what the people's religion, he found that prayer increased activity in the areas of the brain that control communication. It was as if people who were praying were having a conversation with God in the same way they would have a conversation with a friend or family member. In another study, Dr. Newberg found that meditation lowered people's perception of stress.

It's worthwhile to take some time to go to church or synagogue or to pray or meditate during quiet, peaceful times at home to recharge, feel more connected to your family, and let stress slip away.

the things that I liked to do and who also had time off during the week. Letting go of some of my commitments was hard, and I felt as if I was letting someone down. But I was in love for the first (and only) time in my life, and all I wanted to do was spend time with my future husband.

The biggest change for me was that I quickly realized that taking time for me, on a regular basis, to have fun and *rest* and sometimes not even get out of my pajamas for the entire day was vital. My job is so hard. I spend 12 hours completely focused juggling 10 to 15 very sick patients at a time. I rarely get time to take more than a 2-minute break to use the restroom. I never get a meal break. (I've been known to eat my lunch walking to the rest room.) It often gets so busy that my interruptions are interrupted by interruptions.

When I'm off, I need to rest. I need to, literally, zone out and do nothing. My husband has a similar occupation. He takes time to play with model trains. I take time to play on the computer making family videos and movies, and I like to knit. We both take time to just turn off and play, really play with our daughter. It's not uncommon for one or the other of us to be dressed up as her "prince" and dancing around the room with her.

It's hard to carve out time for myself, and it's often taken away from relationships and other commitments. My extended family and friends get frustrated with me because I'm terrible with keeping up socially on a regular basis. But I do what I can.

I think that everyone should significantly limit their involvement in activities and social obligations, no matter how fulfilling, because they often interfere with the mental and physical rest that we need on a regular basis.

—*Lisa Campanella-Coppo, MD, a mom of a three-year-old daughter and an emergency physician with EMCARE and the Meridian Health System, in Monmouth, NJ*

RALLIE'S TIP

Stress can be a tremendous energy zapper, and financial worries can be one of the biggest sources of stress these days.

Spending more than you can afford to, even on the people you love the most, can make a bad situation worse. To ease financial pressure and the stress it causes, put the credit card away, steer clear of the mall, and find creative ways to show your love and affection for the people closest to you. You can start by creating a coupon book. Depending on the recipient, it could include coupons for goodies such as a car wash or a relaxing neck and shoulder rub. For coworkers, you could give the gift of cleaning the break room fridge or dealing with that difficult, dreaded customer. You'll be a hero for sure! Or you can gift your friends and family with your time and expertise. Are you an excellent organizer? Give an hour's worth of your organizational skill. If you're an amateur chef or an avid scrapbooker, you could gift them with a coupon for a gourmet meal or a scrapbooking session.

If you use your imagination, you can come up with dozens of ideas for really neat gifts that you can make or do yourself. These days, most folks have more "stuff" than they could ever want or use. Most would far rather receive the most meaningful gift of all—the gift of your time and interest.

Considering Counseling

If you fell and broke your arm, would you wrap it in duct tape, grin and bear it, and try to heal your broken bone at home until you felt better? Surely not! Then why do so many of us hesitate to see a doctor when our hearts are hurting?

According to the Substance Abuse and Mental Health Services Administration, in 2008, 13.4 percent of adults in the United States received treatment for a mental health problem. This includes all adults who received care in inpatient or outpatient settings and/or used prescription medication for mental or emotional conditions. Yet, that represents only about half of the people who had a serious mental health issue requiring treatment. Clearly our hearts are hurting, and we aren't seeking the help we need.

> **The hardships that I encountered in the past will help me succeed in the future.**
>
> —*Philip Emeagwali,*
> *a Nigerian-born engineer and computer scientist/geologist*

I'm the poster child for counseling. I have seen various counselors at different times in my life.

Counseling has been super helpful to me. I believe it's important to find the right chemistry with a counselor. The right chemistry means if you're with a therapist who seems cold or reserved and who makes you feel self-conscious, think about moving on. Therapy shouldn't be like going to the dentist where you dread it; it should be something that supports you and helps you consider alternatives.

—*Nancy Rappaport, MD*

As a psychiatrist, I have treated many patients who have seen "counselors" of various types. I would recommend being very careful about choosing a mental health professional. Ask for a referral from your family doctor or local hospital, and consider trying more than one counselor if you can, to see whom you find the most trustworthy, helpful, and experienced. Explain your situation and ask for the professional's opinion about what is wrong and what could be done to fix it. Use your own judgment to evaluate whether their response really makes sense to you. For moms, I have found that bringing the dads (and sometimes the kids) into the professional's office as well is often very helpful.

—*Elizabeth Berger, MD, a mom of a 30-year-old son and*
a 29-year-old daughter, a child psychiatrist, and the author of
Raising Kids with Character, *in New York City*

I have seen therapists over the years for multiple issues. I think everyone should see a counselor at some point in their life, especially at times of great transition, such as when you get married or have a baby, or if your mood isn't as good as it should be. A lot of religious institutions do premarital counseling, and that's a great idea. Counseling for new parents is a great idea too. We all need help at times. An ounce of prevention is worth a pound of cure.

—Eva Ritvo, MD

❧

I watch my moods carefully. If I ever felt that my days were pervasively negative or that I wasn't getting joy out of the things that normally make me happy, I would seek counseling.

Considering counseling is especially important for new moms. Couples counseling can be especially helpful. I try to remember that it's so much better for my kids to have a happy, healthy parent than a stressed-out, crabby one.

—Amy Barton, MD

❧

It is super important for moms—especially new moms—to watch out for postpartum depression. After my son was born, I was short-tempered and cried a lot. My husband noticed, and he urged me to seek help. It made a huge difference for me.

I tell moms that if your mood is affecting how you interact with other people, please seek help. It's important to have a primary care physician you trust because that can be a great place to start if you need help.

—Eva Mayer, MD, a mom of a nine-year-old daughter and an eight-year-old son, an associate professor of pediatrics at Temple University, and a pediatrician with St. Luke's Pediatrics Associates, in Bethlehem, PA

❧

About five years ago, I was having a difficult time. I was very busy working and raising my kids. I didn't feel phenomenal about myself. I wasn't really living or enjoying my life.

I knew that there had to be something more. *I can't imagine this is all that there is to life,* I remember thinking.

I was looking online for help and considering counseling. I knew I wasn't depressed, but I wasn't fulfilled either. That's when I heard

FitBit

No doubt about it, mood affects weight, and weight affects mood. A study done in Finland found that people who responded to stress by eating had the highest body weights. More specifically, the study's "stress eaters" consumed more sausages, hamburgers, pizza, chocolate, and alcohol than those who did not respond to stress by eating. And on the flip side, who hasn't stepped on the scale, discovered the needle moved down, and felt a boost of joy? Working to improve your mood will also boost your weight loss efforts and vice versa.

about life coaching. I read about how it can help you to set and implement goals. Rather than finding a life coach, I decided to become one!

I attended the Institute for Professional Excellence in Coaching (iPEC) in New York City to become a Certified Professional Coach and Energy Leadership Index Master Practitioner. I feel fantastic now when I am able to help people with life coaching.

I recommend life coaching for people who recognize that there is more to life and who are looking for a partner to brainstorm with and champion them while holding them accountable for the action steps necessary to live life more fully. Life coaching differs from counseling in that although we explore fears and limiting beliefs that might hold a person back, the focus is on moving forward.

—*Stephanie A. Wellington, MD*

❧

I found I had to let go of the guilt that I was experiencing because I can't be everything to everyone all of the time. A book called *The E-Woman* was very helpful. It said that women who think they must be everything to everyone, every time, suffer from intense stress. We need to accept that we can't always be the wonderful, warm, and nurturing people we think we're supposed to be.

To come to terms with this, it can be helpful to talk with well-centered and supportive friends. Or you can find professional help to get past this. Talking with a trained counselor allows you to open up about topics that you might not want to burden friends with. A counselor will listen without having her own agenda and her own fears. A counselor will also push you harder than a friend will to face your own fears and challenges.

I do have one unique friend whom I can talk about anything with. Nothing is a burden for her. But she lives on the opposite coast, and so the time and space separating us might allow us to do that for each other. We can admit to each other when we're frightened or struggling. I am blessed to have such a friend.

—*Linda Brodsky, MD, a mom of a 30-year-old son and 28- and 25-year-old daughters, the president of WomenMDResources.com, a physician in private practice with Pediatric ENT Associates, and a retired professor of otolaryngology and pediatrics, in Buffalo, NY*

RALLIE'S TIP

If you find that you feel hopeless or in a state of deep despair, it's important to see your doctor. If do-it-yourself remedies and self-help practices don't seem to be working, you might need a little extra help in the form of counseling, or even an antidepressant medication.

I've been very fortunate to have access to wonderful counselors whenever I've felt I really needed the type of help they have to offer. My first experience with a counselor was when I was a single mother, and my son and I were having a difficult time communicating effectively. I knew that we both needed the perspective and guidance of a professional to move forward toward a positive solution and a better relationship. I went about finding a counselor in the same way I would find a good physician, a hairdresser, or a mechanic. I asked the people I trusted whom they would recommend, and then I checked the counselor's credentials.

I think the biggest misperception I had about counseling was that there was going to be a lot of crying, arguing, blaming, and gnashing of teeth. That wasn't the case at all! The counselor wasn't as concerned with what had gone wrong in the past as what we could do in the future to make things work. He had very little interest in rehashing past mistakes. He was all about moving forward and finding positive, win-win solutions. He didn't want to keep us in any type of ongoing therapy for months on end. Instead, he wanted to meet with us for an hour each week for at least a month to teach us tools and techniques that we could use on our own so that we would quickly outgrow the need for his services, and that's exactly what we did.

With his help, my son and I learned to communicate more effectively, and we strengthened the foundation of our relationship at a critical time. My son and I probably didn't spend more than four hours total with our counselor, but that four hours has had an incredibly powerful, positive impact on our relationship, and on our lives.

Identifying Mood Busters

In the '80s, rapper Young MC told us to "Bust a Move." Fast-forward to 2013, and we think more about Bust a Mood.

It can be helpful to do some soul searching to identify what can put you into a funk. Perhaps the weather, crazy drivers on the highway, grumpy people on the phone, or long lines at the store. One surprising cause is low blood sugar. Studies have found that people with low blood sugar tend to be more aggressive and even violent.

You probably can't always avoid bad weather, crazy drivers, and grumpy people, but sometimes a bit of self-awareness can head off a bad mood.

∽◌∾

Being so tied to technology 24/7 can bust my mood. I try to have at least one day each month when I turn my phone and computer off. Try it and see how it goes!

—*Jennifer Hanes, DO*

∽◌∾

When I get sick and can't (or don't) exercise for a few days, I start to feel crummy. I just have to get going again, and it helps. So does chocolate.

—*Lennox McNeary, MD, a mom of a four-year-old son, a specialist in physical medicine and rehabilitation at Carilion Clinic, and a cofounder of the Mommy Doctors Bakery (makers of Milkin' Cookies), in Roanoke, VA*

> **The way I see it, if you want a rainbow,**
> **you gotta put up with some rain.**
> **—Dolly Parton**

Fortunately, bad weather doesn't get me down because it's gray half of the time where I live, in Seattle! What does make me bummed is when my kids get sick. To feel better, I spend as much time as I can with them, reading or watching movies, hunkered down on the couch and drinking hot tea.

—*Katherine Dee, MD*

If I'm working too many hours, it can cause my mood to sink. I try to tell myself, *Life is a marathon, not a sprint. You can't get everything done in one day.*

—*Eva Ritvo, MD*

I have a tendency to overthink everything. This can bring me down. To combat this, I try to focus on what I can do in any given situation and not think about what's beyond my control. When I start to see the results of my hard work, I feel better.

—*Pam D'Amato, MD*

Housework can be truly thankless. You can spend the entire day neatening your home and putting things away. Then the kid comes home, and within moments, it's all a mess again.

So I find it essential to have a time each evening when I call it quits. It's usually around 8:30 pm. I tell myself, *Enough already.* No more! It's when I pick up a book, or simply enjoy my kid.

—*Dora Wang, MD*

When I have a particularly sick patient at work, it can definitely bring me down. But when I get to go home to my family, I immerse myself in *our* life, and that makes me feel better. I focus on what's healthy and "normal" for us: homework, activities, and our bedtime routine. Then I'm able to put whatever happened at work behind me.

—*Amy Barton, MD*

◦∕◦

In my job, I talk with people all day long. Generally, this is a mood booster to me because I love talking to people!

But it can also be a downer if people are mad or sad. I could let it spoil my mood, but I don't. If I talk with someone who threatens my good mood, I shake it off. I tell myself, *You just have to move on,* and I don't let myself dwell on it.

—*Susan Besser, MD, a mom of six grown children, ages 28, 26, 24, 22, 21, and 19, a grandmom of two, a family physician, and the medical director of Doctors Express-Memphis, in Tennessee*

◦∕◦

I'm a very positive person, and not much gets me down. But ugly people—people who are ugly in their souls, who are liars and not nice—drive me crazy. It reminds me of all of the bad things in the world, like Hitler. *Where do these people come from?* I wonder.

The way I fight against these feelings is that I look at the positive, and I strive to be more successful at life than they could ever be.

—*Hana R. Solomon, MD*

◦∕◦

It's my nature to be positive, but sometimes life can be daunting. I rely on my husband to keep me on an even keel. When he's cranky, that's really hard, and it can make me really sad. I don't expect him to be bubbly, but I do expect him to be calm, understanding, and patient.

A few years ago, we decided that we really have to make time for each other to connect. We have a date night every two weeks, without fail. That has helped our relationship so much. My husband realizes now that if I tell him, "You look grumpy," it's not because I'm mad at him. It's because we all have to extend the courtesy of keeping our emotions in check whether we are at work or at home.

—*Tiemdow Phumiruk, MD*

One thing that can really affect my mood is my children's moods. I want them to be happy. If one of my children is unhappy, I try to give him space. My children are quickly turning into young adults. While I like to give them the opportunity to express their feelings, I don't pressure them to feel that they *have* to. If one of my sons is in a mood and has a three-year-old-type tantrum, I give him space and walk away. I try to keep things in perspective and not let it drag my mood down too. It helps to know that later, he'll come around and give me a hug.

—*Leena Shrivastava Dev, MD, a mom of 15- and 12-year-old sons and a general pediatrician and advocate for child safety, in the Baltimore, MD, area*

One thing that can really put me in a bad mood is traffic. I have really bad road rage (at times). I have a 45-minute commute, and bad drivers really upset me—especially when I'm trying to get home after work.

To pull myself out of a traffic-induced bad mood, I often switch on music. I generally listen to upbeat music on my way to work and relaxing music on my way home to decompress.

I know this isn't possible for everyone, but I also bought a new car that I really enjoy driving. It helps make the commute a little bit better.

—*Sonali Ruder, DO*

One thing that can really dampen my mood is when I come home at the end of the day to a house that's a mess. Granted, it looks the same way as it did when I left in the morning. But it's still a big downer. It's stressful to walk into a house of chaos.

I try to make an effort to clean up the house, especially my kids' toys, after my kids go to sleep. And then I try to keep up with it in the morning before we go to work and preschool. This way it's less chaotic when I get home!

—*Jeannette Gonzalez Simon, MD, a mom of four- and one-year-old daughters and a pediatric gastroenterologist at Staten Island Pediatrics GI, in New York*

FitBit

In a funk? Fish for some relief. Fatty fish such as tuna, mackerel, salmon, and herring are rich in omega-3 fatty acids, which appear to protect against depression. Some studies, for example, indicate that fish oil supplements can alleviate depressive symptoms, according to a review article published in the June 2006 issue of the *American Journal of Psychiatry*.

Eating fish is a logical way to get more omega-3s: Aim for several servings a week of omega-3-rich fish, and look for omega-3-fortified foods (listed on the label), including some brands of eggs, margarine, and yogurt.

Or you could go the quicker route: Taking fish oil supplements is another way to boost your intake.

I can't overemphasize the importance of turning off the TV, particularly the news. The world is full of wonderful things, and the world is also full of horrible, terrible things. The news never reports the wonderful things.

I get a quarterly publication from the Nature Conservancy about all of the terrific things they are doing to improve the environment, and I feel good after reading it. I wonder, *Why aren't those things on the news?*

I deal with death, sorrow, other people's anger, frustration, and loss every day. It's hard for me to shut off the constant battery of negativity when I come home and not let it overwhelm me. I'm thankful for my exposure to hardship at my job because it makes me so grateful for my family, and it gives me the insight to cherish all of the wonderful, joyful things in my life.

But, it takes an emotional toll. I can't do what I do every day and then watch the news before bed and be barraged with 60 minutes of murder, civil war, rape, violence, death, destruction, economic loss, and doom and gloom. I haven't watched the news regularly in more than three years. That's not to say that I am uniformed; I read the newspaper regularly, and I read BBC and CNN online. But I *choose* what I want to read.

I truly, deeply feel that the daily horror, violence, and doom and gloom on both the news and in our "entertainment" TV is drastically affecting people, particularly our young people. I often wish we could go back to the days of Beaver Cleaver when TV programming was more responsible and less sensational.

Instead of watching the news, I watch children's shows with my daughter. It's amazing how much calmer I feel after an hour watching *Sesame Street* than an hour of CNN headline news.

—*Lisa Campanella-Coppo, MD*

∽⁄○

My job can be very stressful. When people come to the ER, they are hurt or sick and often not at their best.

Sometimes that can put me in a bad mood. I've found that talking with someone who works in a similar field, who really understands what I'm going through, is helpful. I'm fortunate that this person is my husband. He's also an emergency physician. After work, we'll spend some time talking about our days. I always feel better after talking with him. Sometimes we have to cut our "shop talk" short and say, "Okay, let's talk about something else now" so that we don't spend the whole evening talking about work!

—*Sonali Ruder, DO*

Identifying Mood Boosters

Studies have shown that the most effective mood booster is exercise. It's so powerful that exercise has similar effects as antidepressants for people who have depression. Exercise helps fight depression by triggering the release of endorphins and other neurotransmitters that help you feel good while lowering levels of those that can make depression worse.

If you're feeling so low that a 10-minute walk seems like a climb to the summit of Mount Everest, turn on some music instead. Research shows music is the second most effective mood booster. Our theory is that sometimes the music you loved as a teen is uplifting. We won't tell you what bands that means for us. (Think big hair. A lot of big hair.)

One thing that has made a huge difference for me is that each morning, I read a quote or two from the book *Don't Sweat the Small Stuff*. They are incredible daily affirmations. Reading a few of them each day helps me stay grounded.

—*Eva Mayer, MD*

Consistent exercise boosts my mood. The key is that you have to do it no matter how tired you feel. I try not to go more than two days without doing some cardio training. I find that if I skip two days in a row, I have a problem!

—*Lisa Campanella-Coppo, MD*

I take a large amount of omega-3 combined with vitamin D, both of which are beneficial for improving mood and overall health. I take adaptogens, which are herbs such as rhodiola that reduce the effect of ingrained stress, each morning, which help my mood, and an amino acid called theanine (an extract of green tea) midday to help me focus. I also take bioavailable diindolymethane and chasteberry to keep my PMS under control and stay married.

—*Sara Gottfried, MD, a mom of 13- and 8-year-old daughters, a board-certified gynecologist, and the author of* The Hormone Cure, *in Berkeley, CA*

I make sure to get a good night's sleep, in at least a five-hour chunk. That makes my mood, and my outlook, so much better.

—*Tiemdow Phumiruk, MD*

Practicing my faith helps to boost my mood. I attend Mass every Sunday with my family—my work schedule permitting. It has become a great family routine. On my morning drive to work, I listen to spiritual music. I find it boosts my mood and also my energy. Our spiritual life is healthier when it is nurtured on a daily basis, exactly like our physical life.

—*Aline T. Tanios, MD*

I like talking to people, especially children. I'm fortunate that in my job I interact with children all day. They really boost my mood.

—*Tiemdow Phumiruk, MD*

I started to do a program called Luminosity, at Luminosity.com. Their brain games are helpful to keep cognitive skills from declining as you age. I play them each morning, and my scores are improving! This also helps my mood because they're fun!

—*Eva Mayer, MD*

Doing things with my friends is the best way to keep my mood up. I love taking my kids to playdates at friends' houses because that makes us all happy!

—*Katherine Dee, MD*

> **People are just as happy as they
> make up their minds to be.**
> —*Abraham Lincoln*

Friendships are important for happiness and for health. This is obvious to many of us. It has also been validated in studies. But friendships are probably more important for women, than even for men.

I keep in touch with several of the families from my daughter's first preschool class. Over the past 10 years, they have become very important friends to me. We get together as families, and everyone wins. Mothers get girl-time, kids get playtime, and dads often watch sports.

My daughter loves being at home, which is her base in life. But for me, I often need a break from being at home. There's always a lot of housework when you're a mom.

I like to invite other families over to my house, and I do it often. It makes me stop doing housework for a few hours and enjoy the company of friends, while my daughter does the same.
—*Dora Calott Wang, MD*

Having an attitude of gratitude really boosts my mood. I ran a half marathon at Walt Disney World where spectators lined every street. I was so overwhelmed with gratitude for them that I kept thanking them as I ran by! That feeling of gratitude got me through the entire 13.1 miles!

In contrast, my second marathon didn't have many spectators. I slogged my way through that one. It was awful.
—*Eva Ritvo, MD*

If something is getting me down, I try to find something positive to focus on instead. For example, my daughter flew across the country to visit a friend. She caught a terrible cold and called me to say, "I'm sick as a dog and can't get out of bed."

"Well, thank God you have a warm place to rest," I told her. My message to her and my other kids has always been, "It could always be worse."

—*Hana R. Solomon, MD*

⌒⌒

One strategy I find helpful to boost my mood is scheduling something fun each week to look forward to, such as shopping or going out for dinner and drinks with my friends.

Also, in the bigger picture, I'm always thinking about the next great stage of my life. For example, I looked forward to finishing school, then getting married, buying a house, and having a baby. I'm always thinking, *What's next?* I can hardly wait!

—*Michelle Davis-Dash, MD, a mom of a 19-month-old son and a pediatrician in Baltimore, MD*

⌒⌒

It can be hard for moms to identify things that boost their moods. We're so good at cheering other people up—and calming them down—but we don't always know what works for us. As moms, we need to think about what makes us feel better, and then do that!

For example, I love being of service to other people. That's one of the many reasons why I love my job. Just doing my job and helping people boosts my mood. I feel that it's who I am, not what I do. I also love to take long, relaxing baths.

—*Christy Valentine, MD*

⌒⌒

I'm a very visual person, and so a great way to boost my mood is to look at something beautiful. For example, I love to go to art museums and to take walks in beautiful places such as a wildlife preserve.

It boosts my mood to talk with my children and to see how they're growing up to be wonderful adults.

Another thing that boosts my mood is to look forward to things. For example, I'll plan a small party and look forward to that. I love to entertain close family and friends and enjoy good food and conversation with them.

—*Debra Luftman, MD*

I've learned something very helpful, and I'm trying to teach my kids how to do this. When you're having a bad day, you're usually aware of it. When that happens to me, I try to stop and think about what I could do to make myself feel better, to cheer myself up.

Sometimes it helps me to listen to music or go into my office and shut the door for five minutes so I can have a little quiet time.

I think the act of acknowledging you're in a bad mood is helpful. And if you've identified a few mood boosters ahead of time, then you can choose to use one to help yourself feel better.

—*Kristin C. Lyle, MD, FAAP*

Gear Up for a Belly Laugh

We know that laughter is good for us, but sometimes we need a reminder. One study published in 2012 found that the physical act of laughing released feel-good endorphins and it even heightened people's pain threshold.

This is a good reason to see a comedy movie on date night or rent one to watch after the kids go to bed. Even better, get the whole family giggling with a G- or PG-rated movie or television show that will tickle everyone's funny bone.

Need some ideas? Here's a list of some movies to try.

Kid-friendly:

A Christmas Story

Alvin and the Chipmunks

Dennis the Menace

Elf

The Incredibles

Monsters, Inc.

Mrs. Doubtfire

The Parent Trap

Shrek

I plan something every week to look forward to, such as meeting a friend for coffee or going shopping. It's my me time. I write it down in my calendar to make it a priority.

I also meet about once a month with a group of friends from medical school who are also moms. We all dress up and go for a special lunch in the city. It's a lot of fun!

—*Shilpa Amin-Shah, MD, a mom of a three-year-old son and a two-year-old daughter and an emergency physician and director of the recruiting team at Emergency Medical Associates, in Livingston, NJ*

Wallace & Gromit: The Curse of the Were-Rabbit
Who Framed Roger Rabbit

To watch without the kids:
Ace Ventura: Pet Detective
Airplane!
Anchorman: The Legend of Ron Burgundy
Austin Powers: International Man of Mystery
Best in Show
The Big Lebowski
Bridesmaids
Dodgeball: A True Underdog Story
Groundhog Day
The Hangover
Monty Python's Life of Brian
The Naked Gun
National Lampoon's Vacation
Planes, Trains and Automobiles

When someone in my family needs a pick-me-up, we'll do a backrub trade. It's fun and a great way to reconnect.

Also, my sons are really learning that it feels good to help people. So if I'm not feeling well and I lie down on the couch, one of them will ask me if I'd like a massage or come and sit with me to watch a sports game.

—*Deborah Gilboa, MD*

❧

I tell my patients that just 20 minutes of exercise, three times a week, will decrease their risk for depression, breast cancer, heart disease, and osteoporosis. Those are all great reasons to be active.

Exercise gets adrenaline and endorphins going. It works on some of the same brain receptors as antidepressants. Antidepressants can cause side effects such as sexual dysfunction and weight gain. On the other hand, the side effects of exercise are weight loss and better health. Plus, the mood benefits of exercise are immediate, whereas medications take weeks to begin working.

—*Dora Calott Wang, MD*

❧

A few years ago, I made a concerted effort to spend more time with friends, especially people with different backgrounds from me. I planned time with nonmedical work colleagues and my kids' friends' moms. I enjoyed spending time listening to and talking with them. We shared successes and struggles.

Taking this time helped me to reshape my personality. I started to grow exponentially in my career and in my family life. This was a huge step in taking better care of myself. I don't feel so drained anymore.

—*Aline T. Tanios, MD*

❧

Deep breathing can banish stress and boost mood. Most of us breathe shallowly all day, every day. I used to think deep breathing was a bunch of hooey, but when I read the research, I realized it makes sense. Breathing deeply causes physical changes in your body.

To do it, inhale through your nose as deeply as you can until it causes a bit of discomfort, then slowly breathe out through your nose.

⚫FitBit

Exercise triggers the release of endorphins, which are natural morphine-like brain chemicals responsible for the phenomenon known as "runner's high." Endorphins can dramatically boost your mood, improve your tolerance to pain, and help you cope with stress.

It should fully expand your chest and push out your tummy a bit when you inhale.

—*Jennifer Hanes, DO*

∽⌒∽

I find that what I eat really affects my mood. I've attempted to do a low-carb diet a few times. That was too restrictive for me; I firmly believe in moderation. Now I do a modified low-carb diet. I eat a lot of fruits and vegetables, and I try to limit processed foods. This has helped my mood and also my asthma and my skin.

When I grocery shop, I stick to the perimeter of the stores—the produce, meat, and dairy sections. I avoid the middle of the store where they keep the processed foods.

—*Lisa Campanella-Coppo, MD*

∽⌒∽

When I'm feeling down, I cook, which in the past typically meant cooking—and eating—a heavy meal with comfort foods. Now I love being innovative and experimenting while I'm making good nutritious food, and this really helps me to wind down.

I also love spending time with my kids. They're getting old enough that they can read my mood and tell when I am down—or have had a bad day. It's really sweet.

—*Amy Thompson, MD, a mom of six-, four-, and two-year-old sons and an ob-gyn at the University of Cincinnati College of Medicine, in Ohio*

∽⌒∽

To boost my mood, I like to reach out to someone I haven't seen in years, or connect with an old friend from a past work situation or neighborhood with whom I have lost contact. When you have lived in many places, there are often lots of wonderful people like this. It gives me a lot of joy to reconnect with them through e-mail, phone, or sometimes an old-fashioned letter!

Also, going to the Salvation Army store boosts my mood! I am a thrift store nut. This is a hilarious group project or wonderful solitary activity for me. Even if I don't purchase anything, the thrill of the chase and the nostalgia of those styles-of-yesterday give me a thrill.

—*Elizabeth Berger, MD*

Before having kids, I used to take a walk if I was feeling down. That's not as easy with two kids. Yet of course I still get irritated. I need to find some new coping strategies. For now I admit I do yell and scream a few times!

When I feel tired and grumpy, I tell myself that it's going to get

Mommy MD Guides–Recommended Product
Tony Robbins Get the Edge/Personal Power System

"Because I see the world through 'the glass is half empty' eyes, my sister long ago told me about Anthony Robbins," says Michelle Yagoda, MD, a mom of an 11-year-old son, a facial plastic surgeon, the CEO of Opus Skincare, LLC, and cofounder of BeautyScoop, a patented and clinically proven supplement for skin, hair, and nails, in New York City. "I listened to his Personal Power System. It really helped me to be more positive in my interactions with myself and others. People are more receptive to positive people, and those interactions make you feel good about yourself. This self-help system provides simple steps to learn how to change your internal dialogue and how to recognize positive things in your everyday world."

You can buy the Get the Edge/Personal Power System at online retailers such as **AMAZON.COM** for around $139. Visit **TONY-ROBBINS.COM** for more information.

better. My kids are going to grow up. It's not going to be like this forever! Then I remind myself that I'll miss these days when they are gone. That gives me perspective.

—*Bola Oyeyipo-Ajumobi, MD, a mom of five- and two-year-old sons, a family physician at the Veterans Health Administration, and the owner of SlimyBookWorm.com, in San Antonio, TX*

I think people have a natural tendency to be in a positive—or in a negative—mood. But I also think you do have some control over your mood. I *decide* to be happy. I choose to look at the positive and at the good side of life.

One thing that never fails to boost my mood is being outdoors. Even on a cold day, I love to go outside for a walk in the brisk air. I love to look around for signs of life, such as tiny animal footprints in the snow or leaves budding. Being in nature reminds me that we are all part of something big and beautiful. The world is a beautiful place.

—*Ayala Laufer-Cahana, MD, a mom of 17- and 15-year-old sons and a 14-year-old daughter, a pediatrician, and the founder of Herbal Water Inc., in Wynnewood, PA*

Something that's very uplifting to me is music. I like a lot of types of music—well, anything other than jungle rock anyway! Whatever works to keep you motivated! I like to listen to Pandora radio. It allows you to pick the music that you want to hear without "suffering" through songs that don't suit your tastes.

Also, to boost my mood, I love talking with my husband. My children are grown and most have moved away, so I text them often. I like to keep in touch with them and talk about day-to-day things.

—*Susan Besser, MD*

I find that helping other people outside of my family really boosts my mood and spirit. The more I do for other people in need, the more I appreciate my family and all that I have.

Before my son was born, I worked for a week in a tent in Port-Au-Prince, Haiti, with an organization called Partners in Development.

It was a life-changing experience—like Oprah says, "An aha moment." I realized how much people can do with so little. It really put my life into perspective, and it caused me to realize that I can do so much more with what I have.

Now that my son is a baby, I don't feel that I can pick up and leave for an entire week. So instead we "adopted" a family in need. We donate money, and the program gives it to the family for their needs. Partners in Development is an awesome organization. It has no overhead operating costs like some organizations that use only about five cents of your dollar for the cause you're supporting. I saw with my own eyes the money that was sent from the sponsors for a particular child or family being distributed to that family—in full. (For more information, visit PID.org.) I donate as much as I can. Anything I'm not using, I give to someone who needs it more.

—*Michelle Davis-Dash, MD*

RALLIE'S TIP

If you think of the words you use to describe low moods and feelings (bleak, black, gray, blue, dim, dark, lifeless, silent), you'll realize the importance of surrounding yourself with cheerful sounds, living things, bright light, invigorating scents, and warm, vibrant colors. I keep my curtains and blinds open in my home and office, especially during the short winter days, to let in as much sunlight as possible. I also keep overhead lights and lamps turned on in the rooms I'm using. (You might want to switch to higher-wattage lightbulbs during the dark days of winter.)

If you're really suffering with winter blues, which is also called Seasonal Affective Disorder (SAD), you might consider getting a light box. The results of several studies demonstrate the benefits of light exposure in alleviating symptoms of winter blues. Light boxes offer a safe, effective, and predictable source of light, emitting high-intensity light (2,500 to 10,000 lux, as compared to a normal light fixture that emits a dismal 250 to 500 lux). These boxes are best used daily and early in the morning for periods of 30 minutes to two hours.

Many SAD sufferers find that their mild depressive symptoms begin to improve immediately, and the symptoms often completely resolve after two weeks of use. In some studies, phototherapy, or bright light therapy, successfully alleviated physical and emotional symptoms in 80 percent of subjects.

Although a lot of my home is decorated in soft, neutral colors, I've added splashes of bright, warm color to the rooms I spend the most time in, such as yellow or orange pillows, rugs, and throws and healthy green plants.

I try to sit in a sunbeam whenever I can, and I spend more time in the brightest, cheeriest rooms of my home. I spend less time in dark, dimly light rooms such as a windowless basement.

I always make sure I take my ABCs to help stave off the symptoms of SAD and the winter blues. A good multivitamin and mineral supplement gives my body the nutrients it must have to stay healthy, especially when my diet is less than optimal because of a hectic schedule. The results of several studies suggest that taking extra vitamin D during the winter may be beneficial in the treatment of the winter blues. Vitamin D is manufactured in the skin in response to sunlight. During the dark days of winter, we're normally exposed to less sunlight, and as a result, our bodies don't manufacture as much vitamin D as when we spend more time outdoors basking in the summer sunshine. Recent research suggests that vitamin D is just as important as vitamin C in terms of keeping the immune system fully functional, and studies demonstrate that it isn't a coincidence that most of us tend to be more susceptible to colds and flu during the winter, when our vitamin D levels tend to be lowest. When you're suffering from the winter blues, the last thing you need is to catch a cold or come down with the flu. That's just adding insult to injury!

In addition to vitamin D, I take fish oil or another supplement that offers high-quality essential fatty acids, such as EPA and DHA, which are known to support brain health and help normalize moods. The results of several studies suggest that consumption of fish, fish oil, and other sources of omega-3 fatty acids has an impact on serotonin levels in the brain and can significantly reduce symptoms of depression. Some experts believe that declining levels of omega-3s in the American diet helps explain the increase in the number of Americans suffering from depressive symptoms.

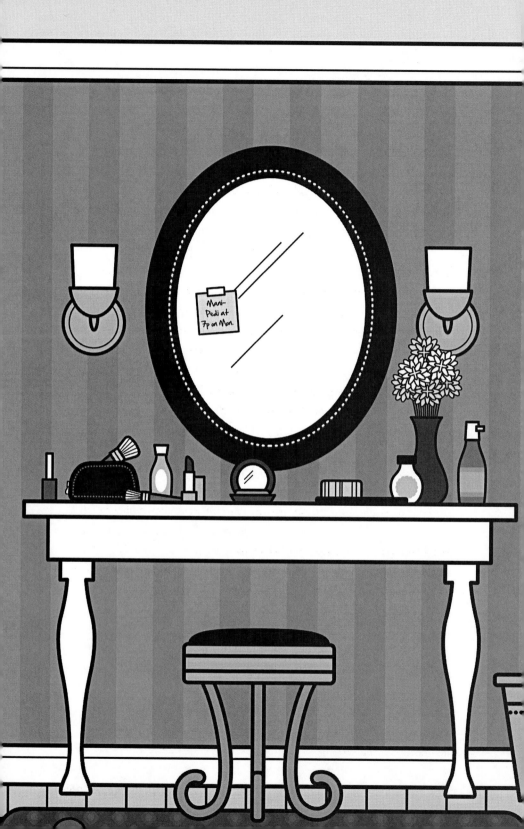

Chapter 7
Boosting Your Self-Esteem

YOUR BODY

A survey conducted by Dove found that only 4 percent of women around the world believe that they are beautiful. Amazingly, that's not just here in the United States, but worldwide. The other 96 percent of women all over the world need some self-esteem soothing.

Having poor self-esteem isn't a trivial problem. It can wreck your self-confidence and well-being. It can hold you back from reaching your full potential.

Wouldn't you like to be the very best you that you could be? Then you could strive harder, achieve more, do better. What would you do if you knew you couldn't fail? Picture that woman: She's confident, strong, beautiful, smart. Look again? It's you!

JUSTIFICATION FOR A CELEBRATION

There's no need to justify it, celebrate anyway! Now is the perfect time to celebrate *you*—warm, wise, witty, wonderful you.

> **You are braver than you believe,
> stronger than you seem, and smarter than you think.**
> —*Christopher Robin*

Assessing Your Self-Esteem

How do you feel about yourself? If you were someone else, would you be your friend? Here's a simple self-esteem quiz. It was developed by Melba W. Benson, PhD, an educator and coach in Arlington, TX. It's reprinted here with her permission.

Rate each of the items below on the following scale:

3 = Always

2 = Over half of the time

1 = Occasionally

0 = Never

When someone compliments me,
I don't have any difficulty accepting the compliment. ☐

When I meet a person for the first time,
I see his/her positive qualities first. ☐

I feel good about myself and my abilities. ☐

When confronted by a new situation,
I view it as an opportunity or challenge. ☐

I can close my eyes and see myself accomplishing my goals. ☐

When confronted with a problem,
I engage in positive thinking and/or planning. ☐

If asked, people would describe me as a positive person. ☐

I develop plans and work toward my goals. ☐

I believe my actions have a great deal
to do with my happiness/success in life. ☐

Total Points: ☐

Interpretation:

23–27: Great self-esteem. You feel good about yourself and your capabilities. You are an optimist with positive attitudes.

18–22: Good self-esteem. Usually you feel good about yourself and your capabilities. Overall you are an optimist with positive attitudes.

14–17: Moderate self-esteem. There are times when you experience self-doubt. You vary between being an optimist and a pessimist, but you tend to be more positive than negative.

9–13: Diminished self-esteem. There are times when you experience self-doubts. You vary between being an optimist and a pessimist, but you tend to be more negative than positive.

0–8: Negative self-esteem. You do not feel good about yourself and your capabilities. You are a pessimist who usually has negative attitudes.

∽◎

I don't think that I have an *excess* of self-esteem, but at this point in my life, I have gained a *healthy* self-esteem. It was won through a lot of blood, sweat, and tears. I've worked very hard to be where I am—both professionally and personally. For me, working toward goals and achieving them has boosted my self-esteem.

> —*Pam D'Amato, MD, a mom of seven- and four-year-old daughters and an interventional pain management physician with University Spine Center, in Wayne, NJ*

∽◎

I think I have good self-esteem. I feel very comfortable in my own skin. This is important for me as a foundation of how I interact with my environment—as a mother, wife, physician, and friend.

> —*Debra Luftman, MD, a mom of a 22-year-old daughter and a 19-year-old son, a board-certified dermatologist in private practice, coauthor of* The Beauty Prescription, *developer of the skincare line of products Therapeutix, and a clinical instructor of skin surgery and general dermatology at UCLA*

For the first time in my life, I would say my self-esteem is a 10 out of 10. My kids are older, and they're doing well in school. I'm confident in my career. I feel like I have so much experience under my belt, I can handle anything!

—*Eva Mayer, MD, a mom of a nine-year-old daughter and an eight-year-old son, an associate professor of pediatrics at Temple University, and a pediatrician with St. Luke's Pediatrics Associates, in Bethlehem, PA*

I had lunch the other day with a friend who treats herself well. We talked about self-esteem for a long time. I think a lot of women take excellent care of other people and not of themselves. We're hard on

When to Call Your Doctor

So much of feeling great and living a healthy, active life that leads to weight loss has to do with how we view and judge ourselves. But people with low self-esteem too often feel badly about themselves, and that interferes with reaching goals and enjoying life.

Low self-esteem can develop when you're struggling with something that's difficult, such as weight loss or changes in your body image, or when someone is treating you badly. If you're experiencing intense work pressure or if someone is being negative toward you, perhaps slinging insults at you on a regular basis, you might find yourself having negative thoughts about yourself. In turn, negative self-talk can lead to negative behavior, such as overeating, drinking too much alcohol, or yelling at people you love.

Low self-esteem also tends to go hand in hand with depression, which needs treatment. Call a doctor or therapist if you find that your mind is swirling with negative thoughts such as the following.

"I am worthless."

"I haven't accomplished anything."

"I always make mistakes."

ourselves: We expect ourselves to be "superwomen" and have it all together, but we don't slow down to recharge our own batteries. I am finally learning to treat myself a little more kindly each day rather than expecting others to supply that boost.

—*Rachel S. Rohde, MD, a mom of a two-year-old daughter, an assistant professor of orthopaedic surgery at the Oakland University William Beaumont School of Medicine, and an orthopaedic upper-extremity surgeon with Michigan Orthopaedic Institute, P.C., in Southfield, MI*

My self-esteem really soared when I was in my thirties. I became very confident in my education and in my roles as a physician, wife, and

"I'm a jerk."

"I don't deserve to be happy and healthy."

"I'm stupid."

While you wait for your appointment with your doctor to talk about low self-esteem, you can work on replacing those negative thoughts with positive ones. You can start by getting into a place of relaxation by doing some deep breathing. Then repeat positive thoughts to yourself over and over again, such as the following.

"I'm valuable."

"I'm accomplished."

"I'm good at many things."

"I'm a great person."

"I deserve health and happiness."

"I'm intelligent."

Also, it helps to question yourself when you have negative thoughts. The next time you think you're worthless, ask yourself, "Is that really true?" And remind yourself of the things that make you anything but worthless. It will take time and practice, but you can get there.

> **People become really quite remarkable**
> **when they start thinking that they can do things.**
> **When they believe in themselves, they have**
> **the first secret of success.**
> —*Norman Vincent Peale,*
> *author of* **The Power of Positive Thinking**

mother. I still fight some of those demons of self-esteem that we all have lingering from high school, but I found that as I got older, my self-esteem really increased. It's important to define yourself, and I don't think it's a bad thing to define yourself in terms of your relationships with others. A positive self-definition that makes you proud is important. I'm proud to be a good wife, good mother, good doctor, and good friend.

> —*Lisa Campanella-Coppo, MD, a mom of a three-year-old*
> *daughter and an emergency physician with EMCARE and the*
> *Meridian Health System, in Monmouth, NJ*

I found having a high self-esteem to be challenging during my pregnancy. I've seen this with other women too. Many times when I tell a mom or mom-to-be that she looks beautiful, she doesn't believe it. I understand why, because I felt the same way when I was pregnant. When you're pregnant, every day when you wake up, you look different. Your body changes so dramatically. Dealing with those changes was difficult for me.

During my pregnancy, I did what I could to stay healthy to feel better. One thing that helped me was moisturizing my skin as much as possible so that it would return to its pre-pregnancy state as quickly as possible.

I found that when I was pregnant, my vision of myself changed. After my baby was born, I really saw myself differently—as a mom.

> —*Christy Valentine, MD, a mom of a seven-year-old daughter,*
> *a specialist in pediatrics and internal medicine, and the founder*
> *of the Valentine Medical Center, in Gretna, LA*

It's important to take stock of how you feel about yourself on the inside because it's so critical in determining how you look on the outside. A few years ago, I traveled to Greece. I noticed that a lot of the Greek women had strong foreheads and long noses. They weren't conventionally beautiful. Yet they walked around perfectly confident and proud! They exuded beauty from their love of themselves, and others took note of their beauty! That was very inspiring to me, and it reinforced how important it is to feel good about yourself. It shines through in your appearance.

—*Michelle Yagoda, MD, a mom of an 11-year-old son, a facial plastic surgeon, the CEO of Opus Skincare, LLC, and cofounder of BeautyScoop, a patented and clinically proven supplement for skin, hair, and nails, in New York City*

After two pregnancies, my body changed, and it probably will never be the same. My hips are wider, and my breasts are gone.

But at the same time, my body image changed. When I was in my twenties, I'd look in the mirror and think, *I'm five pounds overweight!* Today, I'm proud of what my body has done. It has birthed two babies and run half marathons. I feel differently about my body now than I did pre-kids.

I find that reading about stars who bounce back a week after having babies makes women think, *That should be me!* But that's not realistic! Not everyone could—or even should—look like the folks in Hollywood. What's important is doing the best you can to take care of yourself, eat well, and exercise.

—*Heather Orman-Lubell, MD, a mom of 12- and 8-year-old sons and a pediatrician in private practice at Yardley Pediatrics of St. Christopher's Hospital for Children, in Pennsylvania*

Most people form their body image when they're in high school and early college. If you were thin in high school, you think of yourself as a thin person. Even if you gain weight, you'll think of yourself as a thin person who's temporarily gained weight.

On the flip side, if you had a challenge with your weight in

◉FitBit

Perception is reality: The more self-confidence you have, the more likely it is you'll succeed.

Here's a trick to instantly seem more confident: Pick up your pace. One of the easiest ways to tell how a person feels about herself is to examine her walk. People with confidence walk quickly. You have places to go, people to see, and things to do! Even if you aren't in a hurry, put some pep in your step. Walking 25 percent faster will make you look and feel more confident.

adolescence, you'll always think of yourself as a heavy person—one who might be thin at the moment, but a heavy person nonetheless.

I think of myself as a fat person who's thinner now. This fat image is highly ingrained, but you have to face your reality—what you see in the mirror.

—*Marie Dam, MD, a mom of 24- and 20-year-old daughters and an anti-aging medicine specialist in private practice in Naples, FL, and Danbury, CT*

Even though my Body Mass Index (BMI) is right in the middle of the green "healthy weight" zone, and I'm very comfortable there, sometimes I'll see a picture of myself or catch a glimpse of my reflection in a mirror and think, *I need to lose some weight.* Like most women, I'm susceptible to the images I see in pop culture of impossibly thin celebrities.

But I remind myself that I don't have to give in to that pressure. The feeling that I need to lose weight is an emotional response. It's not true. Four pregnancies and being in your forties really changes your body. I'm accepting of that!

—*Deborah Gilboa, MD, a mom of 11-, 9-, 7-, and 5-year-old sons, a family physician with Squirrel Hill Health Center in Pittsburgh, PA, and a parenting speaker whose advice is found at AskDoctorG.com*

One thing that has dramatically helped my self-esteem is that growing up, I had a talent that I could focus on: I was a dancer.

Dance allowed me to express myself creatively, and it gave me a reason to exercise. It also made me different from other people. It really helped me to form the core of my self-worth. Dance made me feel so good about myself, and I carry that great feeling with me today.

If you weren't able to do something like dance as a child, it's not too late! In fact, it might be easier to develop a talent as an adult because you have more resources, and you're in control of your own schedule now! It's not too late to take the time to learn to do something you'd really love to do!

—*Kristin C. Lyle, MD, FAAP, a mom of 10-, 7-, and 5-year-old daughters, the disaster medical director at Arkansas Children's Hospital, and an assistant professor of pediatrics at the University of Arkansas for Medical Sciences, both in Little Rock*

I was born fat. I've had challenges with my weight all of my life. When I look at photos of myself as a baby, I see "Miss Chubette."

This was especially hard growing up because my mother was thin and beautiful. Next to her, I always felt fat. I was teased terribly for my weight as a kid.

I had an "aha moment" with my weight struggles when I read in a book about childhood obesity that if a woman starved herself during pregnancy (as my mother did, only gaining five pounds in her entire pregnancy), the child will store fat more easily. This wasn't an excuse, and I certainly don't blame my mother. But that information made me understand why all of my life I've had to work so hard at managing my weight. That has helped me to make peace with my body.

—*Linda Brodsky, MD, a mom of a 30-year-old son and 28- and 25-year-old daughters, the president of WomenMDResources.com, a physician in private practice with Pediatric ENT Associates, and a retired professor of otolaryngology and pediatrics, in Buffalo, NY*

RALLIE'S TIP

One of the biggest battles of my life has been overcoming low self-esteem. For whatever reason, I never felt good enough, or smart enough, or pretty enough when I was young. As a result, I was always trying to improve myself—and prove myself—and that's part of what drove me to work hard to succeed as a teenager and a young adult.

One of the very best things that happened to elevate my self-esteem was simply being a physician, but not for the reasons you might expect. For some reason, I grew up assuming that other people didn't have the same kinds of challenges that I had—that they were somehow smarter, or that they had happier, better-functioning families, or that success just came more easily to them.

After I became a physician, I began spending a lot of time one-on-one with my patients, listening to the stories of their lives. It didn't take long for me to realize that every person faces obstacles and self-doubt in their life. I learned that you really can't judge a book by its cover! No matter how wealthy, pretty, smart, carefree, or successful someone is, she still has plenty of challenges and problems, and if the truth were known, her challenges and problems might be far greater than the ones that other people face.

This understanding changed my whole perspective about the basis of self-esteem. Now I know that as long as I try my very best to be a kind, generous, sincere, and loving person to everyone I encounter, I am worthy. I don't have to be perfect to earn the right to have high self-esteem.

Identifying Esteem Busters

It's not hard to list things that can bust your esteem. The memory of *that* mean girl back in high school. A pair of jeans that don't zip, despite the fact that they fit. Just last week. (Pesky clothes dryer shrinking clothes again!) Putting on a hat because it's so cold, then looking like a spun-up pencil troll when you take the hat back off. And on and on and on.

⁓◦⁓

Toxic relationships and toxic communication are the worst offenders at depleting women and sending their bad stress hormones through the roof.

—*Sara Gottfried, MD, a mom of 13- and 8-year-old daughters, a board-certified gynecologist, and the author of* The Hormone Cure, *in Berkeley, CA*

⤜⤏

It's always a good idea to spend time with positive people. So I choose to be with people who boost my self-esteem.

Unfortunately, it's not always possible to avoid people who are critical, especially if they are relatives. If someone is being critical, I change the subject and talk about something pleasant and constructive.

—*Dora Calott Wang, MD, a mom of a 10-year-old daughter, historian at the University of New Mexico School of Medicine, a unit director at Las Encinas Hospital in Pasadena, CA, and the author of* The Kitchen Shrink: A Psychiatrist's Reflection on Healing in a Changing World

⤜⤏

Wearing clothes that look unflattering is a guaranteed self-esteem buster. Around twice a year, I go through my closet and donate all the clothes that look unflattering but are still in good condition. An added bonus is I get rid of unwanted clutter. That's just as important to boost my spirits!

—*Jennifer A. Gardner, MD, a mom of a three-year-old son, a pediatrician, and the founder of an online child wellness and weight management company, HealthyKidsCompany.com, in Washington, DC*

⤜⤏

A blow to my self-esteem is when I compare myself to younger women. I'm not in my twenties anymore! Your body changes when you have children, and unfortunately some changes aren't reversible. But you can do the best with what you have. I try to remember that many things make up for lost youth. I've gained experience, wisdom, and a family.

—*Martha Wittenberg, MD, MPH, a mom of an eight-year-old son and a six-year-old daughter and a family physician with Seal Beach Family Medicine, in California*

I have to be careful not to let my esteem take a hit when I put on clothing that I think should look good, but doesn't look as good as I remember. It's not worth keeping those pieces of clothing around. If the clothing is still fairly new, I like to give it to a friend or donate it to a charity that helps women in need of work clothes. I feel this way someone else is getting good use out of it.

—*Leena Shrivastava Dev, MD, a mom of 15- and 12-year-old sons and a general pediatrician and advocate for child safety, in the Baltimore, MD, area*

I have super-high expectations of myself. If I get five compliments and one criticism, I magnify the negative comment, and I'm quick to diminish the positive ones. When I'm giving a lecture, I find it hard not to focus on the one person who's asleep.

I have tried to get better about this as I've gotten older. I practice positive self-talk, and I try to coach myself. This has helped with my self-esteem, but it's taken me a long time to get here.

—*Nancy Rappaport, MD, a mom of 22- and 18-year-old daughters and a 20-year-old son, an associate professor of psychiatry at Harvard Medical School, an attending child and adolescent psychiatrist in the Cambridge, MA, public schools, and the author of* The Behavior Code

I recognize aspects of myself that I want to improve. We're all works in progress. But I learn something from each conversation, friendship, and even each handshake I have.

I have made a choice in my life to let all those who come into my world—whether it's the barista at Starbucks, a patient at my cosmetic center, or a close friend—teach me. They all have positive traits, and I want to learn from them. I seek out their good qualities, and I consider how I can implement them in my own life.

—*Arleen K. Lamba, MD, a mom of a three-month-old son, an anesthesiologist, the medical director of Blush Med Institute, and founder of the Blush Blends Skin Care line, in Washington, DC*

> **If you think you can do a thing or think you can't do a thing, you're right.**
> —*Henry Ford*

We don't often admit it, but I think deep down, all women have moments of great insecurity. In these moments, we feel exactly as we did as teenagers—awkward and uncomfortable. Understanding that even brilliant, successful women battle these feelings brings me great comfort.

The truth is, no one knows anything about you that you don't project. If you project confidence, people think that you feel confident. If you project insecurity, people won't have confidence in you. Even if you're super good at what you do and very well prepared, you sometimes need to fake confidence before you actually feel it.

—*Ayala Laufer-Cahana, MD, a mom of 17- and 15-year-old sons and a 14-year-old daughter, a pediatrician, and the founder of Herbal Water Inc., in Wynnewood, PA*

Having good self-esteem isn't easy. Sometimes I'll see a picture of myself and think, *Oh boy. When did that spare tire arrive?* I'd be lying if I said it didn't upset me, but I try to remind myself that I'm post baby and my body is healthy and capable and allows me to do all of the things that I love to do.

I think of myself as being attractive. I'm not going to walk down a runway or anything, but I keep myself presentable and I take care of myself. I had a horrible self-image in my late twenties. I hated my nose. I hated my shape. I was always too fat. It's amazing how that changes when you fall in love!

—*Lisa Campanella-Coppo, MD*

I turned 40 last year. I had thought that when I got older, having good self-esteem would get easier. I've heard women say that you "grow into yourself." But I still struggle with my self-esteem.

FitBit

You're on a "diet," so you can't "blow your diet." If you eat something you wish you hadn't, forgive yourself immediately, vow not to make the same mistake, and move on! Just because you slip up and eat one cookie doesn't mean you should punish yourself by eating the whole bag.

Sometimes I'm my own self-esteem blocker, talking to myself in a way that hurts my self-esteem. The best advice I've gotten is to talk to myself the way I would talk to my daughter. When I start getting down on myself, I think, *Would you say that to your daughter?* Often, the answer is no. So I think, *Why am I saying it to myself?* That gives me the chance to take a step back and start over.

—*Antoinette Cheney, DO, a mom of a seven-year-old son and a six-year-old daughter and a family physician with Rocky Vista University College of Osteopathic Medicine, in Parker, CO*

The most difficult part of my job in the NICU is when a baby doesn't make it. The feelings of loss linger. Even months later, my colleagues and I ask ourselves, *What could we have done differently?*

It's easy to question our abilities, and it really can hurt our self-esteem. I've come to understand that as much as we do as physicians, there's still a spiritual component and a journey these babies are taking. We impact that journey, but sometimes we can't alter their course. Everyone has to come to terms with this in their own way. For me, I have to make peace with the idea that some souls are here for only a short time.

—*Stephanie A. Wellington, MD, a mom of a 13-year-old son and an 11-year-old daughter, a hospitalist in the Level III NICU at Bellevue Hospital Center in New York City, and the medical coach and founder of PostpartumNeonatalCoaching.com*

After my baby was born, I was heavier than I had ever been. Call me silly, but somehow I thought that after the baby popped out, my six-pack would magically reappear. The first week after I delivered was really hard for me. I still had a bit of a gut and fat in weird places such as my back bra area. I didn't feel like myself. I didn't even want to exercise at the gym because I was too embarrassed to be seen where I had always trained when I was in top shape.

Being a plastic surgeon and specializing in body contouring and mommy makeovers, I know firsthand the challenges that many women face with the body changes that occur with pregnancy. I know that even with maximal effort, sometimes women are unable to get back to their pre-pregnancy states and sometimes have to turn to surgery to get their bodies back. Because I had a C-section, I was not allowed to exercise for six weeks, and that was the longest time I had been away from the gym. During that time, it was hard to have extra weight and fat and not be able to do anything about it.

Once my doctor gave me the okay to exercise, I was grateful to get back into it. Luckily, the weight came off quickly, probably because I also went back to work two weeks after I delivered. The more weight I lost, the more motivated I was. Pretty soon I started to feel more like myself again.

—*Catherine Begovic, MD, a mom of a six-month-old daughter and a plastic surgeon at Make You Perfect, Inc., in Beverly Hills, CA*

I think a big block to self-esteem is guilt. As a parent, you're only as happy as your least-happy child. Whenever one of my children is unhappy, I worry that I could have done something better. This really erodes my self-esteem.

Some of this is useful because it helps me to try to be more balanced in life between work and home. But the reality is that balance for a working mother is an illusion. I feel like I'm one bad grade away from being tossed off the ball I'm balancing on.

I try hard not to focus on my children being perfect and instead focus on their mental equilibrium. I don't get too concerned about each individual performance, but rather I make sure their overall trajectory is good and that their understanding of overall concepts is reasonable.

Because guilt is such an eroder of self-esteem, I try to have more balance in my life. One thing I've realized is that anytime I say "yes" to something, that means I'm saying "no" to something else. This helps me to evaluate new projects and opportunities in a different way.

I've also come to realize that even though I might be the best person to do a task, that doesn't obligate me to do it. For most moms, I think the problem is taking on too many things, and then they feel badly about not being able to do them all as well as they think they should. The solution: Take on fewer things!

I'm somewhat able to do that in my life. For example, I gave up my place on a board for procedural sedation. This was hard to do, but it gave me time to focus on pain research, running my company, Buzzy4Shots, and my emergency department work.

—*Amy Baxter, MD, a mom of 15- and 12-year-old sons and a 10-year-old daughter; the CEO of Buzzy4Shots.com; and the director of emergency research, Scottish Rite, of Children's Healthcare of Atlanta, in Georgia*

I have to admit that I have esteem issues. It's tough because I compare myself to other people—no matter how much I try not to.

One thing that has helped me is the system that our son's school has for grading: Kids don't get grades until fifth grade because the emphasis is on reaching their own goals, not comparing themselves to others. *That's genius,* I thought. I tell myself that I'm competing against my own bar, not anyone else's.

I think keeping my self-esteem high requires finding time to think and enjoy my space and my thoughts. To do this, I love reading novels, magazines, the newspaper, and online information. I'm always amazed at how universal so many of life's experiences are for so many people, especially the feelings and sentiments involved with parenthood. It feels good to know that these emotions are shared and that some writers are so well able to describe the fragility, beauty, and intense effort involved in it. It keeps me grounded and feeling healthier about my own life.

I have a few friends, all moms, who meet for a book club every month or so. Getting together and talking with friends is such a nice way to boost my energy and self-esteem.

I also love painting, making a mess with art with my kids. We have so much fun, and it makes our home a fun place to be.

I also love making beautiful gifts for people. I am a huge fan of diaper "cakes," and I can never wait for the next baby shower that I can make one for.

My favorite episode of *Clifford the Dog* involves Clifford happening upon a dirty city park. He says, "This looks like a great space to make beautiful." I love that! I always try to make the spaces and things around me beautiful and organized because it helps me love my space—and my life.

—Sigrid Payne DaVeiga, MD, a mom of a seven-year-old son and a two-year-old daughter and a pediatric allergist with the Children's Hospital of Philadelphia, in Pennsylvania

Identifying Esteem Boosters

If your internal dialogue has gone from, *I think I can. I think I can. I think I can* to *What the heck was I thinking? I know I can't. I might as well go back to bed*, a major esteem boost is in order!

But how? Simply paying attention to your body and emotions can improve your health and self-esteem. In a study of women who were pregnant with their first babies, those who were trained to be mindful of their physical and emotional feelings reported higher levels of well-being and self-esteem than pregnant women who weren't trained to be mindful.

Even on days when it feels like no one is listening to you, at least you can listen to yourself! What are you telling yourself? Speak a little more kindly, please!

On days when I need an esteem boost, I wear my best-fitting Lucky jeans. That does the trick! But if I am at the hospital (where jeans are not an option), I wear a great pair of shoes instead.

—Jennifer A. Gardner, MD

I'm not big on dressing fancy or wearing a lot of makeup day to day. I usually wear blue jeans and sneakers! When my husband and I go out, it makes me feel extra special. Also, I get my nails and eyebrows done every few weeks, and that makes me feel great and boosts my esteem.

—*Stacey Ann Weiland, MD, a mom of a 14-year-old daughter and 9- and 7-year-old sons and an internist/gastroenterologist, in Denver, CO*

After many years of lecturing and writing, I feel like I have something to stand on now. When I see other people recognize confidence in me, I am able to recognize it in myself.

—*Nancy Rappaport, MD*

In my job, I have to go to court to testify in child abuse cases. The best way to boost my self-esteem is to put on a well-made, well-fitted suit. That always makes me food good. I can get away with wearing an inexpensive T-shirt underneath, as long as the suit is good quality.

—*Amy Barton, MD, a mom of an 11-year-old daughter and 8- and 5-year-old sons and a pediatrician at St. Luke's Children's Hospital, in Boise, ID*

When I started working at the hospital, one of my mentors told me, "You should wear brighter colors." She was right! I started to dress in brighter colors, and that has gone hand in hand with my confidence. My style completely changed. I have a bright red coat, and it's my absolute favorite. Wearing it makes me happy!

—*Eva Mayer, MD*

We moms do plenty of clothes shopping for our kids! I think it's important to do some shopping for ourselves. If you're wearing shabby,
ill-fitting, postpartum clothes, you're not going to feel confident.

Shopping for—and wearing—clothes that fit and flatter my body
makes me feel great!

—*Jeannette Gonzalez Simon, MD, a mom of four- and
one-year-old daughters and a pediatric gastroenterologist
at Staten Island Pediatrics GI, in New York*

One thing that really boosts my self-esteem is completing goals I have
set for myself. Also I find that lots of positive self-talk is helpful.
Self-care such as massage, yoga, Epsom salt baths, and spiritual counseling boosts my self-esteem too.

—*Kay Corpus, MD, a mom of a six-year-old daughter and
a two-year-old son, a family physician, and the director of
Owensboro Health Integrative Medicine, in Kentucky*

My husband is a huge booster of my self-esteem. He has helped me
to feel more confident as a wife and mother. No matter how many
times I ask him if I look fat, he never says that I do! A lot of my self-
esteem comes from his love for me.

—*Lisa Campanella-Coppo, MD*

My close relationships with my family and friends are a big boost to
my confidence. Knowing that I have solid relationships with my husband, my children, and my closest friends gives me the foundation to
be productive and increases my self-esteem. Yes, I can have a bad day
now and then, and I take blows to my esteem. But I draw confidence
and strength from these solid core relationships.

—*Ayala Laufer-Cahana, MD*

Parenting should be a source of self-esteem. Yet the work of parenting
is mostly invisible to others, and it's certainly not rewarding in the
ways a job is. If I were to make one single change in our society, it

would be to make the daily hard work of parenting more visibly rewarding.

As a psychiatrist, I know how important the first few years of a child's life are. So I put a tremendous amount of work into my daughter's first four years. Many of the rewards are only coming now. She's 10 years old, and she recently received a citizenship award at her school. I was so proud of her. I know it's because of work I put in, long ago and all these years.

—*Dora Calott Wang, MD*

I find that when I'm feeling fit, it helps my self-esteem. While it's not always easy to keep the outside of my body fit, I really try to take care of the inside. I make sure I'm in communion with God, and I pray each night before I go to sleep. When I'm at peace, I feel better. And that shows on the outside too.

—*Bola Oyeyipo-Ajumobi, MD, a mom of five- and two-year-old sons, a family physician at the Veterans Health Administration, and the owner of SlimyBookWorm.com, in San Antonio, TX*

Running a half marathon was a tremendous boost to my self-esteem! I was never a runner, but my daughter asked me to run a half marathon with her.

Why not? I thought, and I signed up! I enjoyed it so much I signed right up for another one!

—*Eva Ritvo, MD, a mom of 22- and 17-year-old daughters, a psychiatrist, and a coauthor of* The Beauty Prescription, *in Miami Beach, FL*

I think playing sports is important for women, especially young women. Playing sports gives you a unique perspective, and it makes you competitive. It encourages you to want to achieve more. It makes you stronger, and it builds self-esteem. By playing sports, you learn that you win some and you lose some, and that's okay.

—*Pam D'Amato, MD*

My mother pounded into my head that every human being is special, and I believed her. I have always believed that I'm special, just like everyone else is special. I've always told my patients that they are special too, and an incredibly high percentage of my former pediatric patients are doctors or becoming doctors. That is a wonderful compliment.

—*Hana R. Solomon, MD, a mom who raised four children, a grandmom of three, a board-certified pediatrician, the president of BeWell Health, LLC, and the author of* Clearing the Air One Nose at a Time: Caring for Your Personal Filter, *in Columbia, MO*

⁓

I find that meeting my goals boosts my self-esteem. My main goal in life is to take the best possible care of my children. I want to raise them to be good people who will make the world a better place. But I also set other, smaller goals for myself, such as setting aside time for my hobbies and exercise routine.

I love just about all forms of art, and my daughters know that this is also an important part of me. When I draw or sew, I complete a small project that helps me feel a sense of accomplishment. This helps to show my daughters that mothers can have goals too!

—*Tiemdow Phumiruk, MD, a mom of 13-, 10-, and 7-year-old daughters, a pediatrician in the emergency department of Children's Hospital Colorado at Parker Adventist Hospital, and adjunct faculty at Rocky Vista University College of Osteopathic Medicine, in Parker, CO*

⁓

A very large component of beauty is well within your control. Someone who is confident and happy is beautiful.

I've learned that it's not a perfect nose or beautiful neck that defines beauty. It's an overall glow of health. Think about it: Someone with a perfect nose but dry skin and hair isn't beautiful. Yet someone who takes care of her nutrition and health, who has glowing skin and hair, is beautiful. This type of beauty is contagious.

—*Michelle Yagoda, MD*

My self-esteem is very much tied to exercising and eating well. When I exercise and eat well, I feel like a stronger person.

I also try to surround myself with people who prop me up, rather than people who drag me down.

I'm also a type A person, and so crossing things off of my to-do list makes me feel good. I have come to accept the fact that I will never cross *everything* off of my to-do list, but accomplishing some of it every day keeps me going with a positive attitude.

—*Michelle Spring, MD, a mom of a one-year-old son and two grown stepchildren and a board-certified plastic surgeon with Marina Plastic Surgery Associates, in Marina del Rey, CA*

When I'm eating well and exercising, I feel better about myself. When I'm not eating well and not exercising, I feel bad. It's that simple.

Also, being out of the house and with other people boosts my self-esteem. When I'm home by myself, and around too many mirrors, I feel very self-aware and self-conscious.

—*Judith Hellman, MD, a mom of a 15-year-old son, an associate clinical professor of dermatology at Mt. Sinai Hospital in New York City, and a dermatologist in private practice*

I always try to look well put together. Even when I wasn't at my ideal weight, I made an effort to look good. Sometimes overweight people just give up.

I find that when I dress nicely, do my hair, wear jewelry, and look the best that I can, I feel so much better about myself. And if I feel better about myself, it encourages me to try a little harder to get fit and be healthy. When I wear a flattering color or a nice outfit and someone says, "You look great!" it makes me feel great!

—*Susan Besser, MD, a mom of six grown children, ages 28, 26, 24, 22, 21, and 19, a grandmom of two, a family physician, and the medical director of Doctors Express-Memphis, in Tennessee*

I hate to take the time in the morning to put on makeup and do my hair. I feel that there are many other things I could be doing with that time! But I know that when I've tried to look good, it gives me a confidence boost and the energy to make it through the day.

When I was growing up, my mom didn't believe in makeup, and she always wore her hair in the same, simple style. As I got older, I really enjoyed experimenting and trying out makeup and hairstyles. Sitting down at my vanity table each morning is fun for me now.

—*Kristin C. Lyle, MD, FAAP*

This might seem like a paradox, but I think the best way to boost self-esteem is to not feel like you need to have so much self-esteem!

If you allow yourself to have weaknesses or foibles and not always feel perfectly self-confident, it's very liberating.

I boost my self-esteem by reminding myself that I don't have to be perfect. I tell myself it's okay if I put my foot in my mouth or occasionally say something that's not nice to my family, to a friend, or to my mother-in-law. Then when those things happen, they don't damage my self-esteem. You don't have to be perfect in every area of your life. It's good to be kind to yourself.

—*Linda Brodsky, MD*

To instantly boost my self-esteem, I take a deep breath and adjust my posture. I pull my shoulders down and back. Taking a deep breath releases nitrous oxide—laughing gas!—in small amounts, which is very relaxing. This makes me feel better about myself right away.

To deep breathe, inhale through your nose as deeply as you can; your breath should expand your chest fully and push out your abdomen slightly. When this becomes slightly uncomfortable, slowly breathe out through your nose.

—*Jennifer Hanes, DO, a mom of a seven-year-old daughter and a four-year-old son, an emergency physician who's board certified in integrative medicine, and the author of* The Princess Plan: Shrink Your Waist, Expand Your Beauty, *in Austin, TX*

I start each day with a positive thought of what I like about myself at that moment. I actually say it out loud to myself. It could be something easy like, *I like my hair today* or something deeper like, *I feel smart today.*

People find it hard to say something nice about themselves. They can give compliments to friends and even say nice things about celebrities they don't know. But we rarely take the time to compliment ourselves. Why not? Verbalizing something positive about yourself makes it tangible and helps you realize that only you can make yourself feel good! It's my job to find the good in me, say it out loud, and celebrate it.

Confidence is key. It is the essence of who I am. I am not afraid to say that I am my biggest fan or that I believe in myself. If you don't value yourself and support yourself, it will be hard to convince anyone else of the value you truly hold. And we are all valuable for different reasons.

—*Arleen K. Lamba, MD*

My daughter is so different from me. She's a total flibbertigibbet. At two years old, she owns the world. Everything she picks up is the most fascinating thing she's ever seen. She says goofy things all the time. She's completely her own person, and completely comfortable being herself. I've learned a lot from her about self-esteem.

A huge self-esteem booster for me is when I come home and my daughter greets me with, "Where were you? I missed you so much!" Any insecurities go by the wayside when I'm validated like that.

Having children definitely changes the way you see yourself. All of a sudden, at the moment you think you have no strength left, you're called upon to be someone's superhero.

As my son gets older and faces challenges at school and has

new experiences with his peers, he asks me for advice. When I have to think about what I would tell one of the people I love most in the world about how to handle a tough situation, it makes me a better person, because I can never just take the easy way out. I have to figure out the high road. It is funny how much more completely I understand Ghandi's concept of being the change you want to see in the world.

This year, all of the children in my son's second grade class had to pick a hero, write about him or her, and make a presentation at their weekly assembly. When my son picked me, "Doctor Girl," it was the most wonderful compliment. When your kids see you that way, you feel so good. It's the greatest gift and self-esteem booster that I have ever experienced.

—*Sigrid Payne DaVeiga, MD*

෴

It is good to set a small goal and get to it. I get a charge out of cleaning out a closet or ironing a scarf that has been balled up in a drawer for a year. It amazes me how much it does for my self-esteem to clear out a pile of papers sitting by the computer or finally replace that old mashed Kleenex box languishing in the backseat of the car.

Also, I'm a "fix-it" person, so I always have a project to work on, such as refurbishing an alligator purse I bought for $3 at the Salvation Army or making skinny jeans out of an old pair of boot-cut Levi's from the 1980s. I never throw anything out, which does present a challenge for the top shelves of my closets! Recycling an unusual hair clip or restringing a necklace from my Aunt Clara gives me a sense of accomplishment that's a breath of fresh air from ordinary responsibilities.

—*Elizabeth Berger, MD, a mom of a 30-year-old son and a 29-year-old daughter, a child psychiatrist, and the author of* Raising Kids with Character, *in New York City*

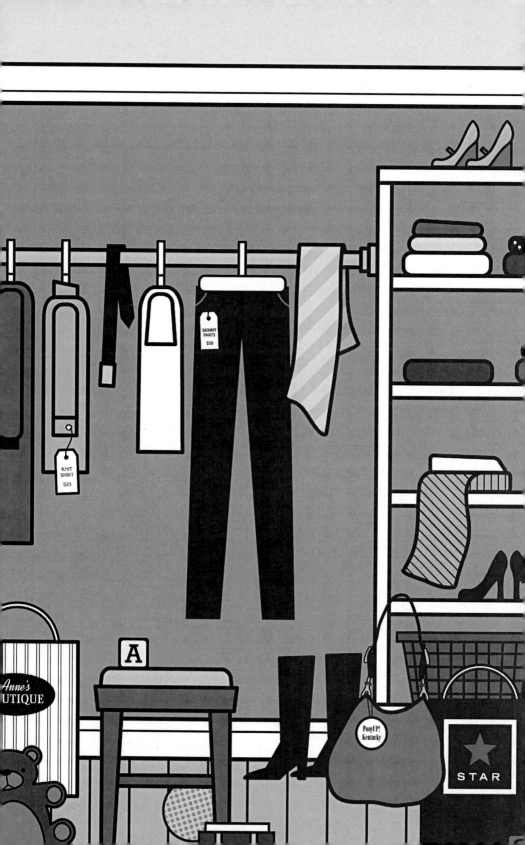

Chapter 8
Looking Your Best

YOUR BODY

The you that you see in your mind's eye—how you think of yourself—is critical to your self-esteem and to your mood. The you that you see in the mirror is important too, of course. It's hard to argue with the logic that if you look your best, you'll likely also feel your best.

A Mint.com survey found that on average, people spend between 15 percent and 23 percent of their discretionary spending on clothing, accessories, and shoes. Not surprisingly, folks in Manhattan spent the most, 21 percent or $362 a month, on fashion. San Francisco was the second-highest spending city, and Dallas came in at number 3.

We all look like super savers, though, in comparison to Catherine, Duchess of Cambridge. She spent more than £35,000 ($54,000!) on clothes in just six months.

JUSTIFICATION FOR A CELEBRATION

Your jeans zipped—without you needing to suck it in, lie on your back, use a pair of pliers, or say a prayer. Way to go!

> **Style is a magic wand, and it turns everything to gold that it touches.**
> —*Logan Pearsall Smith, an American writer*

Assessing Your Style

When people ask "What's your style" it's become somewhat of a sitcom joke. But really, it's helpful to take some time to ask yourself, What is your style? If you don't know where you want to be, how could you ever hope to get there?

Plus, great style goes hand in hand with losing weight and feeling great. Chances are, you don't have a lot of time to spend thinking about your personal style, but this fun and fast quiz can help. Are you all about classic glamor, trendsetting style, free-and-easy elegance, sexy-chic, or business formal?

Take our quiz and find out what approach most complements your personal look and lifestyle preferences. Here's another fun plus: You'll discover the celebrity moms who match your style.

This quiz was written by PonyUPKentucky.com blogger Jennifer Goldsmith Cerra, and it's reprinted here by permission of PonyUP! Kentucky.

My hair color (or closest) is: ☐
    1 = Dark brown
    2 = Red
    3 = Blonde
    4 = Blue/green/pink/wired
    5 = Salt-and-pepper or gorgeous grey

My hair is typically: ☐
    1 = Wavy, loose, and casual
    2 = Voluminous with lots of curls and styling
    3 = Tied back in a chic ponytail

FitBit

Even if you plan to stay at home all day, dress as if you are going out. This changes your attitude toward yourself and makes you more likely to take good care of yourself.

> **What you wear is how you present yourself to the world, especially today, when human contacts are so quick. Fashion is instant language.**
> —*Muiccia Prada, an Italian fashion designer*

4 = Blown out. What else?
5 = Washed, set, and ready for work!

My signature lipstick color is: ☐
    1 = Chanel red
    2 = Lip balm
    3 = Pink lip gloss
    4 = A bold burgundy
    5 = Go-everywhere neutral

My dress of choice for a night out is: ☐
    1 = A little black dress—a staple!
    2 = Something sensational that's either straight off the runway or looks like it is
    3 = Wrap dress with accessories to dress it up
    4 = Halter dress with a plunging neckline and loose-fitting everywhere else—to accentuate the positive
    5 = A pantsuit of luxe fabrics in an inviting and professional color

For me, the ideal way to spend a Saturday night is: ☐
    1= Dancing at the hottest jazz club in town
    2 = An intimate dinner with your closest friends
    3 = Heading to an art gallery opening
    4 = Throwing a fancy party, complete with catered food
    5 = In one of the city's power restaurants, strategizing with work colleagues

My top priority social events typically are: □

1 = Formal dinners and maybe even a fundraising gala, plus cocktail parties

2 = Fab parties and dinners at the hottest restaurants

3 = Cozy dinner parties at our family beach house or vacation time at a ski resort

4 = Cocktail parties and small dinner parties at home with friends

5 = After-work office events and industry parties

The amount of time I spend getting ready for an event is: □

1 = A lot. I'll get my hair done at the salon, along with a mani-pedi and spend an hour on my makeup that evening.

2 = About one hour for hair and makeup. (Wardrobe selection and styling: It might take me up to a week in advance planning, though!)

3 = About 20 minutes: Concealer, bronzer, eye shadow and lip-gloss are all I need. My amazing exercise routine gives me a natural glow, after all! And I'll let my hair do whatever it wants.

4 = As long as it takes to get every detail right and double-check my face and wardrobe from every angle. That usually means listening to the latest Beyonce CD in its entirety.

5 = I'm the expert of office bathroom prep. It'll take me just 10 minutes to brush my teeth, trade my button-down shirt for a cami, and freshen my makeup.

FitBit

As you assess your style and rebuild your wardrobe, each day take a good look in the mirror. Ask yourself: *What do I feel good about? What do I want to update?* Let the changes you make reveal the real you.

> **Nothing makes a woman more beautiful**
> **than the belief that she is beautiful.**
> —*Sophia Lauren*

My personal wardrobe-building philosophy is: ☐
   1 = You can't go wrong investing in designer labels and quality workmanship, no matter what the cost. Avoid the trends and pay more for pieces that will last 10 years—or more.
   2 = It's fun to spend time experimenting and pulling together a unique look, and quality vintage pieces plus inexpensive trend items achieve that nicely.
   3 = Comfort is luxury, so investing in pieces that flatter the body through draping and flowing (as opposed to nipping and supporting) are always a smart approach.
   4 = You should flaunt your assets, so anything fitted, lower-cut, or short fits the bill nicely, in a mix of classic and trendy pieces.
   5 = High-end suits are an investment in your career. Impeccable tailoring shows a woman is inside that suit, while prestige scarves, shoes, and purses show you've arrived.

I never leave home without: ☐
   1 = My favorite scent
   2 = My glitziest jewelry
   3 = My cute and comfy flats
   4 = My gym bag
   5 = My smartphone

My handbag always has: ☐
   1 = Smartphone, iPod, and wallet
   2 = Make-up bag, grocery list, and magazine or book
   3 = What handbag? I have an amazing backpack!

4 = Wallet, comb, and bag of M&M's

5 = Smartphone (and probably some other stuff, though haven't checked lately)

When I open my closet, it has: ☐

1 = Cocktail dresses—you can never have too many!

2 = Bohemian-inspired silk shirts and lots of color

3 = Track suits, T-shirts, sweaters, some jeans, lots of pants, and hardly any skirts

4 = Form-fitting and fun everything

5 = Pant suits in shades of brown, grey, and black

My personal style mantra is: ☐

1 = Good taste is timeless.

2 = Stay ahead of the curve.

3 = Mix comfort and style—fabulously!

4 = Turn heads wherever you go.

5 = A beautifully tailored suit and killer heels will get you through anything.

FIND YOUR STYLE!

Tally up the number of 1s, 2s, 3s, 4s and 5s you chose and read the tips that best match your style.

If you chose mostly 1s, your style is Classic Glamor. You're driven by ideas of timeless femininity and good taste.

FitBit

Invest in a few simple style staples: a good coat, a little black dress, a well cut pair of jeans, a classic pair of black pants, a cashmere cardigan, and a simple stylish ivory or white shirt. You can wear these fom season to season, dress them up or down, and update the looks with accessories.

> **Know, first, who you are;**
> **and then adorn yourself accordingly.**
> **—*Epictetus***

You're not interested in what the "hot thing" today is: You know what looks beautiful on you, and you shop for keeps. That means you don't obsess about your clothing choices; rather, you stick with classic combinations such as tailored white shirts and well-fitting jeans. Finally, you care about your looks, but often keep your beauty regime simple. A touch of blush, a stylish headscarf, and big shades are often all you need before running out the door.

Your celebrity mom matches: Kate, Duchess of Cambridge; Michelle Obama; and Catherine Zeta-Jones

If you chose mostly 2s, your style is Trendsetting, You love what's new, but with a caveat: It can't be what everyone else is wearing. You're an early adopter, and by the time the others have caught up, you've found a new look. One area where you really stand out from the crowd is your love of accessories. Like the legendary Elizabeth Taylor, you're the quintessential diamond icon. Whether they're real or fake, you love to adorn yourself with beautiful jewels. Bangles, big earrings, brooches, anything with color reigns supreme in your wardrobe! You're very confident in your style choices, and you like to go against tradition. Many appreciate your unique and bold take on fashion.

Your celebrity mom matches: Fergie, Madonna, and Gwen Stefani

If you chose mostly 3s, your style is No-Fuss. You're right: If you've got natural beauty and uncontrived style, you're already ahead of the game. Because you like to be easy-peasy, you're just as likely to wear a pair of jeans and a flowy tunic as a billowy gown to a special event. You love pants and flats, and

FitBit

Here's the simplest way to dress to look thinner: Wear clothes that fit well.

Dress like Goldilocks, in clothes that fit just right: If your clothes are too big, they make you look big. If your clothes are too small, they make you look big too. Although it's tempting to try to hide in a long, bulky sweater or to squeeze into skinny jeans, neither of these strategies works when you're trying to look thinner.

you favor a simple ponytail or loose bun over fancy hairdos. You're active, love walking (no stilettos for you), and don't want to be bogged down by accessories or anything too frou-frou.

Your celebrity mom matches: Jessica Alba, Sandra Bullock, and Kate Hudson

If you chose mostly 4s, your style is Sexy Chic. When you enter a room, people's heads turn. You love making a grand entrance and causing some whispers as you saunter by in your stilettos and racy cocktail dresses. You follow the trends and are always on top of what's hot in fashion—as long as it makes you look fabulous! Who cares if it takes you two hours to get ready for a night out on the town? Looking this glamorous is what being a woman is all about! With a hectic schedule of romantic nights and party-hopping to attend to, you need body-flaunting dresses to paint the town red in. Minis are always attention-grabbing, so if you've got what they take, flaunt it!

Your celebrity mom matches: Beyonce, Mariah Carey, and Jennifer Lopez

If you chose mostly 5s, your style is Business Formal. For you, work and play intermingle, so looking your best after hours usually means adapting what you were wearing during work hours too. Business-savvy, you're still a fashionable girl working in a buttoned-up, ultra conservative world, so dressing professionally is an absolute must. These professional settings are not exactly friendly to the fashion forward, but you maintain a level of style by working in fashionable elements through subtle accessories and chic silhouettes.

Your celebrity mom matches: Hillary Clinton, Queen Elizabeth II, and Sheryl Sandberg

❧

I firmly believe that if you look good, you feel good, and if you feel good, you interact with the world in a positive manner. I have found a style that reflects the way I want people to think about me.

> —*Debra Luftman, MD, a mom of a 22-year-old daughter and a 19-year-old son, a board-certified dermatologist in private practice, coauthor of* The Beauty Prescription, *developer of the skincare line of products Therapeutix, and a clinical instructor of skin surgery and general dermatology at UCLA*

❧

It might sound old-fashioned, but I think it's important to look like a woman. I care about my clothing, makeup, nails, and personal upkeep. This is important because when you're feeling confident about your outward appearance, it can give your inner self a boost as well.

> —*Pam D'Amato, MD, a mom of seven- and four-year-old daughters and an interventional pain management physician with University Spine Center, in Wayne, NJ*

❧

My style is ever-changing. I enjoy experimenting and playing in the world of fashion. I believe that fashion is all about choices. My style is all about *my* choices, *my* voice. To me, this is the concept of style. Expressing individual style is far more important than any fleeting fashion trend.

> —*Arleen K. Lamba, MD, a mom of a three-month-old son, an anesthesiologist, the medical director of Blush Med Institute, and founder of the Blush Blends Skin Care line, in Washington, DC*

Style, like confidence, comes from the inside out. I'm in a place in my life where I'm going through a second teenage phase. I wear the same clothes as my daughters! I'm enjoying it immensely.

—Eva Ritvo, MD, a mom of 22- and 17-year-old daughters, a psychiatrist, and a coauthor of The Beauty Prescription, *in Miami Beach, FL*

Browse Fashion Blogs

It's hard to look your best when you haven't gone shopping since before you wore pregnancy pants. And if your toddler's wardrobe is shouting, "Chic!" while you're still wearing jeans you bought in the 1990s, it's time for a little fashion fresh up. There's no question that wearing clothes that fit your body at the weight you are now will make you feel good enough to stick to your weight loss plan.

Before you head out to the store, you might want to see how styles look on real women instead of mannequins, and today that's easy to do, thanks to the hundreds of fashion blogs out there. And thankfully, not all fashion bloggers are stick-thin, wanna-be fashion models. Here are a few to get you started.

- Ain't No Mom Jeans: **AINTNOMOMJEANS.TYPEPAD.COM**
- Momma Go Round: **MOMMAGOROUND.COM**
- The Budget Fashionista: **THEBUDGETFASHIONISTA.COM**
- Perfectly Shaped World: **PERFECTLYSHAPEDWORLD.COM/BLOG**
- Steal the Style: **STEALTHESTYLE.COM**
- Walking in Grace & Beauty: **CYNDISPIVEY.COM**
- All Things Chic: **ALLTHINGSCHIC.NET**

While you're at it, you might want to take some time to try out some new makeup looks. Check out the tutorials on these makeup blogs.

- Makeup Geek: **MAKEUPGEEK.COM**
- Pixiwoo: **PIXIWOO.COM**

> **Fashion fades. Only style remains the same.**
>
> —*Coco Chanel*

It's important to find the style that works for you. Figuring out which colors and outfits make you look best takes time. It evolves over the years. For example, I put on a sweater this morning that made me look dumpy. So I took it off and put something else on, and it was amazing how much better I felt.

> —*Heather Orman-Lubell, MD, a mom of 12- and 8-year-old sons and a pediatrician in private practice at Yardley Pediatrics of St. Christopher's Hospital for Children, in Pennsylvania*

I take care with my wardrobe. Like it or not, we live in a society where you make an immediate impression with your attire. You can influence how people think of you with what you wear.

My clothes are generally simple and classic. I don't go for trends such as skinny jeans because they aren't flattering to my wide hips. Not every trend works for every body shape. Also, I'm mindful of my age. You have to balance the way you dress with what's inside of you.

My clothes provide a simple canvas or background. Then I bring out my best features and my personality with accessories.

> —*Aline T. Tanios, MD, a mom of 10- and 4-year-old daughters and an 8-year-old son and a pediatric hospitalist and assistant professor at the Washington University School of Medicine, in St. Louis, MO*

I used to live in the middle of the woods in Connecticut. I wore ripped barn clothes every day! I'd watch makeover shows on TV and watch plain-looking people become transformed. I remember thinking to myself, *I can do that!*

I gave myself a personal makeover! I went to a new hairdresser and asked for a new look. Then I went to a makeup counter and asked the women there to show me how to do my makeup. And I started to dress better. I realized that it doesn't take any longer to put on something that looks great than it does to put on something that looks horrible!

—*Marie Dam, MD, a mom of 24- and 20-year-old daughters and an anti-aging medicine specialist in private practice in Naples, FL, and Danbury, CT*

RALLIE'S TIP

I spent years trying to master the corporate look, but I always felt like an imposter. Whenever I wear a dress and heels, I don't just feel like an imposter, I feel like I'm practically incapacitated. What if I need to chase a fleeing purse snatcher or perform the Heimlich maneuver on someone who just happens to be choking at the table next to me? Wearing a dress would really make things difficult for me!

It took me years to figure out my style, and it turns out it's nothing more than casual and comfortable, whenever I can get away with it and not seem disrespectful of the environment I'm in or the people I'm with. My style is an extension of my life at home on my farm with my horses. I usually wear jeans and cowboy boots. Fortunately, cowboy boots have made a comeback recently, so I've actually been in sync with the fashion world for a while, even if accidentally! My favorite place to shop for fun, interesting clothes is anywhere that sells saddles, bridles, and boots.

Finding Time to Look Great

If you think about it, it doesn't take any longer to slip on a great-fitting, well-made pair of pants than to throw on sloppy sweats. It takes about two seconds to put on earrings and a necklace. Sure, makeup could take you a few more minutes, and it could take another few more minutes to blow-dry and style your hair. But a few minutes as a trade-off for a full day of looking great sounds worth it!

⟳

I keep my makeup in a case, rather than in a drawer or the counter. This way, I can take it with me. Maybe it's a habit from my teenage years. I grew up in Los Angeles, where teenagers often put makeup on in the car because we spend so much time in cars.

> **Never wear anything that panics the cat.**
> **—P.J. O'Rourke**

In any case, with my makeup in a case, I can carry it anywhere in the house. Sometimes, I bring my makeup to the breakfast table, especially if we're in a hurry. My daughter is entertained by my putting on makeup. It also helps me eat less.

> —*Dora Calott Wang, MD, a mom of a 10-year-old daughter, historian at the University of New Mexico School of Medicine, a unit director at Las Encinas Hospital in Pasadena, CA, and the author of* The Kitchen Shrink: A Psychiatrist's Reflection on Healing in a Changing World

I find that the more effort I put into looking good, the better I feel. Unfortunately, time often is the limiting factor.

Recently I have discovered that waking up 10 minutes earlier to help myself look better gives me more than 10 minutes of energy—or "feel better"—back later in the day.

> —*Rachel S. Rohde, MD, a mom of a two-year-old daughter, an assistant professor of orthopaedic surgery at the Oakland University William Beaumont School of Medicine, and an orthopaedic upper-extremity surgeon with Michigan Orthopaedic Institute, P.C., in Southfield, MI*

I have an interesting challenge to dressing well right now. My daughter doesn't want me to go to work, so I have to kind of hide the fact that I'm getting ready in the morning!

I didn't used to do this, but I've evolved into one of those people who sets out their outfits the night before. That makes getting ready in the morning much quicker. I can get dressed for work in about five minutes!

> —*Sigrid Payne DaVeiga, MD, a mom of a seven-year-old son and a two-year-old daughter and a pediatric allergist with the Children's Hospital of Philadelphia, in Pennsylvania*

Because my thrift store wardrobe is made up of many separate pieces and accessories, I'm constantly recombining them. But it takes time to put together an outfit successfully. I need a try-on period in front of a mirror to make sure the combination really works. Often there's

Take Time to Shop. . .On the Computer

Online shopping is a hot new trend, and one that's oh-so helpful to moms who would rather surf for the perfect outfit during the blissfully quiet hours of naptime than drag tiny, reluctant shoppers to the mall.

There are several reasons why it's worthwhile to take some mommy time to shop from home—the most obvious being that you don't have to be the mom in the dressing room whose little ones are tearing up and down the aisles. But you also have hundreds of options available to you in a myriad of colors and in a bigger variety of sizes than you would in the stores. (Some stores, such as Old Navy, are known for making plus sizes available online but not in their stores.)

You don't even have to limit your purchases to the United States, because there's been an explosion of international retailers that make it easy for you to find whatever you need. And if you choose to buy online from a store with a location near you, often you have the option of in-store pickup. Oftentimes, if you need to return the purchase, you can return the item to your local store, saving return shipping costs.

If you're worried about fit, be sure to read the description carefully, take your measurements, check the size guide for that retailer, and read the comments from other buyers. Some sites even have virtual dressing rooms that give you an idea of what certain clothes would look like on your body. Before you buy, check out the company's return policy and decide if it's worth the risk of having to return an item.

something just "wrong" that needs readjustment. So making sure I have those 5 or 10 minutes to experiment is crucial. Otherwise, I have a tendency to throw on the same black slacks and top with those tried-and-true antique earrings I got in Italy in the '60s and run out the

There are a few things to do to shop smart when you go online. For one, always use a credit card because you'll be protected under the federal Fair Credit Billing Act if something goes wrong. Also, be sure you're shopping on secure websites, which will begin with https:// during checkout. The "s" stands for secure.

Reputable websites will also tell you how your information is processed under its "privacy policy." And when you place an order, give out only the information required for the sale, such as your name and address. Don't give additional information such as your income, and never give your social security number. It's also not a good idea to enter your credit card information when you're on a public Wi-Fi network. It's better to make purchases at home.

Now that your credit card is burning a hole in your pocket, let's get shopping. You can start with your favorite places to shop, or check out some of the following retailers you won't find at your local mall.

- Zappos, which has free shipping and free returns: **ZAPPOS.COM**
- Topshop, which has free shipping on orders of more than $50: **US.TOPSHOP.COM**
- ASOS, which has free shipping both ways: **US.ASOS.COM**
- ModCloth, which has free shipping on orders of more than $50: **MODCLOTH.COM**
- eShakti, which offers custom sizes: **ESHAKTI.COM**
- Kiyonna, which sells plus-size clothes and has free shipping both ways: **KIYONNA.COM**

door. To get out of that rut, I need to take a moment to study the terrain carefully. A new outfit needs a dry run!

—*Elizabeth Berger, MD, a mom of a 30-year-old son and a 29-year-old daughter, a child psychiatrist, and the author of* Raising Kids with Character, *in New York City*

Dressing Well

"I've always believed that clothing is a great way to tell your story," said fashion expert Carson Kressley. What will your clothing say about you?

❧

When I find a particular piece of clothing that's comfortable and acceptable for business attire, I buy a whole bunch of the same item in different colors.

—*Hana R. Solomon, MD, a mom who raised four children, a grand-mom of three, a board-certified pediatrician, the president of BeWell Health, LLC, and the author of* Clearing the Air One Nose at a Time: Caring for Your Personal Filter, *in Columbia, MO*

Mommy MD Guides–Recommended Product
Spanx

"ALL HAIL SPANX! It might not help you lose weight, but it sure helps you feel better while you are trying!" says Rachel S. Rohde, MD, a mom of a two-year-old daughter, an assistant professor of orthopaedic surgery at the Oakland University William Beaumont School of Medicine, and an orthopaedic upper-extremity surgeon with Michigan Orthopaedic Institute, P.C., in Southfield, MI.

You can buy a Spanx undergarment in stores such as Nordstrom and at online retailers such as **SPANX.COM** and **QVC.COM** for around $50. Visit **SPANX.COM** for more information.

FitBit

A simple way to look slimmer, not to mention to pick out your clothes in a jiffy, is to dress all in one color from your top to your shoes. Don't forget to match your tights or stockings to your outfit too. Dark colors are slimming, so try black, navy, charcoal, burgundy, deep green, or purple.

Before I was pregnant with my son, I was on the TV show *Survivor*. One thing I learned from the wardrobe team is to wear solid colors. I avoid wearing clothing with loud prints, patterns, polka dots, and certainly stripes. These patterns and prints break up the lines of your body. Solid colors are generally more slimming and flattering.

> —*Edna Ma, MD, a mom of a six-month-old son, an anesthesiologist at UCLA Olive View Medical Center, and the founder of BareEase pre-waxing numbing kit, in Los Angeles, CA*

The secret to dressing well is to accentuate the positive! I usually prefer outfits that accentuate my legs rather than my tummy. Wrap dresses and empire waist dresses are especially flattering.

> —*Sonali Ruder, DO, a mom of a two-month-old daughter, an emergency physician at Coral Springs Medical Center near Fort Lauderdale, FL, and a recipe developer and blogger at TheFoodiePhysician.com*

I wear scrubs to work. They're comfortable, like pajamas, but they're not especially flattering. I used to wear dark navy blue scrubs, thinking they were more slimming. But lately I've started to wear brighter colors. When I put on a gorgeous color, I feel good!

> —*Stephanie A. Wellington, MD, a mom of a 13-year-old son and an 11-year-old daughter, a hospitalist in the Level III NICU at Bellevue Hospital Center in New York City, and the medical coach and founder of PostpartumNeonatalCoaching.com*

Yes, it's easy to throw on a pair of yoga pants and a T-shirt, but I make a point to dress well even on my days off. I find that V-neck tops are very slimming and flattering. Pretty earrings and necklaces are great to take eyes off of hips and thighs.

> —*Shilpa Amin-Shah, MD, a mom of a three-year-old son and*
> *a two-year-old daughter and an emergency physician and director of*
> *the recruiting team at Emergency Medical Associates,*
> *in Livingston, NJ*

My favorite thing to wear is leggings. They can be slimming if you wear a long shift over them, pulled in with a belt or scarf to give you shape.

> —*Tiemdow Phumiruk, MD, a mom of 13-, 10-, and*
> *7-year-old daughters, a pediatrician in the emergency department*
> *of Children's Hospital Colorado at Parker Adventist Hospital,*
> *and adjunct faculty at Rocky Vista University College of*
> *Osteopathic Medicine, in Parker, CO*

I dress according to how I feel. Some days I want to be casual, so I'll wear yoga pants and a flowy top; other days I want to dress up with jackets and blazers. I love leggings because they're stretchy and

Mommy MD Guides-Recommended Product
Yummie Tummie

"I found a terrific company with great, slimming shapewear: Yummie by Heather Thomson," says Jeannette Gonzalez Simon, MD, a mom of four- and one-year-old daughters and a pediatric gastroenterologist at Staten Island Pediatrics GI, in New York. "They make tops, such as tank tops, that have 'secret' three-panel supports in them. They also sell bottoms, such as leggings, that act as a control top."

Yummie Tummie tank tops cost around $48, and leggings cost $30 to $84. Visit **YUMMIELIFE.COM** for more information.

comfy, and they go with everything! I like simple, ethereal, yoga-ish jewelry.

—Kay Corpus, MD, a mom of a six-year-old daughter and a two-year-old son, a family physician, and the director of Owensboro Health Integrative Medicine, in Kentucky

Because I feel good on the inside, I want to reflect that on the outside. I love reading fashion and makeup blogs and checking out *US* magazine to see what my favorite celebrity is wearing as she picks up her groceries. It's a guilty pleasure.

—Arleen K. Lamba, MD

My overall wardrobe philosophy is to spend money on basics such as classic black trousers and other items that you can wear for years and years. I mix and match those staples with trendy items such as fun costume jewelry. Those pieces jazz up my outfits.

—Heather Orman-Lubell, MD

A lot of department stores offer personal shoppers, but what I find more helpful is going shopping with a friend who has a great sense of style. She doesn't have any vested interest in me making a purchase! When I lost 25 pounds and was ready to replace my "fat clothes," I took a friend shopping. She picked 50 things off of the racks and helped me by saying "yes" or "no" to each one.

—Katherine Dee, MD, a mom of eight-year-old twin daughters and a six-year-old son and a radiologist at the Seattle Breast Center, in Washington

I think it's important to not get too caught up with the number on the tag—the size of your clothes. I've bought clothes based on size alone, even if they didn't look good on me. I've also passed on clothes that fit well, just because I didn't want to wear that particular size.

Now, I try to buy clothes that flatter me, and that I feel great and comfortable in. If I get too caught up in the size, I don't feel pretty.

It's important to remember that those sizes are meaningless.

They're not standardized throughout the fashion industry, and they even change over time!

—*Christy Valentine, MD, a mom of a seven-year-old daughter, a specialist in pediatrics and internal medicine, and the founder of the Valentine Medical Center, in Gretna, LA*

I usually wear every New Yorker's favorite color: black. It's slimming and sophisticated. Anytime I try to put on a different color, I end up tearing it off and putting something black on instead. My closet is so full of black clothing that it's hard to find anything in the sea of black!

I accessorize with other, brightly colored pieces, such as a red scarf. That livens up my wardrobe. But in New York City, you can never go wrong wearing black.

—*Judith Hellman, MD, a mom of a 15-year-old son, an associate clinical professor of dermatology at Mt. Sinai Hospital in New York City, and a dermatologist in private practice*

I try to shop on a budget for sure. I shop the clearance racks, and I'm usually not shopping for something specific. Instead, I browse and look for clothes that are reasonably priced. I find it best to shop and browse for clothes without my kids, in the morning or after lunch when stores aren't crowded.

You can also find really good deals at large warehouse stores, such as Costco. The selection isn't always as great as at clothing stores, but they sell designer clothes at a lower cost.

—*Antoinette Cheney, DO, a mom of a seven-year-old son and a six-year-old daughter and a family physician with Rocky Vista University College of Osteopathic Medicine, in Parker, CO*

FitBit

Just say no to skinny jeans. Instead, choose a pair of dark wash denim with plain pockets and no frills. Straight legs or a slight boot cut are best if you want to look thinner.

> **When in doubt, wear red.**
>
> *—Bill Blass, an American fashion designer*

I feel that it's important to dress like a woman. The body shape that's generally considered to be most beautiful—by both men and women—is one with a waist-to-hip ratio of 0.7. (To find this ratio, divide your hip measurement by your waist measurement.) Think Marilyn Monroe, not Twiggy. It's an hourglass look.

You want to emphasize your waistline, and not worry so much about the width of your hips. To do this, I pull my waist in by wearing belts or scarves. I wear A-line dresses and even skirts with pleats. Dresses with color blocking, with a bright color down the front and black half-moon shapes on the sides, are very slimming.

—Jennifer Hanes, DO, a mom of a seven-year-old daughter and a four-year-old son, an emergency physician who's board certified in integrative medicine, and the author of The Princess Plan: Shrink Your Waist, Expand Your Beauty, *in Austin, TX*

⁓

A few years ago, I made a change in my style: I went from wearing mainly jeans and flannel shirts to more skirts and dresses. One trick I learned is when I find a clothing combo that looks and feels good, I take a picture of myself with my phone! Then I save those photos in a folder on my phone, to refer to on days when I can't decide what to wear.

I also keep photos of my clothes on my phone, especially things that need matching items, such as a pair of pants that need a matching shirt. This way if I'm at a store and see something I think will match, I can check the photo on my phone. This helps me to avoid time-consuming trips back to stores to return things that didn't match!

—Deborah Gilboa, MD, a mom of 11-, 9-, 7-, and 5-year-old sons, a family physician with Squirrel Hill Health Center in Pittsburgh, PA, and a parenting speaker whose advice is found at AskDoctorG.com

I love clothes shopping, and I wish that I had more time to do it. A couple of times a year, or to congratulate myself for a big accomplishment, I splurge and buy a couple of beautiful items at my favorite stores, such as Anthropologie, Boden, and Banana Republic.

Most days, though, beautiful and fragile clothes are just not an option for my lifestyle nor my budget. My kids and my dog are messy, and I have to be comfortable and prepared for anything. I shop a lot at Old Navy and H&M. I love comfortable clothes that are soft and fit well, and if I could live in jeans, I would. When I buy a pair of jeans that I love, I wear them for five years until they literally fall apart.

I think the absolutely most important thing about feeling good in your clothes and shopping wisely is making sure that you buy clothes that fit and flatter your body shape. I find Gap Boot Cut jeans fit me well. I'm slim but hippy, so I need something that flatters curves.

—*Sigrid Payne DaVeiga, MD*

I'm thankful that tailored clothes are in style now, rather than the bloused craziness of the 1980s!

Mommy MD Guides–Recommended Product
Athleta Clothes

"Once you find a brand or style of clothing that works well for you, stick with it," says Heather Orman-Lubell, MD, a mom of 12- and 8-year-old sons and a pediatrician in private practice at Yardley Pediatrics of St. Christopher's Hospital for Children, in Pennsylvania. "My new secret is Athleta. The clothing is inexpensive, wears well, and fits great. I started buying their yoga clothing, but now I buy their casual clothes too. They've quickly become my go-to pieces."

You can buy Athleta clothes online at **ATHLETA.COM** or **AMAZON.COM** and in Athleta stores. Prices vary by style, but tops begin at around $25.

My secret to dressing well is using personal shoppers. Many large department stores have them, such as Macy's. It doesn't cost a thing; you just call ahead to make an appointment. It doesn't have to be for a special occasion; I've worked with a personal shopper just to add to my business casual work wardrobe. The personal shopper works with you to assess your budget, and she helps you select clothes and accessories that will look great on you.

I've met with personal shoppers about four times in my life. It's really helped me to learn what looks good on my body. You'll probably want to buy a few things to avoid seeming rude, but you don't have to buy everything! Once you learn some key style tips, you can apply them at other, less expensive stores. You can take notes in the dressing room or even snap a few pictures while you're there.

Also, I've begun shopping at a great resale boutique here in Cincinnati. I'm not spending a ton of money on clothes now, and it's quick—no mall traffic. If I need a pair of jeans, they're all on one large rack. I can find jeans from different designers, and all in my size. It's far better than trying on two pairs of jeans in one store, and then having to go somewhere else to try on another pair. At my height, I know I have an alteration fee in my future, so it also helps that the price of the garment is reduced. Our store carries some great designer fashions, but not all resale boutiques are created equal. You might have to try several before you find the one that offers the kind of clothes you like.

—*Amy Thompson, MD, a mom of six-, four-, and two-year-old sons and an ob-gyn at the University of Cincinnati College of Medicine, in Ohio*

⌒⌒

I prefer soft and comfortable clothing. If I like the way my clothes look and they feel good, it definitely improves my mood. I try not to wear anything that's too tight or binding—except Spanx now and then!

I used to hang on to clothes that were uncomfortable or didn't fit. Not anymore. I give them to Goodwill. If something doesn't feel good to wear, why keep it around? There are so many options for stylish, fun clothes that actually feel good that I don't think there's ever a need to be uncomfortable just for the sake of fashion.

"I need to wear comfortable heels," says Amy Barton, MD, a mom of an 11-year-old daughter and 8- and 5-year-old sons and a pediatrician at St. Luke's Children's Hospital, in Boise, ID. "The most comfortable ones I've found are Aerosoles. This company makes stylish heels that feel great, and they also last a long time."

You can buy Aerosoles at stores such as Target and Macy's and online retailers such as **AEROSOLES.COM** and **DSW.COM** for around $50. Visit **AEROSOLES.COM** for more information.

Along the same lines, I never wear really high heels. I'm on my feet all day, and I only wear low heels.

—*Michelle Spring, MD, a mom of a one-year-old son and two grown stepchildren and a board-certified plastic surgeon with Marina Plastic Surgery Associates, in Marina del Rey, CA*

As a general rule, I try never to wear sneakers outside of my house! To me, sneakers make me feel sloppy and slouchy. Instead, I wear pumps, or sandals in the summer, and that makes me feel feminine and confident. Then the outfit has to match the shoes, which means I dress up a little more. It is a great change from wearing scrubs.

—*Stephanie A. Wellington, MD*

I love shoes. One thing that has changed over the years is that I now wear more comfortable shoes than I once did. I've learned that the more comfortable I am, the more I relate in a positive way to everyone around me.

—*Debra Luftman, MD*

I found a great website for work shoes: Zappos.com. It has an entire section on "comfort." Because I'm 5 feet 3 inches tall, I need a little height, and I bought shoes with two-inch heels that are the most comfortable shoes ever.

—*Eva Mayer, MD*

In addition to the clothes I wear, I find that another really important thing is shoes! I love heels and tall boots, but my goodness, I cannot wear heels and be on my feet all day seeing patients or as a mom.

My favorite shoes that I cannot live without are my Dansko clogs. They come in many great colors and styles, but a good pair of brown and a pair of black patent leather are so great and versatile. I wear them all of the time.

—*Sigrid Payne DaVeiga, MD*

RALLIE'S TIP

When I need an outfit that makes me look respectable, I go to a wonderful little boutique in town and turn myself over to the fashion experts. I wouldn't dream of trying to go it alone! Before the fashionistas go to work, I tell them my clothing budget so that they don't get carried away.

I love seeing any woman dress in a style that is uniquely her own. It would be a shame if we all showed up to work wearing the exact same outfit. Where's the fun in that? It's far more interesting to see every woman express herself by wearing the kind of clothes and accessories that make her feel beautiful, comfortable, and confident.

The nurses I work with tell me I should be on the TV show *What Not to Wear*. I'm fortunate I work in pediatrics, and I can justify wearing clothes that can be bled on, peed on, and thrown up on—and never need to be dry-cleaned.

—*Amy Baxter, MD, a mom of 15- and 12-year-old sons and a 10-year-old daughter; the CEO of Buzzy4Shots.com; and the director of emergency research, Scottish Rite, of Children's Healthcare of Atlanta, in Georgia*

Mommy MD Guides–Recommended Product
Nordstrom

"In the past few years, I have switched from buying almost all of my clothes at a superstore while I shopped for groceries, to now shopping almost exclusively at Nordstrom," says Jennifer Hanes, DO, a mom of a seven-year-old daughter and a four-year-old son, an emergency physician who's board certified in integrative medicine, and the author of *The Princess Plan: Shrink Your Waist, Expand Your Beauty*, in Austin, TX. "Despite the amazing clothes, I'm spending less money than before. Here are my secrets to saving at Nordstrom."

The huge semi-annual sale. Every six months, Nordstrom has an end-of-season sale that is amazing. The first time I ever shopped there was during one of these sales. On that first visit, I purchased seven clothing items, including a pair of jeans and a dress. My total bill was less than $150. I recall that one of the tank tops was only $7.

The sale racks. The semi-annual sale is the only promoted sale by Nordstrom. However, at other times, there are racks with discounted items. I like to dig into these racks to find treasures. I love the Amber Sun brand of long-sleeved yoga T-shirt. This season, the shirts in fall colors were priced around $35. However, on the discounted rack, the shirts in spring colors were on sale for $13. So I picked up two jewel-tone shirts rather than the autumn-colored shirt.

Quality. This sounds simple, but it's so true. Nordstrom products stand up to the most grueling wear and tear because they're higher quality. As evidence of this, when I was first losing weight, I didn't want to spend a lot of money on bras that I planned to soon "out shrink." So, I bought two bras, one nude and one black. This was a less-than-ideal move when gearing up for the hot Texas summer, because most of my tops are light colored. The point is that I wore the tan bra nearly every day for almost a year, through the heat, the 24-hour hospital shifts, and playing outside. It withstood literally hundreds of washings before I was able to trade it in for a smaller size.

Personal stylist. Even without an appointment, you can shop with a personal stylist who will help you look your very best. She knows the clothing selection and which brands fit your body type best. For example, if you try on jeans but they're too big in the waist, your stylist will bring you other brands that are better suited to your shape. The service is free of charge. As a woman losing weight, I relied on Shari (my stylist extraordinaire) to help me understand the elements of a properly fitting skirt and dress. I had worn baggy clothes for so long, I had no idea how to shop for smaller sizes. The professional service of the stylist means you get clothes that fit your body and your life so your money is not wasted on ill-fitting merchandise.

Nordstrom rewards. They have an amazing rewards program that can be in the form of a credit card or associated with your debit account. With each purchase, you earn points that are then applied to Nordstrom Notes, a gift card to be used at the store. Depending upon how much you spend in a year, you can also earn special rewards such as free alterations. Alterations were new to me until I began shopping at Nordstrom. Getting pants hemmed to the perfect length can give an inexpensive pant a million-dollar look.

Planned purchases. When you buy clothes at a superstore, it's often an impulse buy. You toss a new hoodie or yoga pant into the cart—no need to try it on. Just walk by and grab. I now refrain from that kind of wasteful spending. At Nordstrom, I have developed a relationship with my stylist, and I can e-mail her a list of the items I need. This way, I stop the impulse buys and stick with the essentials.

Customer service. Nordstrom is world-famous for their outstanding customer service. They are very generous about allowing returns. I had worn and washed a blouse when I noticed a snag. They exchanged it at no charge, whereas at other stores, I would have been out the cost of a new blouse. That's definitely a money saver.

Caring for Your Skin and Smile

Good skin care is more than skin deep. How healthy your skin is affects how you look, how you feel about yourself, and how others perceive you. Taking good care of your skin can help you look and feel better—and younger too.

꩜

I always use sunscreen. Along with not smoking, it's the best thing you can do for anti-aging!
　　—*Michelle Spring, MD*

꩜

I wear sunscreen every single day, even in the winter. For a second layer of protection, I always buy makeup with sunblock built in.
　　—*Ayala Laufer-Cahana, MD, a mom of 17- and 15-year-old sons and a 14-year-old daughter, a pediatrician, and the founder of Herbal Water Inc., in Wynnewood, PA*

꩜

I always wear sunglasses. They protect my eyes, and they keep me from squinting, which helps to prevent crow's-feet!
　　—*Katherine Dee, MD*

Mommy MD Guides–Recommended Product
Neutrogena Healthy Skin Anti-Wrinkle Anti-Blemish Clear Skin Cream

"Since college, I've used Neutrogena Healthy Skin Anti-Wrinkle Anti-Blemish Clear Skin Cream with retinol and salicylic acid," says Sigrid Payne DaVeiga, MD, a mom of a seven-year-old son and a two-year-old daughter and a pediatric allergist with the Children's Hospital of Philadelphia, in Pennsylvania. "It helped clear up my acne back then and has worked well ever since. I like to stick with basic things."

You can buy Neutrogena Healthy Skin Anti-Wrinkle Anti-Blemish Clear Skin Cream at stores such as CVS and Target for around $14. Visit **NEUTROGENA.COM** for more information.

I take the time every few weeks to get my nails done. It makes my hands look great, and also it gives me a 45-minute block of time to get a break from everything!

—*Pam D'Amato, MD*

⌁

As we get older, we have to invest a bit more time, and probably even more money, to make our skin look great. When you're younger, you can cover up flaws more easily! But looking radiant and beautiful as you age is also a result of having a positive attitude throughout your life. If you spend your life furrowing your brow and frowning, those lines are going to become set in your face.

—*Eva Ritvo, MD*

⌁

It's important to pay attention to your skin. It will tell your age before anything else. Prevention is the key. Once you see the signs of aging, they're hard to reverse.

Even if your skin is oily, it needs plenty of moisture. Moisturizing your skin helps it to look rejuvenated and fresh. I moisturize my face, my hands, and the rest of my body.

I love Philosophy brand products. This line is awesome! I love the multipurpose cleansing pads, the Purity cleanser, and the Hope in a Jar moisturizer. I've tried more expensive brands, thinking that they'll be better. But they're not. You can buy Philosophy products online at Philosophy.com and in stores such as Ulta.

—*Christy Valentine, MD*

⌁

Because I'm in the cosmetic industry, my patients want to see my skin, not my makeup. I stay on track by washing my face every evening before heading to bed and by using a booster-packed serum to nourish my skin at night when it regenerates.

I use the serum from Blush Blends called Super Star Serum. It allows me to pick my own medical-grade boosters (my personal faves being: luminosity, skin tightening, and anti-redness), and then I choose my aromatherapy scent. (I love Rose for summer and Eucalyptus for winter.)

—*Arleen K. Lamba, MD*

"I've had acne my whole life," says Eva Mayer, MD, a mom of a nine-year-old daughter and an eight-year-old son, an associate professor of pediatrics at Temple University, and a pediatrician with St. Luke's Pediatrics Associates, in Bethlehem, PA. "The only product that has ever helped is Proactiv. I use the Proactiv 3-step system, which includes the Renewing Cleanser, Revitalizing Toner, and Repairing Treatment. I personalized my system by adding the Replenishing Eye Serum and the Refining Mask."

Priced at $19.95 per month for regular shipment members. To purchase, visit **PROACTIV.COM** or call 888-819-2019.

To have healthy skin, you just need a very simple skin care regimen. I use only three products each day. In the morning, I use a gentle exfoliating cleanser, such as Avene Creamy Cleanser. Then I put on a moisturizing sunblock, such as Skinceuticals Moisturizing Sunscreen. In the evening, I put on a product to address any skin care problems I have, such as acne or wrinkles. That's it!

—*Debra Luftman, MD*

My skin care secret is going to a skin care professional called an esthetician. Her husband, who is my colleague and friend, is a plastic surgeon. He removes the moles on my skin, and his wife gives me facials. She recommended a line of vitamin C–enriched skin care products, which work well for me.

—*Linda Brodsky, MD, a mom of a 30-year-old son and 28- and 25-year-old daughters, the president of WomenMDResources.com, a physician in private practice with Pediatric ENT Associates, and a retired professor of otolaryngology and pediatrics, in Buffalo, NY*

I had terrible acne when I was a kid. I went to see an esthetician, and she told me I needed to moisturize my skin.

"You've got to be kidding," I said. But she was right. I started moisturizing, and my skin cleared up.

A side benefit to all of that moisturizing is that even though I'm now pushing 40, I don't have any wrinkles! I moisturize my skin as soon as I step out of the shower each morning when my skin is still damp. I don't use an expensive moisturizer. I buy whatever's on sale at CVS!

—*Lisa Campanella-Coppo, MD, a mom of a three-year-old daughter and an emergency physician with EMCARE and the Meridian Health System, in Monmouth, NJ*

Mommy MD Guides-Recommended Product
BareEase

"I had both of my children without a single speck of pain medication, but send me in for a bikini wax, and I'm climbing the walls freaking out about how much it will hurt," confides Sigrid Payne DaVeiga, MD, a mom of a seven-year-old son and a two-year-old daughter and a pediatric allergist with the Children's Hospital of Philadelphia, in Pennsylvania. "I was thrilled to try BareEase. I applied it at home 30 minutes before my wax appointment as per the package instructions. It worked so well that I could actually tell where I forgot to apply it when my esthetician hit one of those spots! BareEase definitely made the entire experience much more bearable. I think I was actually able to breathe while I got a bikini wax, which has never happened before!

"Even for the rest of the day following the waxing, the area was much less tender and irritated than in the past. I would love it if my salon sold BareEase in case I forgot to apply it at home beforehand. My esthetician and I joked that she should tell her clients to come to the salon early for a glass of wine and their BareEase application. Then they might not even notice the bikini wax!"

You can buy BareEase at **DERMSTORE.COM** for $18. Visit **BAREEASE.COM** for more information.

I joined a spa, and I go there for regular massages and facials. This might seem like an extravagance, but it's really worth the cost. Just having some time to lie down in a quiet, dark room, while listening to soothing music, with no one making demands on me is incredibly relaxing and rejuvenating.

The facial itself is great for my skin, but that's just the icing on the cake.

—*Aline T. Tanios, MD*

The best ways to care for your skin are the same ways you care for yourself in general: Eat a balanced diet, get ample sleep and moderate exercise, have healthy relationships, and minimize stress.

Once you've managed those things the best you can, choose the best skin care products you can find. Generally, the products available on the mass market tend to be less effective than the ones sold at physicians' offices. They don't require a prescription; they're just sold in doctors' offices or spas. Many of these products (with the exception of those that are private label) have undergone scientific testing, while most mainstream products have been tested only through a consumer

Mommy MD Guides-Recommended Product
Nectifirm

"Many younger women ignore their necks and décolleté, until the skin becomes spotted, crepey, and wrinkled," says Michelle Yagoda, MD, a mom of an 11-year-old son, a facial plastic surgeon, the CEO of Opus Skincare, LLC, and cofounder of BeautyScoop, a patented and clinically proven supplement for skin, hair, and nails, in New York City. "Fortunately, there's a cream called Nectifirm by Revision Skin Care that's unrivaled. It firms, tightens, and soothes skin within weeks, and it is utterly addicting!"

You can buy Nectifirm in doctors' offices and online at **AMAZON.COM** for around $70 for 1.7 ounces.

> The beauty of a woman is not in a facial mode, but the true beauty in a woman is reflected in her soul. It is the caring that she lovingly gives, the passion that she shows. The beauty of a woman grows with the passing years.
>
> —*Audrey Hepburn*

advocacy program, which offers subjective comments that can be biased, paid positive results.

One example is a line of skin products called Gly-Derm. Sold in physicians' offices, it is a glycolic acid product line with the lowest pH on the market, making it arguably the most effective.

—*Michelle Yagoda, MD, a mom of an 11-year-old son, a facial plastic surgeon, the CEO of Opus Skincare, LLC, and cofounder of BeautyScoop, a patented and clinically proven supplement for skin, hair, and nails, in New York City*

RALLIE'S TIP

I'm outside in the sun, wind, and rain as often as I can be. I love the outdoors! I live on a small horse farm, and that requires me to be outside to feed, water, and work with my animals every day.

I've been fortunate to know lots of old cowboys and horse trainers in my life, and I've seen what the great outdoors can do to unprotected skin. Lines and wrinkles look okay on the Marlboro man, but I never aspired to have that leathery, weathered look. Before I step foot outside in the morning, regardless of the weather or the season, I put sunscreen on my face and neck, and any other areas of my body that will be exposed to the elements. Then I put on makeup. My horses really don't care a bit if I'm all dolled up, and they probably don't even notice, but I always feel frumpy without makeup, and I also know that those extra layers protect my skin from the sun.

I always wear a baseball cap when I'm outside. The cap protects my hair and scalp, and the visor protects my face, neck, and eyes from the sun. If it's the least bit sunny outside, I wear sunglasses, to avoid getting crow's-feet and also to help prevent the development of cataracts on my eyes.

Kentucky summers are hot and sunny, but I still try to wear long-sleeve, lightweight, sun-protective shirts whenever possible. They make me sweat a little more than short-sleeve shirts or tank tops, but I like knowing that I'm taking care of my skin, and I also like sweating, because it makes me feel like I'm losing weight in the process!

I want my smile to look good, so I rinse with Listerine with peroxide twice a day. I don't drink coffee or too much red wine. The rinse doesn't make your teeth really white, but it removes some of the stains as long as you keep using it.

—*Linda Brodsky, MD*

Mommy MD Guides–Recommended Product
Neutrogena Microdermabrasion System

"I received a Neutrogena Microdermabrasion System as a gift," says Lisa Campanella-Coppo, MD, a mom of a three-year-old daughter and an emergency physician with EMCARE and the Meridian Health System, in Monmouth, NJ. "It's awesome! I use it every week, and it really helps my skin look great."

The Microdermabrasion System is a simple, convenient at-home system that features single-use puffs and the microderm-abrasion applicator. Each puff is pre-dosed with ultra-fine crystals and mild purifiers for the perfect degree of gentle exfoliation. What's more, the massaging micro-vibrations boost surface cell turnover for firmer, younger-looking skin.

You can buy a Neutrogena Microdermabrasian kit at stores such as Walmart and Target for $16. Visit **NEUTROGENA.COM** for more information.

A surprising way to care for your skin that will also help with your weight is to manage stress! Uncontrolled stress can make your skin more sensitive and trigger acne breakouts and other skin problems. To promote healthy skin, try to stress less. Set reasonable limits, scale back your to-do list, and make time to do the things you enjoy. The results—to your skin and your size—might be more dramatic than you expect.

I whiten my teeth at home. I got a custom-molded tray from my dentist as part of the Opalescence whitening system. I use it once or twice a year. You put a tiny drop of gel in each tooth of the tray and wear it. It fits so well that it is not uncomfortable, and it's not difficult to talk. My dentist recommended that I use the gel for about 30 to 45 minutes at a time, twice a day for about a week. But I find that it has a noticeable effect after just a few days. If a special occasion is coming up, I might do a touch-up, and it works great. The custom tray itself costs about $300, but some dentists offer discounts for their patients. $35 worth of the gel lasts me about a year.

I find the Opalescence system much easier to use and less messy than over-the-counter whitening strips. Having whiter teeth boosts my confidence.

—*Tiemdow Phumiruk, MD*

Choosing Makeup

More than 80 percent of women wear makeup. On average, women spend 20 minutes a day putting on makeup. Women without kids must be spending a lot more time to make up for moms who have about 48 seconds each day to spend on it!

୧⁄૭

In terms of makeup, I always make sure to look put together. I can do my hair and makeup for work in about 15 minutes. If I have a TV appearance, it usually takes me about 40 minutes. I always do my hair and makeup the same systematic way—that's the surgeon in me—so I don't waste any time.

—*Catherine Begovic, MD, a mom of a six-month-old daughter and a plastic surgeon at Make You Perfect, Inc., in Beverly Hills, CA*

❧

I'm a true believer that a good lipstick can do wonders. No matter how much I paid for it, I ditch any lipstick that doesn't make me feel good!

—*Jennifer A. Gardner, MD, a mom of a three-year-old son, a pediatrician, and the founder of an online child wellness and weight management company, HealthyKidsCompany.com, in Washington, DC*

❧

I don't wear much makeup. I'm hoping this will help keep my skin looking younger, longer. I wear eyeliner and lipstick but not much more makeup than that. I might put on eye shadow and other makeup to go to a Christmas party!

I choose dark black and navy eyeliner that goes with my complexion. I find that lipstick really brightens my face. I buy lipsticks in more subtle tones that go with my skin tone.

—*Leena Shrivastava Dev, MD, a mom of 15- and 12-year-old sons and a general pediatrician and advocate for child safety, in the Baltimore, MD, area*

❧

I do what I call the "Five-Minute Face." I put on clear mascara, tinted lip gloss, and moisturizer or foundation, and I'm done—out the door.

I like Philosophy makeup. It makes your face look like it's been airbrushed. It's not chalky, and it doesn't rub off. That's important in my job because I'm hugging kids all day. I don't want my makeup to rub off onto their clothes.

—*Michelle Davis-Dash, MD, a mom of a 19-month-old son and a pediatrician in Baltimore, MD*

My makeup is always very light. I use a loose powder to even out my skin tone and take away any shine I might have on my face. I like Maybelline New York ShineFree Loose Powder. I also wear blush, eye shadow, black mascara, and lip gloss. I use eyeliner to spruce up for special occasions. I like makeup that's easy to put on, and also easy to take off. That's a time and money saver!

—*Sigrid Payne DaVeiga, MD*

My sister is getting married, and we went to a department store to have our makeup done before a party. It was fun! I really paid attention to how the salesperson did my makeup. I learned a few tips, such as putting eyeliner on the upper lid to bring out my eyes and using powder to get an airbrushed look. Of course, as soon as I got out of the saleslady's sight, I took off about half of the makeup. Those salesladies put way too much makeup on!

—*Martha Wittenberg, MD, MPH, a mom of an eight-year-old son and a six-year-old daughter and a family physician with Seal Beach Family Medicine, in California*

Mommy MD Guides-Recommended Product
Colorescience

"I love the Colorescience line, especially the line tamer and primer," says Michelle Spring, MD, a mom of a one-year-old son and two grown stepchildren and a board-certified plastic surgeon with Marina Plastic Surgery Associates, in Marina del Rey, CA. "I mix them together. One is a bronzer, and the other helps reduce redness. They both have SPF 20. I use this as a base and then apply other makeup. It really evens out my skin tone and also protects my skin."

You can buy Colorescience makeup products at online retailers such as **DERMSTORE.COM** and **LOVELYSKIN.COM**. Prices start at around $14. Visit **COLORESCIENCE.COM** for more information.

> **The most beautiful makeup of a woman is passion.**
> **But cosmetics are easier to buy.**
> —*Yves St. Laurent, a French fashion designer*

I think that beauty comes from the inside out. I don't feel that you need to do as much on the outside if the inside is healthy and whole.

I'm pretty simple with my makeup. I use a German brand called Dr. Hauschka. It's biodynamic and homeopathic.

You can buy Dr. Hauschka makeup at Whole Foods and some health food stores for around $23. Visit DrHauschka.com for more information.

—*Kay Corpus, MD*

If you invest more time in taking care of your face—your "canvas"—makeup will bring out your beauty and it won't be needed to cover up your "flaws."

My work week makeup "musts" include mascara and a great under-eye concealer. Because I have a newborn, sleep is hard to come by, so I have found creative ways to look fresh-faced. This is where a good regimen with an eye cream can do wonders for you—along with some mascara.

To give my face some color and glow, I put on a blush. (My favorite is Nars Orgasm. You can buy it at Bloomingdales and Saks Fifth Avenue for around $29. Visit Narscosmetics.com for more information.) I put on a colored lip balm or a long-lasting lip lacquer because I don't have time to reapply it throughout the day.

My makeup routine is simple and basic, but it packs a punch on those busy weekdays as I'm rushing to get out of the house in the mornings! And I don't look inappropriate at the office with caked-on makeup.

—*Arleen K. Lamba, MD*

I'm not a makeup person. I wear a little mascara, and that's it!
—*Christy Valentine, MD*

I don't wear makeup every day—only for special occasions or TV appearances. I save a lot of time each day by not putting on, nor taking off, makeup.
—*Deborah Gilboa, MD*

RALLIE'S TIP

I'm always on the lookout for the perfect makeup that's going to make me look at least 10 years younger and at least 10 percent more beautiful, so I'll try a new brand a couple of times a year. Usually it doesn't bring about a dramatic improvement, so I keep going back to my favorite brand, which I've used for years and can apply in my sleep with one hand tied behind my back. To me, the most important factor in a foundation makeup is the SPF. If it doesn't have an SPF of at least 50, I won't buy it.

Maximizing Your Hairstyle

Some things in life are universal, but this isn't one we'd have guessed. An incredible 91 percent of women say they have "serious issues" with their hair, according to a Pantene survey. Frizzy hair was the biggest complaint, followed by "boring" hair. When women were asked which they'd rather have, great hair for life or to boost their IQ by 10 points, more than half chose great hair. Clearly a bad hair day is a big deal.

FitBit

Face-slimming makeup? You bet! Try to plump up your lips. If your lips look small, the rest of your face looks larger by comparison. The best way to beef up your mouth is to dab a shimmery gloss in the middle of your lower lip—on top of a lip-tone lipstick or gloss.

I like the convenience of short hair, but not the look of it. So I wear my hair long enough that I can pull it back in a way that I like.

—*Deborah Gilboa, MD*

When my older son was two years old, I had my hair cut really short. I loved it. I could jump out of the shower, and my hair was ready to go. It just air-dried.

But on the flip side, my hairstyle was always the same. So about a year ago, I asked my hairdresser to help me grow it out. Now it's about shoulder-length, so I have more options. I can wear it down or pulled back into a ponytail with a cinch. That looks very neat and pulled together.

—*Heather Orman-Lubell, MD*

I think all women should have dry shampoo in their bathrooms. I use it when I don't have the time to wash and dry my hair. I know it sounds old-fashioned, but I think dry shampoo is making a comeback! I find that it helps to lift my hair when I can't wash it. It works quickly and effectively.

—*Edna Ma, MD*

To keep my hair looking great, I try to eat very well. I eat a lot of nuts, dairy, and protein foods, which are important for hair growth.

I use sulfate-free shampoos. I have long hair, and I often wear it in a ponytail. This helps keep my hair off my face, which reduces breakouts. I see a lot of patients with acne on their faces caused by oily hair.

—*Debra Luftman, MD*

Having good hair really does help you feel good about yourself. Rollers are a girl's best friend. I often don't have time to fix my hair, so I put it in rollers as I get ready for work. I use both regular dry rollers and hot rollers. The hot rollers are best if you don't have a lot of time: Just roll them in, wait 10 minutes, and voilà!

—*Michelle Davis-Dash, MD*

Early on in life, I realized the value of paying more for a haircut that didn't require me to spend a lot of time styling it on a daily basis. For most of my life, I've never even owned a hair dryer! I have my hair cut short and in a style that falls right into place.

—*Amy Baxter, MD*

I make a hair appointment *before* I really need it. You can never feel your best with bad hair!

My hair is very straight and fine, so I like to use large hot rollers to give it extra body.

When I want my hair to have even more body, I skip applying conditioner, which weighs down fine hair. Instead, I brush out any tangles, and then I wash my hair, gently towel it dry, and brush.

—*Jennifer A. Gardner, MD*

It's very helpful to have a good hairstylist whose opinion you can trust. I asked my stylist to let me know when it was time to start coloring my hair. I used to just put a semipermanent gloss on it,

Mommy MD Guides-Recommended Product
Wen

"I found that after my kids were born, the texture of my hair changed," says Eva Mayer, MD, a mom of a nine-year-old daughter and an eight-year-old son, an associate professor of pediatrics at Temple University, and a pediatrician with St. Luke's Pediatrics Associates, in Bethlehem, PA. "It became more brittle and frizzy. I discovered a great product called Wen Lavender Daily Cleansing Conditioner. I use it as a leave-in conditioner, and it keeps my hair from frizzing."

You can buy Wen hair care products at online retailers such as **QVC.COM** and **AMAZON.COM** for around $40. Visit **WENHAIRCARE.COM** for more information.

> **Some of the worst mistakes in my life were haircuts.**
>
> **—Jim Morrison,**
> *an American singer, songwriter, and poet*

which concealed a little bit of gray with highlights.

As requested, my hairdresser let me know when I needed to actually dye it. "It's time," she said.

I'm fighting that part of aging well. I'm still in denial about needing reading glasses though.

—*Heather Orman-Lubell, MD*

One thing I splurge on is my hair. When my hair looks great, I feel great about myself. I shopped around a bunch of salons until I found a stylist who really understood my hair and knew the best way to cut it.

I get my hair cut every six weeks. I find if I try to push it longer than that, it takes me extra time to style it in the morning and just isn't worth the trouble.

My stylist also puts in highlights. It's nothing drastic, just the sort of color I would get as a kid when I spent a lot of time outdoors. As we age, our hair color can fade. Highlights brighten it back up and help me look and feel younger.

—*Allison Bailey, MD, a mom of a nine-year-old son and a*
five-year-old daughter and founder and director of Integrated
Health and Fitness Associates, in Cambridge, MA

I have fair skin, and I had very dark hair. But I always wanted to be a blonde. Other women said, "No way." But men said, "Go for it!"

The men were right! I started with blonde highlights, and over time I went blonder and blonder. My hair looks better, and I have far more fun as a blonde!

Don't limit your ideas and avoid limiting people. If you want to change your hair, do it!

—*Marie Dam, MD*

I have an easy—and fun—way to style my hair. After I get out of the shower, while I dress and put makeup on, I have a fan blowing on me. It dries my hair slowly and naturally, without overdrying it like a blow-dryer. Plus, I live in Texas, where it's hot, so the fan feels good.

—*Jennifer Hanes, DO*

∽⌒⊙

I have a lot of very wavy hair, which has always been difficult for me to take care of. We currently live in Colorado, and it's a lot drier here than in New York where I grew up. I now only wash my hair every three days or so. (I do bathe daily.) After I wash my hair, I put it up into a twist, and it looks really great the next few days. I don't use any products in my hair other than shampoo or conditioner. I don't blow-dry it anymore either because that really dries it out.

—*Stacey Ann Weiland, MD, a mom of a 14-year-old daughter and 9- and 7-year-old sons and an internist/gastroenterologist, in Denver, CO*

Mommy MD Guides-Recommended Product
Aveda

"I like Aveda hair products, especially the Color Conserve Shampoo and Strengthening Treatment," says Sigrid Payne DaVeiga, MD, a mom of a seven-year-old son and a two-year-old daughter and a pediatric allergist with the Children's Hospital of Philadelphia, in Pennsylvania. "I go to the salon to have my hair dyed. The graying happened more quickly than I would like to admit. I have started to have my hair highlighted about once every six weeks in the past couple of years. My son used to say, 'You don't have any grays, Mom!' Now when I leave for my hair appointment, my son is quick to point out, 'Oh yeah, I can see you have a little gray hair right there.' "

You can buy Aveda Color Conserve Shampoo and Strengthening Treatment at stores such as Aveda and Nordstrom for around $18. Visit **AVEDA.COM** for more information.

I've learned it's best to work with your natural hair type, rather than against it. You should accept who you are. I have naturally curly hair, and I've always had haircuts that allow me to wash it and go. My hair pretty much looks the same all of the time. I never have a bad hair day unless I've slept on it for three weeks without a shower.

Since I had a bout with cancer, I've stopped dying my hair. I'm fine with the gray. First, I'm not 40 anymore, and I don't want to try to look like someone I'm not. Second, the chemotherapy really damaged my hair, and I don't want to put any more chemicals on it.

My husband always says, "I love you for who you are. You don't need another color hair. It won't make you a nicer, better, or smarter person."

—*Hana R. Solomon, MD*

Mommy MD Guides–Recommended Product
Nioxin

"After my daughter was born, I noticed that I had a lot of hair loss," says Shilpa Amin-Shah, MD, a mom of a three-year-old son and a two-year-old daughter and an emergency physician and director of the recruiting team at Emergency Medical Associates, in Livingston, NJ. "It lasted for about three months, and it was very difficult for me. I started to take a vitamin B complex supplement, and that really helped.

"Also, I started to use a thickening shampoo with conditioner called Nioxin. The company also sells a thickening hairspray, which you spray onto your hair before you blow-dry it. It gives my hair fullness and a lot of bounce."

You can buy Nioxin hair loss treatment at online stores such as **AMAZON.COM** and **WALGREENS.COM** for around $35. Visit **NIOXIN.COM** for more information.

🍎FitBit

Drop a few pounds at the salon! Adding a splash of color to just about anything is always a good thing, and your hair is no exception. (Within reason: We're not talking about hot pink or teal highlights here!) Adding some subtle, natural highlights will flatter any face.

I'm pretty low maintenance, especially when it comes to my hairstyle. The key for me is to keep it simple so I can get out the door on time in the morning. I don't wash my hair every day because I find that this way my hair has more lift and body.

One product I love is my Instyler rotating hot iron/brush. (I use the big roller.) It has literally revolutionized the way I style my hair. I spent my entire adult life frustrated with my wavy-frizzy hair and could never figure out how to straighten it, even after stylists gave me pointers and tricks that I could never replicate. This product tames the frizzies, and I actually feel like I can get "grown-up" hair! It works better for me on slightly dirty hair.

—*Michelle Spring, MD*

RALLIE'S TIP

One of my favorite beauty products is Clairol Nice 'N Easy Root Touch-Up. I started going gray far too early in life, at the tender age of 38. I attribute my premature graying to the stress of medical school and having two babies in two years while my oldest son was a wild and rebellious teenager during my medical residency.

I love having my hair colored by my hairdresser, but sometimes it's hard for me to make it to her salon every six weeks on the dot when I'm busy with work and family. If I don't get to my hairdresser on time, the gray roots start to show, and that makes me feel older than my years. Plus, I don't want anyone to know that I have gray hair!

I can apply this product with the little blue brush included in the package in less than five minutes and let it work while I clean the

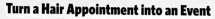
bathroom or put a load of laundry in the washer. Then I just rinse it out and voilà! No more gray roots!

Next to being quick and easy, the best thing about this product is that it's nearly impossible to tell that you've used it. I've used three or four different shades of brown at one time or another, and they have all blended in beautifully with my "natural" hair color. Even my hairdresser can't always tell when I've used it. I told the nurses in my office about this, and they were delighted to learn about it because they have just as much trouble getting to the hairdresser as I do. One of my nurses went out and bought a box on her lunch break so that she could cover her gray "skunk stripe" that evening.

You can buy Clairol Nice 'N Easy Root Touch-Up at drug stores, supermarkets, Target, Walmart, Kmart, and Ulta for around $5 to $7. It's available in 18 shades. Visit Clairol.com for more information.

Accessorizing

Mark Twain once said, "Clothes make the man." Perhaps, but accessories make the *woman*. Make your accessories help, not hinder, your weight loss efforts! Try these slimming styles.

- A long necklace strand that hits just below the bust makes you look taller and leaner.
- Pendant earrings look best on a round or square face.

Studs, buttons, or short drop earrings offset a long or oval face. Hoops? Always a flattering choice.

• Narrow ringbands or ring styles that extend toward the knuckle make your digits appear longer—and thinner.

ᘓ∕◎

Wearing too many accessories can be distracting. I have a few favorite necklaces, and I wear one almost every day. They're pretty, and they dress up an outfit, but they're not too much for work or home.

—*Tiemdow Phumiruk, MD*

ᘓ∕◎

I like to read fashion magazines, such as *Lucky*. I've picked up a lot of great ideas for clothes and accessories. You don't have to spend a lot of money to have a great wardrobe. TJ Maxx and Loehmann's have the same brands as department stores. I also shop at Piperlime.com in the "girl on a budget" section. I like to mix and match cute inexpensive tops with heels and nice jeans or a pencil skirt. Then I use accessories to dress it up or down, depending on where I am going.

—*Martha Wittenberg, MD, MPH*

ᘓ∕◎

I don't have a lot of time, or patience, to fuss with my clothes, so my style is quite simple. But to jazz up my look, I always choose one unexpected accessory. I love to buy unique, artisanal handbags and jewelry when I travel. Those accessories are unique and special, and they also remind me of a wonderful trip. Plus, they're handmade, not mass produced, and they make me feel connected to the art world.

—*Ayala Laufer-Cahana, MD*

ᘓ∕◎

No matter how busy I am, I always have time to accessorize! I wear makeup only on special occasions, but I can't leave my house without accessories. Otherwise I feel boring and flat.

I usually wear earrings, a pendant or necklace, bracelets, a watch, rings, and a scarf or belt. I'm a big fan of belts because they dress up an outfit, and they also cinch and flatter my waist. Even when I have to wear scrubs, I accessorize with fun, colorful socks.

—*Aline T. Tanios, MD*

> **Give a girl the right pair of shoes,**
> **and she'll conquer the world.**
> **—*Marilyn Monroe***

I have learned that my accessories—such as earrings, necklaces, and belts—are really what tie my outfits together. When I try clothes on at the store, I always try to grab a few accessories such as a belt, even if I don't particularly like it, to see how it might look. Often I'm so surprised that I will buy the belt and put the clothing item back. You really have to try things on—both clothes and accessories—because they look differ-ent on than you might imagine. Give yourself permission to try some-thing you ordinarily wouldn't. You might surprise yourself! And don't forget about shoes as well. They set the whole tone of the outfit.

—*Marie Dam, MD*

I wear many hats. Literally. I own about 20 of them. I think I have more hats than shoes.

As an Orthodox Jewish woman, part of my religion is to cover my hair. And so I always wear a hat. I think it's a great idea to adopt some sort of style feature like that. Hats have become my signature style.

—*Susan Besser, MD, a mom of six grown children, ages 28, 26, 24, 22, 21, and 19, a grandmom of two, a family physician, and the medical director of Doctors Express-Memphis, in Tennessee*

I have a very simple style of dress. I don't have a lot of clothes. I buy a few good pieces, and I wear them often. Some last for decades. I keep my jewelry simple and wear my signature pieces. For example, I have a necklace that I helped design. It was made from some emeralds that my husband gave to me as earrings and a diamond from my mother, set in gold from the ring that held the diamond. I wear it every day and get lots of compliments.

—*Linda Brodsky, MD*

I have worn glasses since I was in kindergarten. I actually consider glasses a necessity but not an accessory. I don't have lots of glasses—just one pair—but I did make sure (with my daughter's help) that they are a flattering and neutral style.

Because my glasses are so critical to my looks, I always take my daughter with me to pick them out. She has a good sense of style, and she helps me to pick out the best frames for my face.

—*Susan Besser, MD*

RALLIE'S TIP

Fortunately, it's really easy to accessorize casual clothes! I can usually manage to keep up with one pair of earrings and a necklace at any given time. I love wearing simple silver hoop earrings and a simple silver chain with a charm in the shape of a horse's head made by a jeweler I love. I've always admired women who wear beautiful, interesting, elaborate jewelry, but I just can't seem to carry it off. In the end, I think the most

Mommy MD Guides-Recommended Product
PonyUP! Kentucky Handbags

You've been working so hard buying, organizing, and cleaning your child's clothing and shoes for years now. It's a great time to treat yourself to something, such as a new outfit, pair of shoes, or a handbag.

We love PonyUP! Kentucky handbags, which are unique, fun, and hardworking, just like you! These beautiful, high-quality handbags are made in the United States, and 100 percent of profits are donated to help horses in need.

PonyUP! Kentucky handbags are perfect for the mom who needs to carry all of her stuff, her kids' stuff, and likely her husband's stuff too. They come in beautiful, durable fabrics and genuine leather.

PonyUP! Kentucky hobo handbags start at $125. For more information, visit **PONYUPKENTUCKY.COM**.

important thing about the accessories you choose is how they make you feel when you wear them. The ones I choose always end up being simple and straightforward—which is probably a good reflection of my style and my personality.

Organizing Your Closet and Supplies

Do the words "organized closet" sound like an oxymoron to you? Maybe you need some justification for organization. According to the super-organized minds at ClosetMaid, most people wear 20 percent of their clothing 80 percent of the time. With some organization, you might wear more of the clothing you've bought with your hard-earned money.

Plus, some of those "80 percent" items could probably vacate your closet entirely, freeing up space for new "20 percent" items. Check out the donation value guide at http://www.goodwill.org/wp-content/uploads/2010/12/Donation_Valuation_Guide.pdf. (Click on "our donation value guide.") Who knew a suit that's gathering dust in your closet could be worth $30?

∽⌒∾

My body changed so much during my pregnancies, and after my two babies were born, that I had amassed a ton of clothing. I had a few years between the births of my two kids, and I think I held onto my maternity clothes, my pre-pregnancy clothes, and my post-pregnancy clothes because I just sort of felt like I never knew what state my body was going to be in. I wasn't wearing 70 percent of the clothes hanging in my closet, and if I tried to get dressed in something I hadn't worn in a while, I would hate it, and I would hate how I felt in it.

I started trying on everything in my closet that I hadn't worn in more than two years and also the clothes that I didn't like but had kept as "just-in-case" items. I put the clothes into two piles: one to donate and one to consign. I called a charity called Purple Heart and asked them to pick up several bags of old clothes. Having an emptier closet actually feels great! Now I know that when I pull clothes out, they'll fit and that will make me feel good.

—*Sigrid Payne DaVeiga, MD*

༻✿༺

I'm a very efficient and decisive person. I guess that's the surgeon part of me. When I need to get dressed, I pick an outfit quickly, and I stick with it. I don't change my mind and my outfit 10 times.

It helps that my closet is very organized. Work clothes are on one side of my closet, and everyday clothes are on another side. I have a giant section for workout clothes, and another section for dresses. Everything is color coordinated to allow me to find whatever I need quickly. Because I'm usually in surgery during the week, I wear scrubs most of the time. That makes choosing what to wear easy!

—*Catherine Begovic, MD*

༻✿༺

Doesn't everyone have an organizer on retainer? Seriously, I have ADD, and I'm a disaster at this stuff. As a woman married to a neatnik with OCD, I pay people to keep me organized, and their fees are far

> **Don't agonize, *organize*.**
>
> —*Florynce R. Kennedy,*
> *an American lawyer, activist, civil rights advocate, and feminist*

FitBit

Is there a connection between organizing, losing weight, and feeling great? You bet! Good organization and good health go hand in hand. Take the time to clean out your closets, and you'll free up time and brainpower to have more time to eat right and exercise more.

If it feels too daunting to take on your whole closet at once, break it up into smaller tasks, such as cleaning out one drawer or shelf at a time. Group similar things together, and put things where you'd look for them.

Carefully evaluate every item in your closet. If you don't use it, don't need it, don't love it, get rid of it. When you've identified items you can get rid of, take them away immediately, such as to a clothing donation box, so they don't creep back into your closet.

After you've met each goal, such as cleaning out a drawer, be sure to reward yourself for a job well done!

less expensive than couples therapy. Fortunately, I live in Berkeley, CA, so I don't have a lot of makeup or clothes to organize. Whenever my beloved and extremely hip sister visits, she is stunned by the lack of beauty products and clothing, and she tries to bring me into the current century. She asks hilarious questions, such as: "Um, Sara, when exactly did you buy those jeans?" I'll smile sheepishly and say in my weird, passive-aggressive voice, "I dunno. Maybe five years ago. Aren't they size 7, and don't they make my butt look small?" Yeah, let's just call that a work in progress!

—*Sara Gottfried, MD, a mom of 13- and 8-year-old daughters, a board-certified gynecologist, and the author of* The Hormone Cure, *in Berkeley, CA*

It's important to clean your beauty tools. I wash my hair brushes and makeup brushes once a week.

Also, I only use makeup brushes for about six months. Using disposable ones is even better for your skin.

It's also important to avoid storing your razor in the shower. It can get rusty and cause you to get folliculitis, which is an inflammation around a hair follicle. I usually use a razor only once, then throw it away.

—*Debra Luftman, MD*

RALLIE'S TIP

Organizing? My closet and bathroom cabinets? Surely, you jest!?!

Index

Note: <u>Underlined</u> references indicate boxed text.

A

Accessories, fashion, 395, 414, 440–44

Acne, <u>422</u>, 424, <u>424</u>, <u>429</u>, 434

Adaptogens, as mood booster, 356

Adrenal burnout, 274–75

Aerobic exercise. *See also* Cardio training

    health benefits of, 154

    recommended amount of, 84

    target heart rate zone for, 154, 158, <u>158</u>

    teaching, 91–92

    types of, 97, 154

Aerosoles, <u>418</u>

Age, self-esteem and, 379, 381

Aging

    cognitive health and, 357

    weight gain and, 112, 113, 159

    weight maintenance and, 228

Alcohol, 71, 76, <u>76</u>, 83, 340

Alzheimer's disease, <u>213</u>, <u>294</u>, <u>321</u>

Amazon, shopping from, 333–34

Amin-Shah, Shilpa, 17, <u>55</u>, 56, 93, <u>98</u>, 227–28, 263, 277, 286, 361, 412, <u>438</u>

Anemia, 268

Antibiotics, <u>213</u>, <u>301</u>

Antidepressant medications, 262, 349, 355, 362

Anti-inflammatory diet, 60

Apple body shape, 135

Apples, health benefits of, <u>186</u>

Apple sandwich snack, 234

Apps

    for food and exercise tracking, <u>11</u>, <u>38–39</u>, 84, 233

    hypnosis, <u>34</u>

    journaling, <u>49</u>

    for keeping to-do lists, 287–88

    on nutrient content of foods, 149

    for weight tracking, 9

    Weight Watchers, <u>40</u>

Arc Trainer, <u>96</u>

Arnold, Jennifer, i

Arnold Sandwich Thins Rolls, <u>59</u>

Aromatherapy, 280, 283, 287

Artichoke Hearts and Sun-Dried Tomatoes, Chicken with, 208

Artificial sweeteners, 103, 275

Ashwagandha, for better sleep, 285

Asian dishes, 63–64

Asprey, Dave, 294

Asthma, preventing, <u>197</u>

Atherosclerosis, preventing, <u>197</u>

Athleta Clothes, <u>416</u>

Au Bon Pain, <u>63</u>

Aunt Joy's Curried Chicken Salad, 305

Aveda Color Conserve Shampoo and
Strengthening Treatment, <u>437</u>
Avene Creamy Cleanser, 424
Avocado snack, 234

B

Back support, Belly Bandit for, <u>122</u>
Bailey, Allison, 15, <u>40</u>, 60–61, 98–99,
203, 246, 258–59, <u>259</u>, 265–66,
436
Balance, as esteem booster, 383, 384
Balance ball, situps on, 88
BareEase, <u>425</u>
Barefoot time outdoors, as energy
booster, 282–83
Barton, Amy, 30–31, 75, 84–85, 110,
258, 335, 347, 351–52, 386, <u>418</u>
Baths, 250, 251, 277, 286, 287, 387
Baxter, Amy, 5, <u>11</u>, 46–47, 54, 55,
71–72, 106–7, 123, 224, 246,
281–82, 383–84, 419, 435
Beans, protein in, 141, 142
Beauty, 359, 369, 375, 385, 389
Beef, as protein source, <u>179</u>
Beer, calories in, <u>76</u>
Begovic, Catherine, 32–33, 70–71,
106, 119, 123, 336–37, 382–83,
429–30, 445
Belly Bandit, <u>122</u>
Belts, 412, 415, 441, 442
Benson, Melba W., 370
Berger, Elizabeth, 226, 270, 287, 346,
363–64, 393, 408–10
Berna, Judy, i–ii
Besser, Susan, 69–70, 120, 128, 233,
279, 352, 365, 390, 442, 443
Biking, 89, 90, 95
Bikini waxing, <u>425</u>
Bikram yoga, 85
Billy Blanks DVDs, <u>92</u>
Bipolar disorder, 325
Bird-watching, 278
Birthday cake, 66–68

Black Bean "Lasagna," 203
Blogs, 280
fashion and makeup, <u>404</u>, 413
JudeOnFood.com, 206, 210, 304, 322
Blood pressure reduction, with
dark chocolate, <u>65</u>
exercise, 154
omega-3 fatty acids, <u>307</u>
potassium, <u>297</u>
weight loss, 3, <u>111</u>, 135
Blood sugar
artificial sweeteners and, 103
foods raising, 80, <u>131</u>, 137, 138
low, effects of, 137, 257, 350
regulating, with
breakfast, 230
cinnamon, 100
complex carbohydrates, 139, 141
exercise, 31, 154
fiber, <u>302</u>
olive oil, <u>299</u>
protein, 141, <u>281</u>
psyllium, 102
weight loss, 3, <u>111</u>
Blueberry Crumble, 217
Blueberry-Zucchini Muffins, 322–23
Blush Blends Super Star Serum, 423
BMI. *See* Body Mass Index
Body changes, with pregnancy, 18,
120, 374, 375, 383, 444–45
Body fat
from high insulin levels, 137–38
location of, health risks and, 135
strength training reducing, 159
Body image, self-esteem and, <u>372</u>,
374–76, 377, 381, 382–83
Body Mass Index (BMI)
acceptable range of, 6, 7, 10–12, 13
clinical programs for lowering, <u>39</u>
determining, 6, <u>6–7</u>, 134, <u>134</u>
fast food increasing, 114
interpreting, <u>7</u>, <u>134</u>
purpose of, 133–34

Stationary bike, 90
Strawberry-Yogurt Pudding, 215
Strength, weight loss improving, 4
Strength training, 84, 91, 95, 158–59
Stress
 adrenal burnout from, 274–75
 as energy buster, 270
 from financial worries, 344–45
 overeating from, 129, 140, 161, 348
 as sign of energy levels, 240
 weight gain from, 44, 129, 161
 as weight loss challenge, 121
 When to Call Your Doctor about,
  339
Stress reduction
 for better skin, 426, 429
 methods of, 338–45
  deep breathing, 362–63
  exercise, 270
  hypnosis, 34
  journaling, 49
  yoga, 85, 93
 Natural Calm for, 341
String Beans, Roasted French, with
  Toasted Sesame Seeds, 312
Strokes
 preventing, 54, 297, 299
 risk factors for, 3, 134, 135, 239
Stuffed Peppers, 210–11
Style assessment quiz, 396–403
Subway foods, 126
Sugar
 avoiding, 71, 72, 229, 269
 in complex carbohydrates, 139
 increasing blood sugar levels, 131
 overconsumption of, 102–3
 in simple carbohydrates, 136–38
 in soda, 75
 spices replacing, 100
Sugar alcohol, xylitol as, 103–5
Sugar Busters diet, 44
Sunblock, makeup with, 422, 431, 433
Sunglasses, 422, 427–28

Sun protection, 427
Sunscreen, 422, 424, 427
Super Chocolatey Cookies, 320–21
SuperTracker online food plan, 16, 39
Supplements
 bedtime, 284, 285
 energy-boosting, 267–68
 fish oil, 354, 367
 mood-boosting, 354, 356, 357
 multivitamin, 83, 99, 267, 367
 for weight loss help, 98–105
Supporters, for weight loss, 23, 105–9
Support group, weight loss, 16, 108,
  112
Sweet and Salty Trail Mix, 318
Sweeteners
 artificial, 103, 275
 natural, 275
Sweet potato snack, 234
Sweet treats, 14, 119, 120. See also
  Desserts
Swimming, 32, 94, 95

T

Tabbouleh, 26, 303
Take Five! program, xiv, 161
 Daily Food and Exercise Log for
  for days 1 through 21, 163–83
  sample, 155
 daily menu planning for, 149
 numbers to know in, 147–49
 recipes used with, 185, 293
 sample menu for, 152–53
 Success Tracker for, 162
 worksheets for, 150–51, 156–57
Take Off Pounds Sensibly (TOPS), 39
Tanios, Aline T., 9–10, 38, 43, 77–78,
  90–91, 121, 258, 269, 288–89,
  332–33, 342–43, 356–57, 362,
  405, 426, 441
Tank tops, 412
Target heart rate zone, for aerobic
  exercise, 154, 158, 158

About the Authors

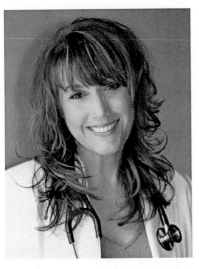

RALLIE McALLISTER, MD, MPH, MSEH

Dr. McAllister is a family physician and nationally known health expert. She is also a cofounder of Momosa Publishing LLC, publisher of MommyMDGuides.com and DaddyMDGuides.com and the Mommy MD Guides book series. She is a coauthor of *The Mommy MD Guide to Pregnancy and Birth, The Mommy MD Guide to Your Baby's First Year,* and *The Mommy MD Guide to the Toddler Years.*

Dr. McAllister's nationally syndicated newspaper column, Your Health, appeared in more than 30 newspapers in the United States and Canada and was read by more than a million people each week.

A nationally recognized health expert, Dr. McAllister has been the featured medical expert on more than 100 radio and television shows. She recently appeared on *Good Morning America Health*. She's the former host of *Rallie on Health*, a weekly regional health magazine on WJHL News Channel 11 with more than one million viewers in a five-state area, and *No Bones about It*, a weekly radio talk show. A dynamic public speaker, Dr. McAllister educates and entertains audiences from coast to coast with her upbeat, down-to-earth delivery of the latest health news.

Dr. McAllister is the author of several other books, including *Healthy Lunchbox: The Working Mom's Guide to Keeping You and*

Your Kids Trim, and the founder of PonyUP! Kentucky, a company that creates unique, equestrian-style handbags and accessories and donates 100 percent of profits to support rescued and retired horses (PonyUPKentucky.com). She is also a mother of three sons and a grandmother of two toddlers.

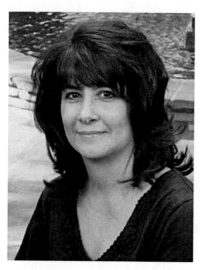

JENNIFER BRIGHT REICH

Jennifer is a cofounder of Momosa Publishing LLC, publisher of MommyMDGuides.com and DaddyMDGuides.com and the Mommy MD Guides book series. She is a coauthor of *The Mommy MD Guide to Pregnancy and Birth*, *The Mommy MD Guide to Your Baby's First Year*, and *The Mommy MD Guide to the Toddler Years*.

Jennifer is a writer and editor with more than 15 years of publishing experience. She has contributed to more than 150 books and published more than 100 magazine and newspaper articles.

Jennifer's credits include writing *The Babyproofing Bible*, contributing writing to 12 books in the *How to Survive Guide* book series, including *How to Survive Your Baby's First Year*, project editing the *New York Times* bestsellers *The South Beach Diet Cookbook* and *The South Beach Diet Good Fats/Good Carbs Guide*, copyediting *Kitty Bartholomew's Decorating ABCs*, cowriting *The Outwit Your Weight Journal*, and writing more than a dozen articles for *Prevention* magazine, as well as articles for various newspapers.

Jennifer honed her planning and organizing skills during four years in the Reserve Officer Training Corps at the Univer-